Neighbourhoods and Public Health

This book examines the concept of neighbourhood over space and time and understands how neighbourhoods can impact human health and well-being. It discusses the identification of neighbourhood boundaries, features of individual neighbourhoods, and the concept of neighbourhood in some major world as well as Indian cities. Based on extensive research, this study refers to both primary as well as secondary sources of data using various statistical and geo-spatial techniques. The first section of the book focuses on the concept of neighbourhood, concept of neighbourhood unit, methods used in the identification of neighbourhood boundaries and theories related to neighbourhood effects on health. The subsequent section of the book deals with a case study on neighbourhood effects on health in an Indian city. The case study is followed by a comparison of its results with other global studies.

This book will be useful to the departments of Geography, Public Health, Sociology and Social Work. It will also be of use to professionals and practitioners like city planners, architects, NGOs, Environmentalists, and urban policy makers.

Uzma Ajmal is an ICSSR Post-Doctoral Fellow at Department of Geography, Aligarh Muslim University, Aligarh. She has completed B.Sc. (2012), M.Sc. (2015) and Ph.D. (2020) from Aligarh Muslim University. She has been a topper throughout her University career and has received University Gold Medals in B.Sc. and M.Sc. Geography. She qualified UGC Junior Research Fellowship (2014) in her first attempt. She has received "Young Geographer Award" by Rajasthan Geographical Association (2017) and "Commendation Certificate" in Young Geographer Competition by National Association of Geographers of India (2017). She has more than eight years of research experience in the field of urban and environmental geography. She has also worked as a Research Associate in an ICSSR project. She has published nineteen research papers with National and International publishers of repute like Taylor and Francis, Springer, and Elsevier.

Saleha Jamal, Associate Professor, Department of Geography, Aligarh Muslim University completed her B.Sc. (2006), M.Sc. (2008) and Ph.D. (2012) from

Aligarh Muslim University. Throughout she had a brilliant academic career having obtained University Gold Medal for first position in B.Sc. and M.Sc. She has more than ten years of teaching experience at UG and PG level. She has been awarded with various prestigious scholarships like PG Merit Scholarship (2007), INSPIRE Fellowship (2010), Young Geographer Awards (2010, 2010, 2012) Best Researcher Award (2011) Special Recognition Award on World Wetland Day (2021) and Best Geography Teacher Award (2023). She specialises in the field of Environmental issues-urban, health etc. She is an active researcher and a prolific writer and has published five books and more than 55 research papers in National and International journals of repute. She has completed one major project and presently working with another major project awarded by ICSSR.

Neighbourhoods and Public Health

The Impact of Place in Urban Areas

Uzma Ajmal and Saleha Jamal

Routledge
Taylor & Francis Group

LONDON AND NEW YORK

First published 2024
by Routledge
4 Park Square, Milton Park, Abingdon, Oxon OX14 4RN

and by Routledge
605 Third Avenue, New York, NY 10158

Routledge is an imprint of the Taylor & Francis Group, an informa business

Disclaimer: The international boundaries, coastlines, denominations, and other information shown in the maps in this work do not necessarily imply any judgement concerning the legal status of any territory or the endorsement or acceptance of such information. Maps used in this book are for representational purposes only.

Trademark notice: Product or corporate names may be trademarks or registered trademarks, and are used only for identification and explanation without intent to infringe.

British Library Cataloguing-in-Publication Data
A catalogue record for this book is available from the British Library

ISBN: 978-1-032-49981-9 (hbk)
ISBN: 978-1-032-58089-0 (pbk)
ISBN: 978-1-003-44248-6 (ebk)

DOI: 10.4324/9781003442486

Typeset in Times New Roman
by SPi Technologies India Pvt Ltd (Straive)

Contents

Figures

Tables

Preface

Worldwide, there is a rising apprehension about climate change and the global environment degradation. Scholars are mostly concerned about global warming, ozone depletion, acid rain, sea-level rise, etc. However, generally, people are not aware of the fact that it is the immediate housing environment which exercises the most significant and most immediate impact on their health and well-being. Neighbourhood environment or immediate housing environment represents a routine setting for the residents which can both enhance or limit their physical, mental and social well-being. Neighbourhoods or localities have emerged to take an important place in health studies as they possess both social and physical characteristics that can affect the health of its residents. Impact of neighbourhood environment on human health has slowly been recognised as potentially crucial factor in health differences among population. Now there is an increase in the awareness that people's health is not only determined by their own characteristics like age, sex, race, socio-economic status, etc., rather than by the characteristics of the neighbourhood too in which one lives.

It is a well-known fact that apart from biological factors, health is also affected by several factors known as social determinants of health. These are non-biological factors affecting health and they include circumstances in which people are born, grow, live and work. They can be grouped into five categories like education, health and health care, economic stability, social and community context as well as neighbourhood and built-environment. This is where neighbourhood environment enters into domain of health.

Environmental problems that are found in the neighbourhood environment have immediate and threatening effects on the health of the residents. Though these problems are not long term, but they do induce unanticipated threat to the environmental basis for human survival. Many cities are presently burdened by infectious diseases namely typhoid, malaria, diarrhoea, etc., supported by poor living conditions. These are the results and a combined interaction of social determinants of health with neighbourhood environment playing a crucial part.

It has been found that there is lack of books dealing with the theme "neighbourhood" that cover both conceptual backgrounds of the theme as well as empirical evidences. Therefore, the current book is presented which will be focusing on the theme and will also cover an empirical study. Here, an attempt is made to understand the concept of neighbourhood and its impact on human health with the help of a case study in Azamgarh city, an urban centre, from India. This book is based on both conceptual as well as empirical aspect of neighbourhood and human health. Major objectives of the book are to understand the concept of neighbourhoods and health over time, to get an overview of neighbourhood environmental characteristics and problems in Azamgarh city, India, to examine the relationship between neighbourhood environmental problems and human health, to find solution to the problems of vulnerable neighbourhoods and finally to compare the results of the current study with other global studies. In this book, an attempt has been made to mix traditional research methods and techniques with modern ones. Apart from using conventional techniques to examine neighbourhood impact on health, attempt is made to use satellite data, GIS and GPS techniques and field monitoring to support the results.

Dr. Uzma Ajmal
Department of Geography,
Aligarh Muslim University, Aligarh, India

Dr. Saleha Jamal
Department of Geography,
Aligarh Muslim University, Aligarh, India

Acknowledgements

Authors would like to express their sincere gratitude to the Department of Geography, Aligarh Muslim University, Aligarh, for providing infrastructural support, University Grants Commission for providing fellowship grant, Maulana Azad Library, Aligarh Muslim University and Seminar library, Department of Geography, Aligarh Muslim University, for providing relevant literature and Municipal Office, Azamgarh City, for providing all the required data. Thanks are also due to all the persons who have helped in one way or the other in completion of this work.

Dr. Uzma Ajmal
Dr. Saleha Jamal

Glossary

Harijan	Scheduled caste
Mallah	Boatman (backward caste)
Harijan basti	a locality of Scheduled caste
Mallah basti	a locality of boatmen (backward caste)
Prajapti	Pottery making community (other backward caste)
Kachcha	uncemented
Pucca	cemented
Nali	drain
Qasaibada	slaughterhouse
Nalas	big drain
Chowraha	roundabout
Chowk	An open market at the junction of two roads
Sabhasad	An elected member of municipal council
PM	Particulate matter
beedi-making	making of local cigarette
Mohalla	Division of a ward

Introduction

Concept and Significance of the Study

According to the simplest definition, a neighbourhood is a locality in which people reside. Neighbourhood is the immediate surrounding area around one's house. Neighbourhood can also be a socially distinguished area which is perceptionally recognised by people. According to renowned urban geographer "Lewis Mumford" neighbourhoods are "Fact of nature" and they exist wherever a group of people lives. A neighbourhood is also a sector of any urban or rural area like villages, towns and cities (Meenakshi, 2011). A city, town or village is simply cluster of neighbourhoods. The major identifying features of neighbourhoods are its geographic, demographic and social characteristics, i.e. whether it is rural or urban, what is the density of households, what is the function of neighbourhood like residential, commercial, retail or mixed and what is the ethnic group that resides in it. Two neighbourhoods could be different in its area, size of population and density of population according to local conditions. However, the size of neighbourhood is not much so that daily needs of the life, mostly in the centre, would be of walking distance for its residents. There are facilities like bus stop, shopping and retail, cultural and recreational activities in the centre of neighbourhood. There could also be a number of large and small residential units, grocery shops, eateries, workplaces, community buildings like educational institutions, theatres, places of worship, clubs, community parks and play yards in the centre of the neighbourhood. A neighbourhood possesses any peculiar physical, social, cultural or demographic feature that differentiates it from the remaining settlement. Residents of a neighbourhood may have a similar type of families, income and education level. According to George Galster, the neighbourhood is defined as follows: "Neighbourhood is the bundle of spatially based attributes associated with clusters of residences, sometimes in conjunction with other land uses" (Galster, 2001).

Attributes of a neighbourhood include geographic as well as social features such as environmental, i.e. topography and pollution, proximity, i.e. location and transport, buildings and its type, density, infrastructure, i.e. patterns of roads and streets, demography, i.e. age and sex profile, social status, ethnic group and adjustability of the population, social-interaction, i.e. friend and family networks, etc. (Galster, 2001). The whole scheme of introduction has been shown in Figure 0.1.

DOI: 10.4324/9781003442486-1

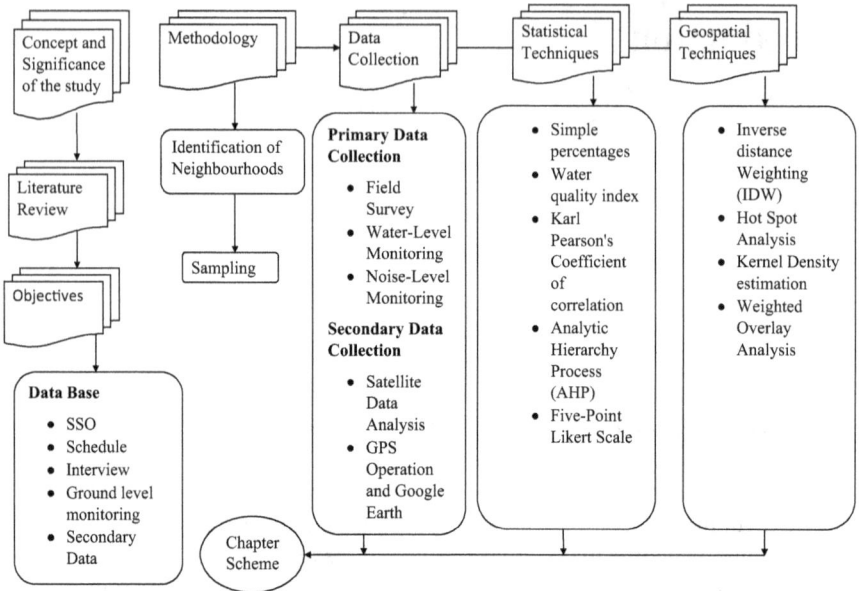

Figure 0.1 Flowchart of Whole Scheme of Introduction.

It has been suggested by studies that apart from people's socio-economic conditions, it is the socio-economic status of their neighbourhoods that separately affects their health (Lemstra et al. 2006). People living in socio-economically backward neighbourhoods are often found facing several health problems than that of the residents of socio-economically sound neighbourhoods (Diez-Roux, 1998; Kawachi and Berkman, 2003; Mushir and Khan 2007; Lakshman et al. 2011). The serious neighbourhood environmental problems associated with supply of drinking water, sanitation, solid waste management as well as air and noise pollution are although present in all types of neighbourhoods, but their particular prevalence is found in socio-economically weaker neighbourhoods (Songsore and McGranahan, 1993) and health impact of the environmental problems is now an established fact. It has also been proved by other studies that people living in socio-economically weaker neighbourhoods are prone to the problems of local environment than that of high- and middle-income neighbourhoods (Rahman, 2008).

Now there is an increase in the awareness that an individual's health is not only determined byhis/her own characteristics (age, sex, race, socio-economic status) but also by the characteristics of the neighbourhood in which one lives. Neighbourhoods or localities have emerged to take an import place in health studies as they possess both social and physical characteristics that can affect the health of its residents (Roux, 2007). Impact of neighbourhood environment on human health has slowly been recognised as potentially crucial factor in health differences among population (Messer et al., 2006).

Worldwide, there is a rising apprehension about climate change and the global environmental degradation. Scholars are mostly concerned about global warming, ozone depletion, acid rain, sea-level rise, etc. However, generally, people are not aware of the fact that it is the immediate housing environment which exercises the most significant and most immediate impact on their health and well-being (Rahman, 1998). Neighbourhood environment or immediate housing environment represents a routine setting for the residents, which can both enhance or limit their physical, mental and social well-being.

It is a well-known fact that apart from biological factors like micro-organism and pathogens, genetics, age and gender, health is also affected by several factors known as social determinants of health. These are non-biological factors affecting health and they include circumstances in which people born, grow, live and work. They can be grouped into five categories like education, health and health care, economic stability, social and community context as well as neighbourhood and built-environment (Figure 0.2). This is where neighbourhood environment enters into domain of health.

People's health is affected by their neighbourhood environment in the form of unsafe water and sanitation conditions, outdoor smoke from industries, indoor smoke from solid fuels, toxic exposures and haphazard patterns of development that adds to air pollution, traffic issues and other forms of urban

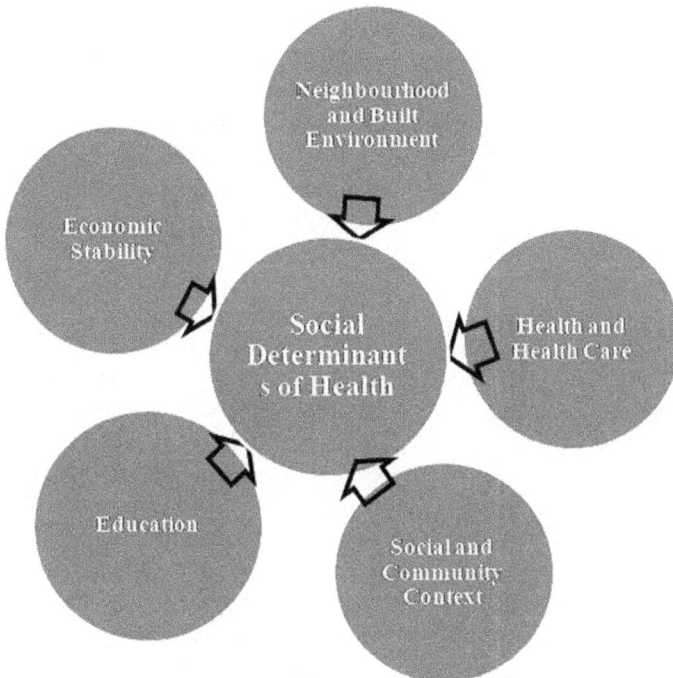

Figure 0.2 Social Determinants of Health.

environmental deterioration. Many cities are presently facing infectious diseases, namely typhoid, malaria, diarrhoea, etc., culminating from poor living conditions. These are the result of combined interaction of social determinants of health, including insufficient infrastructure and services as well as harmful use of alcohol, road accidents, violence and crime that mainly impact the health of the poor and slum inhabitants (WHO, 2010).

From long-lasting to emergent hazards, environmental factors are the underlying cause of a considerable burden of death and disease, particularly in developing countries. As estimated, 25% of all avoidable illnesses are caused by environmental factors including environmental threats in the work, home and broader community/neighbourhood environment. Environmental hazards and related diseases kill millions worldwide every year (WHO, 2004). It was estimated that of the worldwide deaths in the year 2012, around 23% (12.6 million) happened due to environmental factors. These environmental risk factors included sum of all the physical, chemical and biological factors to which men are exposed. It has also been found that environmental factors associated with deaths and disease burden are mostly prevalent in low- and middle-income countries. This can hamper their achievement of sustainable development goals that are related to environment like good health and well-being, clean water and sanitation, sustainable cities and communities and climate action (United Nations, 2017; Dhimal et al. 2017). WHO has estimated that from the year 2030 to 2050, climate change can cause 2,50,000 deaths annually from malnutrition, malaria, diarrhoea and heat-related diseases only (WHO, 2016).

Environmental problems that are found in the housing environment have immediate and threatening effects upon the health of the residents. Though these health impacts are not long lasting, as compared to impacts caused by global environmental problems, they do pose a severe threat to human life. Therefore, in those areas where water supply is inadequate, drainage system is poor, streets are laced with litter, priority setting must be formed and proper attention should be provided.

0.1 Literature Review

An exhaustive survey of literature and research works done on the study of neighbourhood environment and health reveals that extensive studies have been conducted by environmental geographers, health geographers as well as the sociologists. A lot of research work has been done in different countries all over the world in this regard.

A review of the development of modern public health shows an early awareness of a relationship between the incidences of communicable diseases with the surrounding environment. Various studies have been conducted worldwide regarding the association between neighbourhood environment, i.e. housing environment or residential environment and incidence of various health problems. Some prominent works contributed to the issue of neighbourhood environment, and related health problems are given below.

Although worldwide medical geography has received great attention of scholars; however, this field has been somewhat neglected in India when coming to neighbourhood environment and health.

Literature related to the impact of environment on the health can be traced back from the era of Hippocrates in the 4th century B.C. Hippocrates described the impact of environmental factors on incidence of diseases in an area. He has also highlighted the relationship between the quality of water and the occurrence of various diseases. His famous quote is *"If you want to learn about the health of a population look at the air they breathe, the water they drink, and the place where they live"*. John Snow (1813–1858) demonstrated the water-borne origin of Cholera (Stamp, 1964). He inspected the outburst of cholera in London in which more than 500 deaths happened in a small area within ten days. Atiqur Rahman (1998) analysed the environmental conditions of households, their association with income and their effect on health and found that with decreasing income the household environment deteriorates and the risk of health problems related to environment like diarrhoea, respiratory diseases, jaundice, etc. increases. He further added that low-income households have environment-related health problems while high-income households have problems related to wealthy lifestyle like heart diseases, hypertension, diabetes, etc.

M. Sambasiva Rao (1999) studied the morphological land-use changes with time and social and physical environmental problems in Madurai city and suggested remedial measures for the improvement of urban environment and quality of life. Mariana Malmström et al. (1999) in their research work regarding cardiovascular risk factors and neighbourhood environment pointed out that people residing in the deprived neighbourhoods have higher cardiovascular risk factors. Ana V. Diez Roux (2001) has documented links between resident's health and a wide range of conditions in neighbourhoods. According to her people's level of income, education and occupation is dependent upon the socio-economic characteristics of the neighbourhoods in which they live. Therefore, people's health indirectly depends upon the socio-economic characteristics of neighbourhoods as it is directly dependent upon their level of income, education and occupation. She added that it is socio-economic difference among population which gives birth to residential segregation, and living in disadvantaged neighbourhoods leads to poor health.

Andrew McCulloch (2001) tried to investigate how people's lives are affected by the socio-economic condition of the neighbourhoods in which they live. The study concluded that also people's individual socio-economic condition is important; however, socio-economic condition of the neighbourhood is also significantly associated with people's health status, income level, financial position as well as social support. The study maintains that to reduce socio-economic inequality among population groups, it is needed to focus on the socio-economic inequality among neighbourhoods. Hayley Christian et al. (2015) have also maintained that in those neighbourhoods where ample of safe open green spaces are available, young children are more engaged in outdoor playing activities. Evidences are also found that child-friendly neighbourhood services are

associated with overall development of children in terms of physical development, well-being and social capabilities.

Macintyre et al. (2002) while measuring place effects on earth suggested that
there should be a distinction between the compositional and contextual explanation for spatial variation in health and hypotheses should be developed
about the impact of local social and physical environmental features on human
health. Sunil Kumar Karn et al. (2003) have done a remarkable work regarding
impact of the living environment and socio-economic conditions on the health
of urban poor taking four different poor settlements, i.e. slums, squatters and
pavement dwellers from different areas in Mumbai. They found a direct contribution of poor living and socio-economic conditions in the prevalence of diseases. They also added that it is poor socio-economic conditions, i.e. poverty
and unemployment, that people live in slums and squatters.

Roux et al. (2004) in their cardiovascular health study tried to relate neighbourhood environment and mortality in elderlies and documented that among
white elderly adults, the ones residing in most deprived neighbourhoods face
50% more risk of death due to cardiovascular factors even after controlling their
income, education and occupation. Damodar Pokhrel and Viraraghavan (2004)
have worked on impact of water supply and sanitation on diarrhoeal diseases
and found that apart from factors like inaccessibility of safe drinking water,
poor hygiene and sanitation etc. there are various other factors like literacy rate,
social and economic status as well as religious and cultural factors that are
responsible for deaths and morbidities due to diarrhoeal diseases. They have suggest that people are needed to educate about environmental influences on health,
causes and spread of diseases as well as behavioural changes as well as provided
with improved water supply and sanitation to fight with water-borne diseases.

Cummins et al. (2005) emphasised that features of the neighbourhood environment, unhealthy residential environment, abundance of unemployed individuals, poor access to transport facilities have a negative impact on self-rated health.
Jason Corburn et al. (2006) identified neighbourhoods with elevated concentration of asthma and revealed the contribution of inadequate housing environment, ambient air pollution and presence of establishment releasing harmful
substances. Nancy A. Ross et al. (2004) tried to document the impact of neighbourhood environment on health in an urban centre in Canada. The findings
revealed that effect of neighbourhood on health cannot be overlooked as it works
beyond the people's socio-economic, behavioural and demographic characteristics.

Ariane L. Bedimo-Rung et al. (2005) in their study emphasised the importance of the presence of recreational activity centre and parks on public health.
Their main focus was on the benefits of parks in terms of physical health of
people, environmental health as well as social and psychological benefits in
terms of community interaction at the parks.

Jolanda Maas et al. (2006) tried to examine the relationship between green
spaces in the neighbourhood (urban green space, agricultural space, natural
green space) and self-rated general health. The results suggest that presence of
open green spaces within 1 km and 3 km radius has a strong impact on the self-
rated general health.

Konstantinos Tzoulas et al. (2007) tried to put together the theoretical framework of relationship between urban green spaces, environment and human health. They critically reviewed the potential role of urban green spaces on human health and environment.

Debashis Das and Angshuman G. (2007) observed that densely populated areas inhabited by poor, illiterate and immobile people generate a considerable amount of solid waste while the municipal services in these areas for waste collection are inadequate as compared to high-income counterparts. This situation results in unhygienic environment in low-income areas with heaps of garbage which become breeding sites of numerous insects and pests leading to transmission of various infectious diseases.

Sulata Maity et al. (2007) have worked on the quality of water and health status and found that diseases like diarrhoea, skin diseases, worm infestation and liver problems were highly associated with contaminated water.

Alon Unger and Lee W. Riley (2007) examined the unhygienic living conditions and their adverse health outcomes on slum dwellers and suggested the ways to meet the challenges of slums. They emphasised that the promotion of urban health in the 21st century must take neighbourhood-centred as well as person-centred approaches. Seemin Mushir and Firoz Khan (2007) made a comprehensive study of urban quality of the environment in Saharanpur city and documented that it is underdevelopment and poverty that result in deterioration of the environmental quality. The findings of the study also lead to the conclusion that livability in sub-city areas also goes to socio-economic status and political power of the residents, and these are the people at the bottom of status hierarchy who are both economically and politically deprived and face most of the environmental problems. They also emphasised the strength of local bodies and their role in improving the environment to develop a sustainable urban environment.

Sacoby Wilson et al. (2008) in their work focused on the contribution of planning and zoning to unfair development, environmental injustice and neighbourhood health and described how the distribution of resources within and between neighbourhoods has an impact on neighbourhood health.

Abdul Shaban (2008) appraises the relationship between urbanisation and environment, searching empirical evidences from India and attempted to explore and explain the issues and challenges in water supply and sanitation, air-quality management and solid waste disposal in urban India.

Mitra (2008) has discussed the impact of urban environment on human health, particularly on the urban poor living under impoverished conditions. She suggested that eco health research concerned with close interaction between environment and human health is particularly important in developing countries. Cubbin et al. (2008) stated that living in a poor neighbourhood can be bad for one's health, even if one is not poor. They further added that kids may be predominantly in danger to poor conditions in neighbourhoods, with ill effects on health both in present and even in their future life.

Paul R. Hunter et al. (2010) in their study revealed existing relationship between water supply and health conditions emphasising on water's direct link with health, i.e. association with diarrhoeal and non-diarrhoeal disease as well as indirect link like malnutrition.

Dr. A. Munian (2010) studied the residential water demand and supply in Chennai and found that nearly two fifth of the households are not connected to house supply, and hence they depend on the public water distribution system to meet their own needs, which is very unreliable. The study also revealed that these are the urban poor especially the slum dwellers who bear the water unreliability cost to the maximum. Aggarwal and Kumar (2010) examined the environmental risk factors like air pollution, faulty dietary habits, lack of exercise, behavioural and psychological changes due to rapid urbanisation and their association with cardio vascular diseases. They suggested that these factors can be modulated by how we design and build our environment, so urban planning should incorporate measures like preserved green spaces, mixed land use with walkable neighbourhoods, more contiguous development and effective coordinated regional planning.

WHO (2010) focused on the impact of urbanisation on human health and claimed that health of the city residents differs unjustly. The study suggests that to overcome this problem, participatory urban governance is needed to make cities inclusive that are accessible to all irrespective their class, age, sex or race. This can be achieved by making improvements in the urban environment, i.e. houses should be located at safe places, both ambient and indoor air pollution should be checked and safe water and sanitation to every citizen should be ensured.

Rajalakshmi Lakshman et al. (2011) studied neighbourhood deprivation, individual socio-economic factor and its association with behavioural risk factors and found that with people living in disadvantaged neighbourhoods have more chances to be engaged in smoking and less chances to consume full meal.

Tasneem Shazli and Abdul Munir (2016) conducted a study in Azamgarh city regarding urban environmental conditions and socio-economic conditions. The study revealed that housing pattern is quite old in central upland area and also very conjusted. Socio-economic conditions of households are better in southern and northern parts than the central part. The Civil Lines areas of Azamgarh city are well built and economically sound.

Manuel Franco et al. (2018) in their recent work discussed the requirement of well-aware citizens, policy makers, urban practitioners and researchers to achieve sustainable neighbourhood and public health.

0.2 Objectives

The primary aim of this study is to develop a framework for evocative environmental health intervention in Azamgarh city. The study attempts to provide a framework for strong understanding of how environment affects the health of its residents. For this, an attempt has been made to assess the influence of neighbourhood environment on the health of residents in Azamgarh city. Earlier work had been done on the health impacts of neighbourhood environment in larger cities of developed and developing countries, but the medium and smaller cities were neglected. For example, we can find neighbourhood effect studies in New York city (Corburn et al. 2006); Berne, Biel-Bienne, and Payerne, Switzerland (Bringolf-Isler et al. 2010), Philadelphia (Matthews and Yang, 2010) Los Angeles (Nagami et al. 2007), Brazilian cities (Giatti et al. 2010) in case of foreign cities, and in India some recent studies are conducted in Mumbai and Chennai (Adlakha et al. 2020), Kolkata (Mistry et al. 2022, Saha et al. 2022), Nagpur (Bahadure and Kotharkar, 2015, 2018). These studies have no doubt helped in forming a literature base for the current study; however, as already mentioned, medium and smaller cities are left out. Also studies conducted in developed countries have focused on issues prevalent in developed countries only, and in case of studies conducted in Indian cities, they are very few and have picked very few aspects of neighbourhood environment while neighbourhoods can impact health in a variety of ways. In the current study, an attempt has been made to measure all the forms of neighbourhood environment like physical, social and service environment and their impact on health. The Azamgarh city has been selected as study area because smaller cities like Azamgarh are on the way of becoming an urban nightmare like an urban area with pathetic environmental condition. Persistent urbanisation and lack of investment in urban infrastructure development have made disastrous impacts. Attention should also be given to the smaller cities like Azamgarh city which are no longer small but are fast developing as big cities with challenging urban issues of massive garbage, overcrowding, poor urban planning, ageing infrastructure, etc. In Azamgarh city, streets are littered with garbage, waste can be seen disposed to various illegal sites and water logged sites serving a prime habitat for rodents, mosquitoes and flies. Distribution of municipal services is also highly uneven in the city with respect to garbage collection, supply of drinking water, drainage and sanitation, etc. Continuous in-migration from rural counterparts of the district to city has resulted in unplanned and chaotic development of residential areas with narrow streets, crowding, congestion, serious problems of drainage and waste accumulation. Resident's socio-economic conditions are also playing an important role in respect to their household and neighbourhood environment. Keeping in view the above facts, Azamgarh city was selected as study area for the present analysis. The study has certain specific research objectives.

The major objectives of this study are as follows:

1. To understand the concept of neighbourhoods over time and space.
2. To examine the pathways by which neighbourhoods affect human health.
3. To get an overview of neighbourhood environmental characteristics and problems in Azamgarh city.
4. To examine the relationship between neighbourhood environmental problems and human health.
5. To deal with vulnerable neighbourhoods in Azamgarh city.
6. To compare the results of the current study with other global studies.

0.3 Database

The study used both primary as well as secondary sources of data. However, it is mainly based on primary sources of data. Primary data collection techniques involved the following:

0.3.1 Systematic Social Observation (SSO) of Different Neighbourhoods

This method involved walking through the neighbourhoods to make observations about general physical condition i.e., overcrowding, road facilities, water facilities, traffic flow, street lighting and availability of various public services like parks, schools, malls and cinemas, public toilets, etc. A checklist (questionnaire, Appendix I) was used and presence and absence of criteria were marked on it.

0.3.2 Schedule Method

In this method, a questionnaire (Appendix I) was prepared regarding neighbourhood environment, socio-economic conditions of respondents and prevalent diseases in the city. Respondents were selected and explained with the nature and importance of the survey and their responses were filled in by the researcher herself.

0.3.3 Interview Method

In this method numerous responsible members of the city, i.e., municipal officers, *Sabhasad* of different wards, local representative members of different communities, as well as health practitioners from different hospitals and clinics (OPDs of Sadar Hospital, Mahapandit Rahul Sankrityayan Mahila Hospital, Lifeline Hospital, Vedanta Hospital) in the city were interviewed regarding environmental and health conditions in Azamgarh City.

0.3.4 Noise Level and Water Quality Monitoring

Noise pollution monitoring involved the use of sound level meter to measure the level of noise at a particular location. Total 16 locations including, residential, commercial, traffic intersections as well as silence zones were selected and noise levels were recorded. For water quality monitoring, water samples from nine locations were collected and were transported to Environmental Engineering Lab, Civil Engineering, Aligarh Muslim University for analysis. GPS operation was involved to record the coordinates of monitoring stations.

Fieldwork was conducted from the year 2016 to 2019. Observations for each neighbourhood were recorded and for schedule method a senior person (Head of the household or a responsible person of a considerable age and experience) was selected from selected households. For recording accurate information, sampled households were visited frequently. Visit of municipal and other related offices, hospitals and clinics was also made during that time. Secondary data has been collected from the following:

1. Azamgarh Municipal Office, Azamgarh City
2. Azamgarh Development Authority (ADA), Vikas Pradhikaran, Azamgarh city
3. Public Works Department (PWD), Azamgarh City
4. Water Works Department, Azamgarh
5. District Urban Development Authority (DUDA), Azamgarh
6. Chief Medical Office, Azamgarh
7. Basic Shiksha Adhikari (BSA) Azamgarh
8. SP Office, Azamgarh
9. Regional Office, U.P. Pollution Control Board, Azamgarh
10. Census of India, 2011
11. District Census Handbook of Azamgarh (2011)
12. *Sankhikiya Patrika* (Statistical Bulletin, year-wise from 2001 to 2011) published by District statistical office
13. Master Plan 1998–2011, 2011–2031, Azamgarh City
14. "Air Kills, Measuring Crisis of Air Pollution in Uttar Pradesh", Report by Climate Agenda, 2019
15. Maulana Azad library, Aligarh Muslim University; Seminar library of the Department of Geography, Aligarh Muslim University; Library, Department of Geography, Shibli College, Azamgarh; Environment Research Lab, Shibli College Azamgarh
16. Sentinel Satellite 2A data for the year 2017 (10 m spatial resolution) has been used to prepare land use map of the city
17. GPS operation and Google Earth version 7.1.5.1557

0.4 Methodology

To achieve the research objectives, the following methodology has been adopted:

0.4.1 Statement of the Problems

In the cities of underdeveloped countries, population is growing faster than the city's capacity to provide the basic infrastructure and facilities. Here the major environmental problems can be expected in the neighbourhoods in which people live. Inadequate supply of water, accumulation of waste and heaps of garbage in the neighbourhoods, inadequate sanitation facilities and improper housing conditions are responsible for millions of deaths worldwide. Apart from that, urban areas in developing countries are also facing worst air and noise pollution in the world. The present study is concerned about neighbourhood environmental problems in Indian cities and chooses a medium-sized city for the study. Health impacts of the neighbourhood environmental conditions and vulnerable neighbourhoods are the major focus of the study.

0.4.2 Research Approach and Design

Research approach could be quantitative or qualitative and mixed type of approach. For the present study, quantitative approach has been used. This approach is efficient for testing causal relationship between variables. Quantitative approach is used when statistical conclusions are needed to collect operative insights. Numbers provide a clear perspective to take important decisions.

The design used in the research is cross sectional. In cross-sectional research data is taken from a population at a specific point of time. This type of research is used to depict the characteristics that exist in a community. Cross-sectional studies are observational and are known as descriptive research. In descriptive research, a researcher is exclusively interested in describing the situation or case under his/her research. It is typically concerned with describing the problem and its solution.

0.4.3 Identification of Neighbourhoods

Historically, three important approaches are common to examine the neighbourhood effects on health; ecological studies, contextual or multilevel studies and a comparative study of several well-defined neighbourhoods. For the present analysis, third strategy, i.e. comparison of several well-defined neighbourhoods has been adopted as it is best suited for local area investigations (Diez Roux, 2001). Direct information is collected about characteristics and health outcomes of different neighbourhoods. Due to direct collection of primary data from different neighbourhoods, this method gives a first-hand experience of how neighbourhoods affect health of the residents. The study assumes that the local environment people face on daily basis cannot be generalised or predicted until and unless direct exposure of local people is studied. This method seeks what local environment people experience on daily basis. Macintyre et al. (1993) advocate examination of local area characteristics to get more detailed and empirical information about what people of different classes experience in different areas so that social policies could be formed accordingly (Macintyre, 1993). This method has been used to analyse difference across neighbourhoods in services and resources and to associate these differences to different health outcomes (Phillimore and Morris, 1991 and Forsyth et.al, 1994). For the current study, neighbourhoods are taken as unit for analysis. Therefore, first of all defining neighbourhoods and identifying neighbourhood boundaries has been focused on.

Defining Neighbourhood – A neighbourhood is basically the locality in which people reside. The term neighbourhood can be used for a small cluster of dwellings in the immediate surroundings of one's home or a more substantial area with a similar type of housing and market value. Neighbourhoods can also be based on ward boundaries, either part of a ward, a single ward as a neighbourhood or several wards forming a single neighbourhood. For the present study, a group of wards having similar socio-economic characteristics has been taken as a neighbourhood.

Defining Neighbourhood Environment – The term neighbourhood has been used to refer to an individual's immediate living environment, possessing both physical and social characteristics (Diez Roux, 1998). Amerigo (2002) clarified that residences and neighbourhoods are usually examined into two forms: one deals with physical and service features associated with facilities and amenities and the other one deals with social features associated with community bonding in the common areas of the residences as well as in the neighbourhood (Amerigo, 2002). Cubbin et al. (2008) studied neighbourhood environment into three forms, i.e. neighbourhood physical environment, neighbourhood social environment and neighbourhood service environment. The present considers neighbourhood environment as physical, social and service environment in the vicinity.

Identifying Neighbourhood Boundaries – In the present analysis, cluster of wards is identified as neighbourhood. It is basically due to the fact that neighbourhoods differ from each other with their certain physical and social characteristics. And since several wards have similar kind of population composition (income group) and density characteristics, it was feasible to group them into certain neighbourhoods of similar characteristics. In the previous studies also, neighbourhood boundaries have been defined by combining census tracts having similar population composition (income groups) as well as population and household density (King, 2008; Furr-Holden et al., 2008).

This stage involved grouping of 25 wards (Table 0.1 and Figure 0.3) into 7 neighbourhoods on the basis of the following:

- Income-wise dominance in the wards, i.e. high income (>25,000) to medium income (10,000–25,000) and low income (<10,000). A neighbourhood was considered as low income when more than 30% families of the neighbourhood belong to the low-income category and vice-versa (Lemstra et al., 2006) (Table 0.2)

Table 0.1 Azamgarh City: Administrative Wards

Ward Number	Ward Name	Ward Number	Ward Name
1	Farashtola	14	Mukeriganj
2	Sidhari west	15	Heerapatti
3	Seetaram	16	Sarfuddinpur
4	Badarka	17	Raidopur
5	Jalandhari	18	Narauli
6	Gurutola	19	Matbarganj
7	Sidhari East	20	Paharpur
8	Arazibagh	21	Civil Lines
9	Bazbahadur	22	Pandey bazaar
10	Katra	23	Ailval
11	Asifganj	24	Sadavarti
12	Harbanshpur	25	Madya
13	Ghulami ka pura		

Source: Municipal Office Azamgarh City.

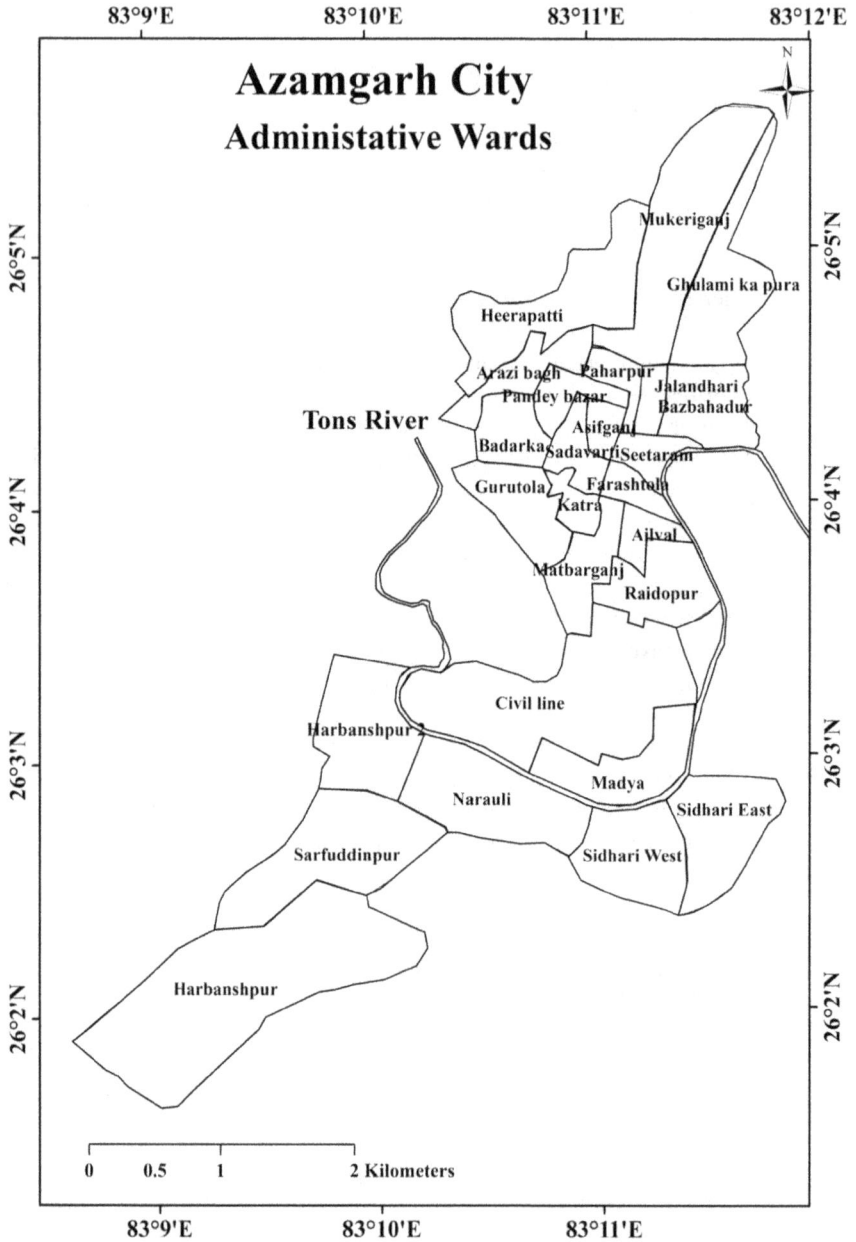

Figure 0.3 Azamgarh City: Administrative Wards.

Source: Municipal Office, Azamgarh City.

- Population density of the ward, i.e. high density (>20,000 persons per sq.km), medium density (10,000–20,000 persons per sq.km) and low density (<10,000 persons per sq.km) (Table 0.3)
- Household density of the ward, i.e. high density (>2700 households per sq.km), medium density (1400–2700 households per sq.km) and low density (<1400 households per sq.km) (Table 0.4)

By combining all these three criteria like income-wise dominance in the wards, population density and household density, all the 25 wards of the city are grouped into 7 wards. These are High-Income High-Density Neighbourhood (HI/HD), High-Income Medium-Density Neighbourhood (HI/MD), High-Income Low-Density Neighbourhood (HI/LD), Medium-Income High-Density Neighbourhoods (MI/HD), Medium-Income Low-Density Neighbourhood (MI/LD), Low-Income High-Density Neighbourhood (LI/HD). Low-Income Medium-Density Neighbourhood (LI/MD) (Figure 0.4). Details of the wards categorised into different neighbourhoods are presented in (Table 0.5).

Table 0.2 Ward-Wise Categorisation On the basis of Dominant Income Group

Income Group Category	Income Range*	Wards included	Total Wards
High	>25,000	2,21,25,17,14,15,11,8,9,17	10
Medium	10,000–25000	10,4,12,16,18	5
Low	<10,000	3,9,5,20,22,13,24,1,6,13	10

Source: Municipal Office Azamgarh City, *Rs./month (1$ = 81.42 Rs., January, 2023).

Table 0.3 Ward-Wise Categorisation on the Basis of Population Density

Population Density Category	Range*	Wards included	Total Wards
High	>20,000	12,14,18,21,25,16,15,2,17	9
Medium	10,000–20,000	13,8,7,24,1,22,6,19,23	9
Low	<10,000	20,10,4,5,3,11,9	7

Source: (i) Census of India, 2011, * (persons per sq.km).

Table 0.4 Ward-Wise Categorisation on the Basis of Household Density

Household Density Category	Range	Wards included	Total Wards
High	>2700	12,14,18,21,16,15,2,17	8
Medium	1400–2700	13,8,7,24,1,22,6,19,23,25,20	11
Low	<1400	10,4,5,3,11,9	6

Source: (i) Census of India, 2011* (households per sq.km).

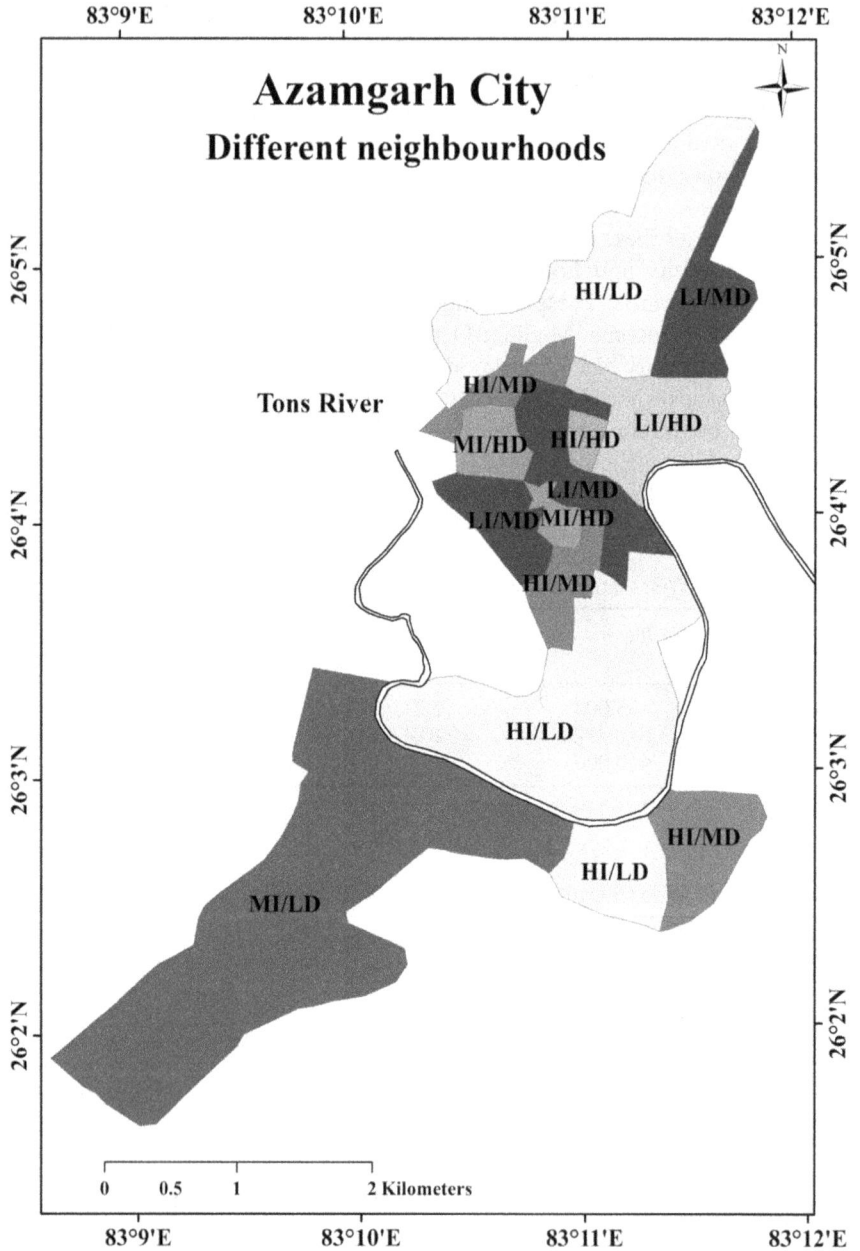

Figure 0.4 Azamgarh City: Different Neighbourhoods (2016–17).

Source: (i) Census of India (ii) Municipal Office, Azamgarh City (iii) Based on City Survey.

Introduction 17

Table 0.5 Design for Survey Adopted for Selection of the Samples from Different Neighbourhoods in Azamgarh City

S. no.	Neighbourhoods	Acronyms	Ward numbers	Total number of wards	Name of the wards	Number of total population	Percentage of total population	Number of total households	No. of selected households (10% of total households)
1	High income with high density	HI/HD	11	1	Asifganj	3727	3.36	523	52
2	High income with medium density	HI/MD	8,19,7	3	Arazibagh, Matbarganj, Sidhari East	15392	13.87	2281	228
3	High income with low density	HI/LD	2,21,25,17,14,15	6	Sidhari West, Civil Lines, Madya, Raidopur, Mukeriganj, Heerapatti	28324	25.53	4506	451
4	Medium income with high density	MI/HD	10,4	2	Katra, Badarka	9800	8.84	1446	145
5	Medium income with low density	MI/LD	12,16,18	3	Harbanshpur, Sarfuddinpur, Narauli	14322	12.9	2197	219
6	Low income with high density	LI/HD	3,9,5,20	4	Seetaram, Bazbahadur, Jalandhari, Paharpur	18635	16.79	2410	241
7	Low income with medium density	LI/MD	22,23,24,1,6,13	6	Pandey bazar, Ailval, Sadavarti, Farashtola, Gurutola, Ghulami ka pura	20756	18.71	2931	293
Total 7			25	25	25	11983	100	16294	1629

Source: (i) Census of India, 2011 (ii) Municipal Office, Azamgarh City (iii) Based on City Survey.

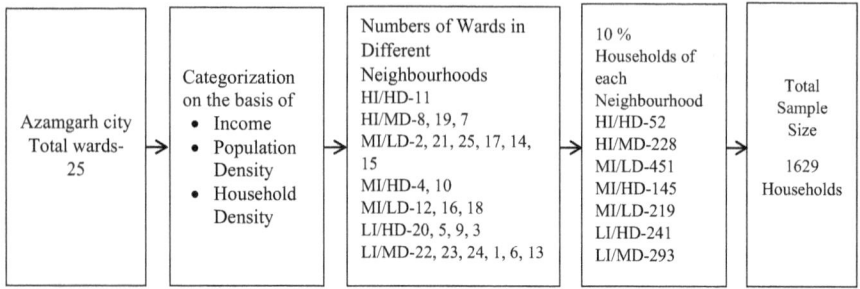

Figure 0.5 Sampling Design.

Source: Authors.

0.4.4 Sampling Procedure

Stratified random sampling was used to select 1629 households from 7 neighbourhoods. First of all, all 25 wards of the city were grouped into 7 neighbourhoods based on some common characteristics (dominant income group, Population density and household density), then further, 10% households from each neighbourhoods were randomly selected for surveying (Figure 0.5 and Table 0.5).

0.4.5 Selection of Indicators and Preparation of Schedule

Selection of indicators is one of the most important tasks in research. Indicators were chosen considering the objectives of the study, consulting relevant literatures and discussion with experts in urban environmental geography as well as public health specialists. The experts included senior professors of environmental geography from various universities (Aligarh Muslim University, Aligarh; Jamia Millia Islamia. New Delhi; Shibli National PG college, Azamgarh), Chief Environmental Officer (Regional Office, U.P. Pollution Control Board, Azamgarh), Chief Medical Officer (District Hospital, Azamgarh), Superintendent of Police (SP Office, Azamgarh), Town Planner, Azamgarh city, officials from municipal office Azamgarh city as well as several doctors from private clinics. They were selected based on their expertise and experience in the current research interest. Except from geographers from different university and private doctors of city, all the officials and specialists from Azamgarh were predominately males. Environmental geographers helped in constructing base for environmental research, environmental officers helped in understanding pollution condition in Azamgarh city; police officer helped in understanding law and order and prevalent crimes in the city; municipal officials helped in understanding distribution of municipal services in the city, while health professionals helped in clearing base for health-related researches. Schedule for the residents was prepared based on previous information. Indicators from the three major categories of neighbourhood environment were selected and further their variables were analysed. List of the indicators chosen that were relevant for the study is given in Table 0.6.

Table 0.6 List of Total Selected Variables for the Current Study

Category	Indicators	Variables
Neighbourhood Physical Environment	Residential density	No. of houses per square km
		Sense of overcrowding
	Built-up density	Percentage built-up area per neighbourhood
		Narrow/congested streets
	Open green spaces	Percentage open/green area per neighbourhood
		Presence of parks/playgrounds
	Quality of housing	Substandard housing/slums
	Air pollution	Prevalence of PM2.5
		Prevalence of PM10
	Noise pollution	Noise level in dB
	Drinking water quality	pH
		TDS
		EC
		Chloride
		Alkalinity
		Total Hardness
		Ca
		Mg
		Chlorine
		TSS
Neighbourhood Service Environment	Water supply	Source of water supply
		State of water supply
		Duration of water supply
	Solid waste management	Disposal/Collection of solid waste
		Frequency of waste collection
		Presence of waste segregation
		Waste accumulation in the neighbourhoods
		Site of waste accumulation
		Presence/absence of stray animals due to waste
		Satisfaction with waste collection services
	Waste water management	Existence of drainage facility around houses
		Presence of water logging
		Type of water logging (rain/sullage)
		Place of water logging
	Connectivity and accessibility	Type of road
		Width of road
		Road density
	Presence of amenities and facilities	Health facilities
		Educational facilities
		Recreational facilities
		Religious facilities
		Markets
		Shopping malls

(*Continued*)

Table 0.6 (Continued)

Category	Indicators	Variables
Neighbourhood Social Environment	Social cohesion and connectedness	Residents visit each other
		Willing to help each other
		Trustworthy
	Neighbourhood disorder	Theft
		Robbery
		Pick pocketing
		Drunk people
		Drug dealing
		Liquor stores
		People loitering
		People smoking
		Fighting
		Safety
		Prostitution
		Rowdy groups and street fighting
	Residential segregation	Presence of segregation in neighbourhoods

The questions for schedule were developed by keeping in mind the indicators and variables of the study and by taking help from the questionnaires in the previous studies (Perkins et al., 1992; Singh et al., 1996; Ross and Mirowsky, 1999; Karn et al., 2003; Rahman, 2008; Jamal, 2012; Christian et al., 2015; Baba, 2015 etc.). The schedule consisted of about 193 questions divided into 4 heads such as checklist of systematic social observation (SSO) (15), neighbourhood environmental conditions (54), socio-economic condition of the households (82) and health profile of the households (42). Checklist involved physical condition of the neighbourhoods, i.e., overcrowding, road facilities, water facilities, traffic flow, street lighting and availability of various public services like parks, schools, malls and cinemas, etc. The second part consisted of neighbourhood environmental problems like water supply, sanitation, drainage and water logging, noise pollution, water pollution, air pollution, social environment, neighbourhood disorder, etc. In the third part, socio-economic and housing conditions of households were incorporated. The last part focused on the prevalent diseases in different neighbourhoods.

0.4.6 Data Collection Methods

0.4.6.1 Field Survey

Primary data was collected through field survey with the help of schedule. Different neighbourhoods and household were visited and selected households were interviewed. Respondents were selected and explained with the nature and importance of the survey and their responses were filled in by the researcher herself. Respondents were explained with the nature and scope of survey and were further asked about their neighbourhood condition, socio-economic status, housing and health conditions. Frequent visits were performed to each neighbourhoods and households to verify the information provided. Different government offices like municipality, Azamgarh Development Authority, regional office of pollution control board, Basic Shiksha Adhikari, CMO office and various hospitals and clinics were also visited frequently to collect data. The questionnaire survey took the researcher nearly a year. The data collected were then tabulated and entered in excel sheets. Afterwards analysis was performed.

0.4.6.2 *Water Quality Monitoring*

To assess the quality of drinking water in Azamgarh city, nine samples were collected for physico-chemical analysis in the month of August 2019. Out of the nine samples, two samples were taken from municipal taps (Matbarganj and Sarfuddinpur), three samples from public hand pumps (Harbanshpur, Bazbahadur, Paharpur) and four samples from submersible pumps installed inside the houses (Arazibagh, Civil Lines, Heerapatti and Sidhari). For collecting the water sample, taps and hand pumps were operated for about 5 minutes to flush out stagnant water in it. Then the samples were collected in sterilised polythene bottles and labelled with adequate information. The samples were placed in thermocol box and transported to Environmental Engineering Lab, Civil Engineering, Aligarh Muslim University, Aligarh. Tests were performed by the researcher in Environmental Engineering Lab under the guidance of lab attendant and technicians.

0.4.6.3 *Noise Level Monitoring*

Noise level monitoring was done with the help of Precision Sound Level Meter, Model Number GM1351, which was capable of measuring noise levels within the range of 30–130 dB. For the present study, a sample time of 5 minutes was selected. Noise samples were collected in dB (A) scale at every 10 seconds interval (6 counts per minute) or total 30 reading in a sample. Average of all the readings were taken as representative of the particular area/zone. Total 16 locations, 5 residential, 2 commercial, 5 silence and 4 traffic stations were chosen to monitor sound levels (Table 0.7). For the present analysis, insights from some previous researches were taken (Firdaus and Ahmad, 2010; Bano et al. 2018).

0.4.6.4 *GPS Operation and Google Earth*

Google Earth version 7.1.5.1557 was used to map the location of health, educational and recreational etc. facilities in the city as well as water and noise quality monitoring stations. GPS was used to record coordinates of facilities in the city. Further, Kmz files of facilities and amenities were prepared in the Google Earth and they were converted into shape files by using Arc Map version 10.2.1.

Table 0.7 Location of Noise Monitoring Stations in Azamgarh City

S. No	Category of Area/Zone	Noise Monitoring Stations
1	Residential	Sidhari East, Millat Nagar (HI/MD); Badarka (MI/HD); Rahmat Nagar (LI/MD); Sarfuddinpur (MI/LD)
2	Commercial	Chowk (MI/HD); Takiya (HI/HD)
3	Silence	Shibli College (LI/HD); DAV College, Lifeline Hospital(HI/LD), Sadar Hospital (LI/MD); GD Global School (Outskirts)
4	Traffic Intersections	Hydel Intersection, Bus Station (HI/LD), Narauli, Pahalwan Sukhdev Tiraha (MI/LD)

Source: Based on Field Survey.

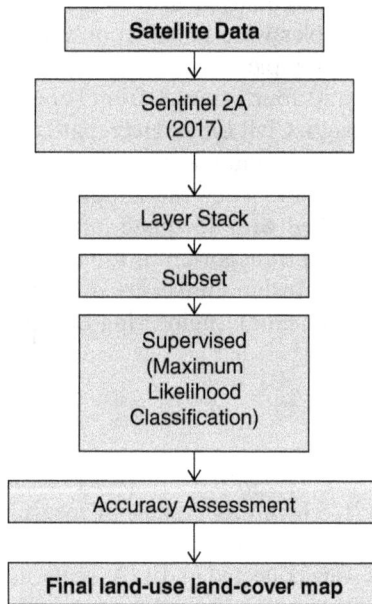

Figure 0.6 Flowchart of Methodology for Land-Use Land Cover Map Preparation.
Source: (Authors).

0.4.6.5 Satellite Data Analysis

Sentinel 2A data for 2017 has been used to prepare land use map of the city to compute built-up area, open green spaces and tree cover in the city (Figure 0.6).

0.4.6.6 Health Data Collection

According to World Health Organization, Health is "[a] state of complete physical, mental and social well-being and not merely the absence of disease or infirmity". Apart from this holistic concept of health, there are several other concepts, i.e. biomedical, ecological and psychological concepts of health. The current study lies on ecological concept of health. According to ecological concept, "Health is a dynamic equilibrium between man and his environment and diseases is maladjustment of human to the environment". Although the current study has touched upon the mental and social well-being of the residents as well, our major focus is on the diseases result- ing from the maladjustment of human to their environment. For the current study, primary data of diseases has been collected through direct interview. Respondents were asked to report and identify the diseases that they have experienced during last two years. Their responses were recorded in the standard questionnaire. The data of prevalent diseases was also verified by health professionals of various government hospitals and private clinics in the study area.

0.4.7 Statistical Techniques Applied

0.4.7.1 Simple Percentage Method

The data used for the study are in percentage form. The formula of percentage is as follows:

$$Simple\ Percent = \left(\frac{n^{th}}{n}\right)100$$

where n = numerical value of the whole commodity
n^{th} = the part of that commodity n (Table 0.8).

0.4.7.2 Water Quality Index Calculation

Although there are a number of methods used for WQI calculation, but most of them are used for WQI calculation of surface water bodies especially rivers (Uddin et al. 2021). For the present study, water quality index has been calcu- lated by using the arithmetic index proposed by Ramakrishnaiah et al. (RWQI) as it was developed to assess ground water quality for drinking use (Ramakrishnaiah et al. 2009). Another rationale behind selecting this method was that it was developed in India so that it will be more suitable for the current study. The method has also been used by various researchers in the previous studies (Batabyal and Chakraborty, 2015; Cooray et al. 2019; Ali and Ahmad, 2020, etc.)

WQI determination involves a number of methods; however, for the current study the current method was adopted which has widely been used by previous researchers (Batabyal and Chakraborty, 2015; Cooray et al. 2019; Ali and

Table 0.8 Details of Methods Applied in the Present Study

Type of analysis	Purpose in the study	Methods used	Formula	Application in the study
Land-use land-cover classification	Land-use land-cover map of Azamgarh city	Maximum likelihood supervised classification	—	LULC map of Azamgarh city, Study Area (Chapter 2)
For Ordinal data Collection	Social relation among residents	Five-point Likert scale	—	Neighbourhood Social Environment (Chapter 3)
To determine the water quality	To determine the overall quality of collected water samples in the city	Arithmetic index method	$WQI = \sum_{i=1}^{n} Si$	Quality of drinking water, Neighbourhood Physical Environment (Chapter 4)
To create Interpolation map	Interpolation map of Air, water and Noise Pollution	Inverse Distance Weighting (IDW)	$vp = \dfrac{\sum_{i=1}^{n} \frac{1}{d} vi}{\sum_{i=1}^{n} \frac{1}{d}}$	Air, water and noise pollution, Neighbourhood Physical environment (Chapter 4)
To find-out the presence of clustering in data	To find out hot and cold spots of SC population (Residential Segregation)	Hot Spot Analysis	$G_i^* = \dfrac{\sum_j wij(d)\,xj - W_i^* \bar{x}}{s\left\{\left(nS_1^* - W_i^*\right)/(n-1)\right\}^{\frac{1}{2}}}$	Residential Segregation, Neighbourhood Social Environment (Chapter 4)
To measure the density of any variable	Density of various facilities in Azamgarh city	Kernel Density Estimation	$\lambda_k(y) = \sum_{k=}^{n} \dfrac{1}{\tau^2} K\left(\dfrac{y-y_i}{\tau}\right)$	Educational, health and recreational facilities density, Neighbourhood Service Environment (Chapter 4)
To determine relationship between two variables	Relationship between risk factors in neighbourhood environment and prevalent diseases	Karl Pearson's Coefficient of Correlation	$r = \dfrac{n\sum x_i y_i - \sum x_i y_i}{\sqrt{n\sum x_i^2 - (\sum x_i)^2} \times \sqrt{n\sum y_i^2 - (\sum y_i)^2}}$	Relationship between neighbourhood environmental problems and health (Chapter 5)
To identify and map vulnerable areas	Identification of environmentally vulnerable neighbourhoods	Analytic Hierarchy Process, Weighted Linear Combination	$M = \sum_{i=1}^{n} WiXi$	Identification and mapping of vulnerable neighbourhoods (Chapter 6)

Ahmad, 2020, etc.). Determination of Water Quality Index involved following steps:

First of all, all parameters are given weights (w_i), based on their relative significance in the quality of water (range, 1–5).

Secondly, relative weight (W_i) of the parameters is calculated using the given equation $$Wi = \frac{wi}{\sum_{i=1}^{n} wi}$$

where Wi = relative weight,

wi = weight of individual parameter

n = number of parameters

Further quality rating is calculated for every parameter by dividing concentration of parameter in each sample to its respective standard chosen for the study (BIS in current study) and the outcome is multiplied by 100.

$$qi = \frac{Ci}{Si} \times 100$$

where qi is the quality rating,

Ci is concentration of each parameter in each sample expressed in mg/L;

Si is Index drinking water standard for the each parameter in mg/L.

For computing WQI, the sub-index (SI) is first determined for each parameter, as:

$$SI_i = W_i \times q_i$$

Water Quality Index $$WQI = \sum_{i=1}^{n} Si$$

where SI_i is the sub index of ith parameter;

Wi is relative weight of ith parameter;

Qi is the rating based on concentration of ith parameter, and n is the number of chemical parameters.

0.4.7.3 Karl Pearson's Correlation Coefficient

This method was used to analyse the association between risk factors in neighbourhood environment and associated diseases.

$$r = \frac{n\Sigma x_i y_i - \Sigma x_i y_i}{\sqrt{n\Sigma x_i^2 - \left(\Sigma x_i\right)^2} \times \sqrt{n\Sigma y_i^2 - \left(\Sigma y_i\right)^2}}$$

where r = coefficient of correlation

x, y = the two given variables

Student's t test is used to examine the significance of the relationship.

$$t = r\sqrt{\frac{n-2}{1-r^2}}$$

where t = test of significance
n = no of observations
r = computed value of coefficient of correlation

0.4.7.4 Analytical Hierarchy Process (AHP)

AHP is a method of multicriteria decision-making which can be applied within GIS. It calculates criterion weights and also possesses the capability to solve problems of unreliable judgements, having been used in various studies to make decision in urban environment (Belton and Stewart, 2002).

This step involves the following procedures:

1) Calculating the priority vector for each criterion using Saaty's scale of pairwise comparison (Table 0.9).
2) Calculating the Principal Eigenvalue (λmax).
3) Deriving the Consistency Index (CI).
4) Selecting the suitable value of the Random Index from the table of Random Index numbers (Table 0.10).
5) Calculating consistency ratio (CR) (Saaty, 1980).

Table 0.9 Saaty's Scales for Pairwise Comparison (Analytic Hierarchy Process)

Variables	Verbal Items
1	Equal Importance
3	Moderate Importance
5	Strong Importance
7	Very strong Importance
9	Extreme importance
2,4,6,8	Intermediate values between adjacent scales values

Source: Saaty, 1980.

Table 0.10 Saaty's Table of Random Index (Analytic Hierarchy Process)

Size of Matrix (n)	2	3	4	5	6	7	8	9	10	11	12	13	14	15
Random Consistency Index (RI)	0.00	0.58	0.90	1.12	1.24	1.32	1.41	1.45	1.49	1.51	1.48	1.56	1.57	1.59

Source: Saaty, 1980.

In the present study, AHP is used to determine weights of the criteria to generate environmental vulnerability maps.

0.4.7.5 *Five-Point Likert Scale*

Likert scale was used to collect the primary data towards the attitudes of the respondents. In the present study, it has been used to measure social cohesion and connectedness among residents. The scale was developed by a sociologist, Dr. Rennis Likert at the University of Michigan. Likert scale is defined as a psychometric response scale primary used in questionnaire or schedules to obtain participant's preference or degree of agreement with a statement or a set of statements (Likert, 1932). These scales are non-comparative scale techniques and also one-dimensional in nature. The most common scale is five-point Likert scale which segments the option to the residents in five parts, i.e. strongly agree, agree, neutral, disagree and strongly disagree.

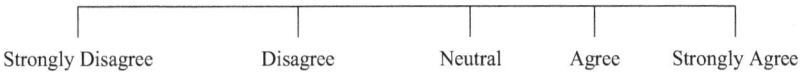

| Strongly Disagree | Disagree | Neutral | Agree | Strongly Agree |

0.4.8 Geo-Spatial Techniques Applied

0.4.8.1 *Inverse Distance Weighting (IDW)*

IDW technique was used to generate interpolation map of Azamgarh City for air pollution, noise pollution and water quality index. IDW is the most popular method of interpolation to calculate values of unknown points using a known set of scattered points. The main idea behind this method is that any two given points have similar kind of attributes, but this similarity decreases as the distance between those points increases, i.e. there is an inverse relationship between similarity and distance. IDW has been accepted as one among the standard interpolation methods in GIS (Burrough et al., 1998; Longley et al., 2005). The basic formula for IDW interpolation is

$$vp = \frac{\sum_{i=1}^{n} \frac{1}{d} vi}{\sum_{i=1}^{n} \frac{1}{d}}$$

where vp = value to be estimated
  v_i = Known value
  d_1-d_n = distances from the data point to the point estimated n

0.4.8.2 Hot Spot Analysis

Hot spot analysis is used to identify presence of clustering in the data. Clustering identifies the patterns where high proportions of attributes are concentrated. In the present study, hot spot analysis has been used to identify clustering of scheduled caste population to measure residential segregation. Hot spot analysis tool in ArcMap was used to calculate the Getis-OrdGi* statistic for identifying wards with high values neighbouring other wards with similar/high values. The equation is

$$G_i^* = \frac{\sum_j wij(d)xj - W_i^* \bar{x}}{s\left\{(nS_1^* - W_i^*)/(n-1)\right\}^{\frac{1}{2}}}$$

Source: Rogerson, 2010

In the present study, hot spot analysis has been conducted with the null hypothesis that proportion of SC population in each ward compared to the entire wards within the city is equal. The hot spot analysis compares a particular ward from its neighbourhood and to the entire study area. If all surrounding neighbouring wards contain high values, then the selected ward is considered as hot spot.

0.4.8.3 Kernel Density Estimation

Kernel Density Estimation (KDE) tool in the Arc Map has been used to measure the density of educational, health, recreational as well as religious facilities in different parts of Azamgarh city. KDE tool calculates density of point features around its neighbourhood. The main idea behind this method is that any feature exhibits a density at any place in the study area not just at the place where it has occurred or displayed (O'Sullivan and Unwin, 2002; Lloyd, 2010). It defines the density surface for each individual point. The formula is

$$\lambda_k(y) = \sum_{k=}^{n} \frac{1}{\tau^2} K\left(\frac{y - y_i}{\tau}\right)$$

where $\lambda_k(y)$ denotes the total estimated density calculated for all features located at y_i around y, τ is the kernel bandwidth which determines the search radius and K is an indicator for the degree of smoothness.

0.4.8.4 Weighted Linear Combination (WLC)

WLC method is used when we need to make decision while dealing with multiple criteria or attributes. Each attribute here is called criterion which is allocated a weight depending on its significance. The output will be multi-attribute feature with a final value.

WLC is dependent on the notion of a weighted average. It was performed after standardisation and calculation of weightage for each criterion using Analytical Hierarchy Process. The weights were then allocated to every criterion layer on the map. The total score for each option was calculated by multiplying the weight assigned to each attribute by the scaled value given for that attribute to the alternative and then summing the products over all attributes. The scores were calculated for all the alternatives and the attributes with the highest and lowest scores were chosen.

The method has been used to identify environmentally vulnerable neighbourhoods of Azamgarh city. In this method, criteria are combined after assigning weights to them and the final map is achieved.

$$M = \sum_{i=1}^{n} WiXi$$

where M is the Final neighbourhood environmental vulnerability map;
n is the number of criteria;
W_i are weights of the criteria i;
X_i is the sub-criteria score of the criteria i (Drobne and Lisec, 2009).

Weighted overlay tool in Arc Map is the best tool for overlay analysis to solve multicriteria problem. It generates final suitability map while taking into consideration the individual weights of all the criteria.

0.4.9 Hypothesis of the Study

The hypothesis that needs to be tested in the present study is as follows:

- There is a significant effect of neighbourhood environment on resident's health.

0.4.10 Limitations of the study

Despite the well-planned strategy and research methodology formulation, the research work faced several limitations during data collection whether primary or secondary and during selection of methods.

0.4.10.1 Limitations in the Data Collection

- Lack of existing researches on smaller and medium-sized cities in general and study area in particular.

- Unavailability of secondary data regarding prevalent diseases in Azamgarh city. We could barely find data of existing diseases in the city therefore had to rely on primary data only.
- Data regarding air pollution was not available in the regional office of Pollution control board, Azamgarh city. Due to unavailability of instruments and financial constraints, it was hard to carry out the experiment by the researcher herself; therefore, we had to rely on the data collected by an NGO which was also available for two parameters only.
- Regarding water sampling, very few samples were collected from the city keeping in mind the distance between the sampling location and the laboratory to which samples were to be transported for chemical analysis.
- For ordinal data collection, five-point Likert scale was used which also has several limitations, i.e. results might not be objective. There are chances of acquiescence bias as people sometimes tend to agree to the given statements. Also, neutral options provided are difficult to treat.
- Non-communicable diseases like diabetes, obesity and cardio-vascular diseases were excluded from the final analysis as during survey very weak association was observed between these diseases and neighbourhood environment while vector-borne and water borne-diseases were found more prevalent and significantly associated with neighbourhood environmental problems in the study area.
- Qualitative data like observations and interactions are absent as this is basically a quantitative study based on numerical data and correlations.

0.4.10.2 Limitations of the Methods Used

Despite the care taken while choosing the methods for analysis, there are certain limitations in methods which are basically due to the fact that each method comes with certain limitation and no method has been proven perfect. Attempt has been made to choose the best suitable methods among all the methods available; however, their limitations are as follows:

- **Limitation behind WQI method used** – There may be several limitations in using one type of water quality index method, i.e. different standard values given by different agencies produce different results. Different methods of WQI calculations may give different results. A water sample which may be good according to one method can fall into poor category in a different method. Another case could be that same WQI is used but classification is different; this can also lead to different results (Kachroud et al. 2019).Yadav et al. 2010 have also developed WQI calculation method which uses the same method of WQI as Ramakrishna et al. (2009); however, further both of them use different classification scales (e.g., the category of excellent water ranges from 0 to 25 for Yadav et al. while it is 0–50 for Ramakrishna et al.). It is also a limitation that most of the WQI models are developed for surface water quality (Uddin et al., 2021).

- **Limitations behind interpolation method used** – There are several limitations in the interpolation method: Inverse Distance Weighting (IDW) used, i.e. for interpolation distribution of sample data point, should be even, or it can decrease the quality of interpolation result. Interpolation results show maximum and minimum values as peaks and pits and do not show proper spread of high and low values. This method is sensitive to outliers and it highlights isolated points of extreme values. It cannot estimate results below and beyond minimum and maximum value. It does not smooth the results and presents result as exact.
- **Limitation behind density estimation method used** – Kernel density estimation (KDE) method has been used to calculate the density of facilities and amenities in the city. One of the major drawbacks of Kernel density estimation is edge or boundary effect as it can estimate densities with bounded support only.
- **Limitation behind method of correlation used** – Karl Pearson's coefficient of correlation was used, which is a very lengthy and time-consuming method. A crucial limitation of Karl Pearson's correlation is that it cannot differentiate between dependent and independent variables. Although it does calculate the relationship between two variables, it cannot suggest which variable is cause and which one is effect. It also cannot determine non-linear relationships. Another limitation of Karl Pearson's correlation is that it gets affected by extreme values/outliers.
- **For identification of most and least vulnerable neighbourhoods** – Analytic hierarchy process has been used to assign weights to criteria related to neighbourhood vulnerability. However, it is not suitable to complex scenario due to the absence of flexibility of its hierarchical structure. AHP also uses accurate judgements; however, in many cases human judgements are incomprehensible.
- **For land-use-land-cover map preparation** – Maximum likelihood supervised classification method was used to prepare LULC map. The major limitation of maximum likelihood classification is that it is vulnerable to division of categories and collection of samples. If the division of categories is discrete, or collected samples do not represent properly, the classified map might deviate considerable from actual situation on the ground.

The study could have been better with better resources like government data on prevalent diseases, more information on neighbourhood amenities and more data on features of neighbourhoods associated with non-communicable diseases, etc. Addition of qualitative data could also have made the arguments stronger.

0.5 Chapter Scheme

The book is divided into six chapters apart from introduction and conclusion.

Chapter 1 – The first chapter deals with different concepts of neighbourhood over space and time as well as an understanding of how neighbourhoods can impact health of its residents. The chapter is divided into two sections. The first section deals with the concept of neighbourhood while the second section deals with the ways by which neighbourhoods can affect health of its residents. The analysis reveals that neighbourhoods have been identified since early times; however, their official recognition as a planning unit has started only after publication of the idea of "Neighbourhood Unit" by Clarence Perry and "Neighbourhood" by Stein and Wright in 1929. The second section of the chapter deals with different forms of neighbourhood environment, i.e. neighbourhood physical environment, neighbourhood social environment as well as neighbourhood services environment and ways by which they can influence residents' health. Further various methods used to measure neighbourhood impact on health have been discussed ranging from ecological studies to contextual or multi-level studies and a comparison of certain number of well-defined neighbourhoods.

Chapter 2 – This chapter deals with details about study area Azamgarh city. This chapter has been divided into two sections. The first section deals with geographical and other characteristics of study area Azamgarh city, while the second section deals with identification and mapping of different neighbourhoods in Azamgarh city. In the first section, origin and evolution in medieval, British and modern period; physical setting in terms of terms of site and situation, drainage, soil, climate; demographic setting in terms of population growth, literacy level and sex ratio, occupational structure as well as land use pattern in the city are discussed in detail. In the second section, first of all criteria selected for identification of different neighbourhoods like income-wise dominance, population density as well as household density are discussed. Further, each neighbourhood of the city, along with its picture, is discussed in detail.

Chapter 3 – This chapter is devoted to characteristics of neighbourhood environment in Azamgarh City. Characteristics of neighbourhood environment have been discussed under three heads, i.e. neighbourhood physical environment, neighbourhood service environment as well as neighbourhood social environment. Neighbourhood physical characteristics involved residential density, built-up area, open green spaces, parks and play grounds; service environment involved water supply, solid waste management, waste water management, safety/street lighting, availability of health facilities, educational facilities, recreational facilities, shopping facilities and religious sites while social environment involved social cohesion and connectedness among residents. An analysis of neighbourhood physical environment in the city revealed that residential density and proportion of built-up area is the highest in the old central part of the city. Most of the parks are located in the high-income counterparts. Water supply pipelines of the city do not cover all the houses of the city and out of the total household waste generated in the city only about 80% waste is collected by the municipality, about 32.29% reported presence of open drains around their houses. There are 31 government, 93 private schools and 3 degree colleges in the city and 6 parks, 6 gyms, 3 cinema halls and 2 libraries which are inadequate for the population. It was found that overall social environment in the city was good.

Chapter 4 – In Chapter 4, specific problems found in the neighbourhood physical environment like overcrowding, narrow and congested streets, air pollution, noise pollution and water quality problems; in neighbourhood service environment like inadequate water supply, improper drainage and water logging, accumulation of solid waste and unequal distribution of amenities and facilities; and in neighbourhood social environment like neighbourhood disorder and residential segregation have been discussed. The study revealed that sense of overcrowding was found the highest in the old central parts of the city where problem of narrow streets was also seen. Values of PM_{10} and $PM_{2.5}$ at all the monitored stations were higher than national standards for ambient air quality. Water Quality Index of the drinking water samples revealed that the water quality of five samples was poor out of nine samples. Problems of inadequate water supply, inadequate drainage system as well as accumulation of solid waste in the neighbourhoods were also prevalent. Problems in the neighbourhood social environment include the problem of residential segregation and neighbourhood disorder. Hot spot analysis to measure residential segregation revealed that significant hot and cold spots of Scheduled caste population are prevalent in the city. Neighbourhood disorder was mainly prevalent in the central, congested, old parts of the city and major problems are theft, robbery, pick pocketing and people drunk.

Chapter 5 – In the fifth chapter, an attempt has been made to examine the health impacts of neighbourhood environment on residents' health. The chapter has been divided into three sections. In the first section, most frequent diseases in the city that have occurred during the last two years have been identified and analysed thoroughly. In the second section, an attempt has been made to identify risk factors in the neighbourhood environment and to understand their association with the prevalent diseases. In the third section, hypotheses of the study are tested using Karl Pearson's coefficient of correlation. The results revealed that most common diseases in the city were cold and flu, malaria, diarrhoea, cholera, skin infections, jaundice, dengue, typhoid, chicken pox, measles, tuberculosis and asthma. In the second section, prevalent diseases in the city are identified. Karl Pearson's coefficient of correlation has been used to study the association between these risk factors in the neighbourhood environment and prevalent diseases. It has been found that risk factors related to water and sanitation were associated with diseases like typhoid, cholera, jaundice, diarrhoea and skin infections. Neighbourhood disorder was associated with the prevalence of stress; air pollution was associated with shortness of breath; noise pollution was associated with annoyance; sleep disturbances and headache. In the third section, hypothesis testing has been performed by using Karl Pearson's coefficient of correlation. It has been found that null hypothesis of the study, i.e. "There is insignificant effect of neighbourhood environment on resident's health", failed to be accepted as suggested by "r" and "p" values of correlation.

Chapter 6 – The sixth and last chapter is divided into three sections. In the first section, socio-economic profile of the sampled households has been discussed. In the second section, an attempt has been made to identify most vulnerable neighbourhoods of Azamgarh city, while in the third section an attempt has been made to tackle major environmental problems of the city. Environmentally vulnerable neighbourhoods in the city are identified using 14 environmental problems of the city like irregular supply of water, water quality problem, open drains, poor cleaning of drains, waterlogging, inadequate waste collection, waste accumulation in neighbourhood, overcrowding, narrow streets, air pollution, noise pollution, substandard housing, and neighbourhood disorder as well as unequal distribution of facilities. Weighted linear combination technique has been used to divide neighbourhoods into three categories, i.e. most vulnerable, moderately vulnerable and least vulnerable. It has been found that mostly low-income neighbourhoods lie in the most vulnerable category and environmental problems are at their worst level in them. Medium- and high-income neighbourhoods are in somewhat better condition. In the second section, an attempt was made to address all the major problems identified in the city, i.e. drainage and water logging, solid waste management, neighbourhood overcrowding, water supply and quality problem, air pollution, noise pollution, neighbourhood disorder and unequal distribution of amenities and facilities. Policy suggestions have been provided while considering existing schemes and policies running in the city.

Finally, a brief conclusion based on the results has been given.

References

Adlakha, D., Krishna, M., Woolrych, R., & Ellis, G. (2020). Neighbourhood supports for active ageing in urban India. *Psychology and Developing Societies*, *32*(2), 254–277.

Aggarwal, A., & Kumar, P. (2010). "Urban Environment and Health: Chronic Cardio Vascular Diseases". Ed. Dubey, R. N. *Urbanisation and Urban Planning in India Vision and Reality*. Shree Nataraj Publication New Delhi, pp. 290–295.

Ali, S. A., & Ahmad, A. (2020). Analysing water-borne diseases susceptibility in Kolkata Municipal Corporation using WQI and GIS based Kriging interpolation. *GeoJournal*, *85*(4), 1151–1174.

Amerigo, M. (2002). "A Psychological Approach to the Study of Residential Satisfaction". Eds. Aragones, J.I., Francescato, G., & Gärling, T. (Eds.), *Residential Environments. Choice Satisfaction and Behavior*. Bergin & Garvey, Westport, CT, pp. 81–100.

Baba, S. A. (2015). *Residential environment and related health problems in Srinagar city Jammu Kashmir*. Unpublished Thesis. Aligarh Muslim University, Aligarh.

Bahadure, S., & Kotharkar, R. (2015). Assessing sustainability of mixed use neighbourhoods through residents' travel behaviour and perception: the case of Nagpur, India. *Sustainability*, *7*(9), 12164–12189.

Bahadure, S., & Kotharkar, R. (2018). Framework for measuring sustainability of neighbourhoods in Nagpur, India. *Building and Environment*, *127*, 86–97.

Bano, N., Ahmad, A., & Shamim, S. K. (2018). Environmental impact assessment of noise quality: a health based study of Firozabad City (India). *The Geographer*, *65*(1), 1–9.

Batabyal, A. K., & Chakraborty, S. (2015). Hydrogeochemistry and water quality index in the assessment of groundwater quality for drinking uses. *Water Environment Research : A Research Publication of the Water Environment Federation, 87*(7), 607–617. https://doi.org/10.2175/106143015X14212658613956

Bedimo-Rung, A. L., Mowen, A. J., & Cohen, D. A. (2005). The significance of parks to physical activity and public health: a conceptual model. *American Journal of Preventive Medicine, 28*(2), 159–168.

Belton, V., & Stewart, T. (2002). *Multiple Criteria Decision Analysis: An Integrated Approach.* Springer Science & Business Media, Dordrecht.

Bringolf-Isler, B., Grize, L., Mäder, U., Ruch, N., Sennhauser, F. H., & Braun-Fahrländer, C. (2010). Built environment, parents' perception, and children's vigorous outdoor play. *Preventive medicine, 50*(5–6), 251–256.

Burrough, P. A., McDonnell, R., McDonnell, R. A., & Lloyd, C. D. (1998). *Principles of Geographical Information Systems.* Oxford University Press, New York.

Census of India, (2011).

Christian, H., Zubrick, S. R., Foster, S., Giles-Corti, B., Bull, F., Wood, L., ... & Boruff, B. (2015). The influence of the neighborhood physical environment on early child health and development: a review and call for research. *Health & Place, 33*, 25–36.

Cooray, T., Wei, Y., Zhong, H., Zheng, L., Weragoda, S. K., & Weerasooriya, R. (2019). Assessment of groundwater quality in CKDu affected areas of Sri Lanka: implications for drinking water treatment. *International journal of Environmental Research and Public Health, 16*(10), 1698.

Corburn, J., Osleeb, J., & Porter, M. (2006). Urban asthma and the neighbourhood environment in New York City. *Health & Place, 12*(2), 167–179.

Cubbin, C., Egerter, S., Braveman, P., & Pedregon, V. (2008). *Where We Live Matters for Our Health: Neighborhoods and Health.* Robert Wood John Foundation, New Jersey.

Cummins, S., Stafford, M., Macintyre, S., Marmot, M., & Ellaway, A. (2005). Neighbourhood environment and its association with self rated health: evidence from Scotland and England. *Journal of Epidemiology & Community Health, 59*(3), 207–213.

Das, D., & Angshuman, G. (2007). "Some Issues Associated with the Municipal Conservancy Services to Dispose Of Solid Waste in a Small Town of Birbhum District, W.B". Ed. Ghosh, A. *Environment Drinking Water and Public Health Problems and Future Goals.* Daya Publishing House, c, pp. 48–71.

Dhimal, M., Dhimal, M., Karki, K., Montag, D., Groneberg, D., & Kuch, U. (2017). Tracking health-related Sustainable Development Goals (SDGs) in Nepal. *Journal of Health and Social Sciences, 2*(2), 83–86.

Diez Roux, A. V. (2001). Investigating neighborhood and area effects on health. *American Journal of Public Health, 91*(11), 1783–1789.

Diez-Roux, A. V. (1998). Bringing context back into epidemiology: variables and fallacies in multilevel analysis. *American Journal of Public Health 88*(2), 216–222.

Drobne, S., & Lisec, A. (2009). Multi-attribute decision analysis in GIS: weighted linear combination and ordered weighted averaging. *Informatica, 33*(4), 459–474.

Firdaus, G., & Ahmad, A. (2010). Noise pollution and human health: a case study of Municipal Corporation of Delhi. *Indoor and Built Environment, 19*(6), 648–656.

Forsyth, A., Macintyre, S., & Anderson, A. (1994). Diets for disease? Intraurban variation in reported food consumption in Glasgow. *Appetite, 22*(3), 259–274.

Franco, M., Díez, J., Gullón, P., Margolles, M., Cofiño, R., Pasarín, M., & Borrell, C. (2018). Towards a policy relevant neighborhoods and health agenda: engaging citizens, researchers, policy makers and public health professionals. SESPAS report 2018. *Gaceta sanitaria, 32*, 69–73.

Furr-Holden, C. D. M., Smart, M. J., Pokorni, J. L., Ialongo, N. S., Leaf, P. J., Holder, H. D., & Anthony, J. C. (2008). The NIfETy method for environmental assessment of neighborhood-level indicators of violence, alcohol, and other drug exposure. *Prevention Science*, *9*(4), 245–255.

Galster, G. (2001). On the nature of neighbourhood. *Urban studies*, *38*(12), 2111–2124.

Giatti, L., Barreto, S. M., & César, C. C. (2010). Unemployment and self-rated health: neighborhood influence. *Social Science & Medicine (1982)*, *71*(4), 815–823. https://doi.org/10.1016/j.socscimed.2010.05.021

Hunter, P. R., MacDonald, A. M., & Carter, R. C. (2010). Water supply and health. *PLoS Medicine*, *7*(11), e1000361.

Jamal, S., (2012). Health impacts of indoor air pollution from household energy used in Aligarh city, published thesis, Aligarh Muslim University, https://hdl.handle.net/10603/12905

Kachroud, M., Trolard, F., Kefi, M., Jebari, S., & Bourrié, G. (2019). Water quality indices: challenges and application limits in the literature. *Water*, *11*(2), 361.

Karn, S. K., Shikura, S., & Harada, H. (2003). Living environment and health of urban poor: a study in Mumbai. *Economic and Political Weekly*, *38*, 3575–3586.

Kawachi, I., & Berkman, L. F. (Eds.). (2003). *Neighborhoods and Health*. Oxford University Press, New York.

King, D. (2008). Neighborhood and individual factors in activity in older adults: results from the neighborhood and senior health study. *Journal of Aging and Physical Activity*, *16*(2), 144–170.

Lakshman, R., McConville, A., How, S., Flowers, J., Wareham, N., & Cosford, P. (2011). Association between area-level socioeconomic deprivation and a cluster of behavioural risk factors: cross-sectional, population-based study. *Journal of Public Health*, *33*(2), 234–245.

Lemstra, M., Neudorf, C., & Opondo, J. (2006). Health disparity by neighbourhood income. *Canadian Journal of Public Health/Revue Canadienne de Sante'ePublique*, *97*, 435–439.

Likert, R. (1932). *A Technique for the Measurement of Attitudes*. Archives of Psychology, New York.

Lloyd, C. D. (2010). *Local Models for Spatial Analysis*. CRC Press, Boca Raton.

Longley, P. A., Goodchild, M. F., Maguire, D. J., & Rhind, D. W. (2005). *Geographic Information Systems and Science*. John Wiley & Sons, New York.

Maas, J., Verheij, R. A., Groenewegen, P. P., De Vries, S., & Spreeuwenberg, P. (2006). Green space, urbanity, and health: how strong is the relation?. *Journal of Epidemiology & Community Health*, *60*(7), 587–592.

Macintyre, S., Ellaway, A., & Cummins, S. (2002). Place effects on health: how can we conceptualise, operationalise and measure them?. *Social Science & Medicine*, *55*(1), 125–139.

Macintyre, S., Maciver, S., & Sooman, A. (1993). Area, class and health: should we be focusing on places or people?. *Journal of Social Policy*, *22*(2), 213–234.

Maity, S., Dutta, S., & Paul, T. (2007). "Quality of Water and Health status in Tribal Villages of Santiniketan". Ed. Ghosh, A. *Environment Drinking Water and Public Health Problems and Future Goals*. Daya Publishing House, New Delhi, pp. 120–131.

Malmström, M., Sundquist, J., & Johansson, S. E. (1999). Neighborhood environment and self-reported health status: a multilevel analysis. *American Journal of Public Health*, *89*(8), 1181–1186.

Matthews, S. A., & Yang, T. C. (2010). Exploring the role of the built and social neighborhood environment in moderating stress and health. *Annals of Behavioral Medicine, 39*(2), 170–183.

McCulloch, A. (2001). Ward-level deprivation and individual social and economic outcomes in the British Household Panel Study. *Environment and Planning A, 33*(4), 667–684.

Meenakshi (2011). 'Neighbourhood unit and its conceptualization in the contemporary urban context', Institute of Town Planners. *India Journal, 8*(3), 81–86.

Messer, L. C., Laraia, B. A., Kaufman, J. S., Eyster, J., Holzman, C., Culhane, J., ... & O'Campo, P. (2006). The development of a standardized neighborhood deprivation index. *Journal of Urban Health, 83*(6), 1041–1062.

Mistry, R., Kleinsasser, M. J., Puntambekar, N., Gupta, P. C., McCarthy, W. J., Raghunathan, T., ... & Pednekar, M. S. (2022). Neighbourhood tobacco retail access and tobacco use susceptibility in young adolescents in urban India. *Tobacco Control, 31*(e2), e162–e168.

Mitra, K. (2008). "Environment and Urbanisation: The Impact on Human Health". Ed. Singh, A. L., & Fazal, S. *Urban Environmental Management*. B.R. Publishing Corporation, New Delhi, pp. 135–149.

Munian, A. (2010). *Dynamics of Residential Water Demand and Supply in India: A Case Study of Chennai City*. Gyan Publishing House, New Delhi.

Mushir, S., & Khan, M. F. (2007). *Quality of Urban Environment*. Idarah-i-Adabiyat-i-Delhi, New Delhi.

Nagami, S., Cohen, D. A., & Finch, B. K. (2007). Non-residential neighborhood exposures suppress neighborhood effects on self-rated health. *Social Science & Medicine (1982), 65*(8), 1779–1791. https://doi.org/10.1016/j.socscimed.2007.05.051

O'Sullivan, D., & Unwin, D. (2002). *Reducing the Number of Variables: Principal Component Analysis*. Geographic Information Analysis; John Wiley & Sons, Hoboken, NJ, USA, pp. 343–355.

Perkins, D. D., Meeks, J. W., & Taylor, R. B. (1992). The physical environment of street blocks and resident perceptions of crime and disorder: implications for theory and measurement. *Journal of Environmental Psychology, 12*(1), 21–34.

Phillimore, P. R., & Morris, D. (1991). Discrepant legacies: premature mortality in two industrial towns. *Social Science & Medicine, 33*(2), 139–152.

Pokhrel, D., & Viraraghavan, T. (2004). Diarrhoeal diseases in Nepal vis-à-vis water supply and sanitation status. *Journal of Water and Health, 2*(2), 71–81.

Rahman, A. (1998), *Household Environment and Health*, B R Publishing Corporation, New Delhi.

Rahman, M. (2008). *Urban environmental problems in Bangladesh: a case study of Chittagong city* (Doctoral dissertation, University of Hull).

Ramakrishnaiah, C. R., Sadashivaiah, C., & Ranganna, G. (2009). Assessment of water quality index for the groundwater in Tumkur Taluk, Karnataka State, India. *E-Journal of Chemistry, 6*(2), 523–530.

Rao, M. S. (1999). "Environmental Impact Assessment for Sustainable Urban Environment and Morphological Transformation in the cities: A Case of Madurai". Eds. Rao, R. R. M., & Simhadri, S. *Indian Cities: Towards Next Millenium*. Rawat Publicatons, Jaipur pp.133–143.

Ross, C. E., & Mirowsky, J. (1999). Disorder and decay: the concept and measurement of perceived neighborhood disorder. *Urban Affairs Review, 34*(3), 412–432.

Ross, N. A., Tremblay, S., & Graham, K. (2004). Neighbourhood influences on health in Montreal, Canada. *Social Science & Medicine, 59*(2004), 1485–1494.

Roux, A. V. D. (2007). Neighborhoods and health: where are we and were do we go from here?. *Revue d'epidemiologie et de santepublique, 55*(1), 13–21.

Roux, A. V. D., Borrell, L. N., Haan, M., Jackson, S. A., & Schultz, R. (2004). Neighbourhood environments and mortality in an elderly cohort: results from the cardiovascular health study. *Journal of Epidemiology & Community Health, 58*(11), 917–923.

Saaty, T. L. (1980). *The Analytic Process: Planning, Priority Setting, Resources Allocation*. McGraw, New York.

Saha, S., Basu, S., & Pandit, D. (2022). A framework for identifying perceived quality of life indicators for the elderly in the neighbourhood context: A case study of Kolkata, India. *Quality & Quantity, 57*, 1–33.

Shaban, A. (2008). "Urban Environmental Management in India: Issues and Challenges". Eds. Singh, A. L., & Fazal, S. *Urban Environmental Management*. B.R. Publishing Corporation, New Delhi, pp. 107–134.

Shazli, T., & Munir, A. (2016). Quality of urban indoor environment and socio-economic condition in Azamgarh City: a case study of Azamgarh City, Uttar Pradesh. *Journal of Global Resources, 1*(1), 35–47.

Singh, A. L., Fazal, S., Azam, F., & Rahman, A. (1996). Income, environment and health: a household level study of Aligarh City, India. *Habitat International, 20*(1), 77–91.

Songsore, J., & McGranahan, G. (1993). Environment, wealth and health: towards an analysis of intra-urban differentials within the Greater Accra Metropolitan Area, Ghana. *Environment and Urbanization, 5*(2), 10–34.

Tzoulas, K., Korpela, K., Venn, S., Yli-Pelkonen, V., Kaźmierczak, A., Niemela, J., & James, P. (2007). "Promoting ecosystem and human health in urban areas using Green Infrastructure: a literature review" *Landscape and Urban Planning*, 81 (2007), 167–178.

Uddin, M. G., Nash, S., & Olbert, A. I. (2021). A review of water quality index models and their use for assessing surface water quality. *Ecological Indicators, 122*, 107218.

Unger, A., & Riley, L. W. (2007). Slum health: from understanding to action. *PLoS Medicine, 4*(10), e295.

United Nations. (2017). *The Sustainable Development Goals Report 2017*. United Nations, New York.

WHO. (2004). Health & Environment Tools for Effective Decision-Making.

WHO. (2010). *Why Urban Health Matters*. World Health Organisation.

WHO. (2016). Public health and environment. https://www.who.int/data/gho/data/themes/public-health-and-environment

Wilson, S., Hutson, M., & Mujahid, M. (2008). How planning and zoning contribute to inequitable development, neighbourhood health, and environmental injustice. *Environmental Justice, 1*(4), 2008.

Yadav, A. K., Khan, P., & Sharma, S. K. (2010). Water quality index assessment of groundwater in Todaraisingh Tehsil of Rajasthan State, India – A greener approach. *E-journal of Chemistry, 7*(S1), S428–S432.

1 Understanding the Neighbourhood Concept and Its Health Impacts

Neighbourhood is simply the vicinity in which people live. It can be understood as groups of families and houses, whether used for dwelling or for commercial uses, generally consisting of buildings and conveniences, providing opportunities for work, leisure, education and shopping. Neighbourhood is an area where one can find residential, commercial, leisure, education and health services within walking distance (Narad et al., 2014). The built environment of a neighbourhood interconnects and allows neighbours to share infrastructure and services.

Since ancient times, settlements of people have been geographically separated into numerous zones and neighbourhoods (Friedmann, 2010; Smith, 2010), which indicates the significance of neighbourhoods in the structure of a city. According to Arnold Whittick (1974), a neighbourhood is an incorporated and properly designed urban area, a part of a broader district, comprising dwelling units, educational institutions, shopping centres, religious places and open spaces (Whittick, 1974).

A neighbourhood represents an everyday-landscape, which can either support or limit the physical, mental and social well-being of the residents. Neighbourhood, as a basic unit of planning, has always been of particular interest to planners and urban thinkers (Rohe, 2009). Neighbourhoods can be taken as a physical entity in planning because a neighbourhood which is sound in design and services is believed to nurture healthier and more socially interactive communities. Since the early 20th century, various theories and models have been developed to create better and more liveable neighbourhoods.

1.1 Understanding Neighbourhoods

The term neighbourhood has several interpretations and usages. For example, a neighbourhood could be a cluster of several houses in the surroundings of one's home or a more substantial region with a similar type of houses. It can also be defined as a census ward. A neighbourhood can also be used to refer to an area encircling a small establishment like school, church or any other social agency utilised by residents. The above interpretations can lead to a healthy debate on neighbourhood boundaries. Every field has a different reason for its

DOI: 10.4324/9781003442486-2

definition. City planners often define neighbourhood boundaries along with census boundaries while generally resident communities have an entirely different mental map of their neighbourhood than the census boundaries. When a neighbourhood combines with other neighbourhoods, it becomes a town.

In the words of the urban scholar Lewis Mumford, "Neighbourhoods, in some annoying, inchoate fashion exist wherever human beings congregate, in permanent family dwellings; and many of the functions of the city tend to be distributed naturally—that is, without any theoretical preoccupation or political direction into neighbourhoods" (Mumford, 1954).

In the words of Warren (1981), a neighbourhood can be defined as "a social organisation of a population residing in a geographically proximate locale" while Hallman (1984) defined neighbourhood as "a limited territory within a larger urban area, where people inhabit dwellings and interact socially" (Warren, 1981; Hallman, 1984). Some other definitions of neighbourhood are as follows:

"ward, or one sixth part of the city....in some sense a complete town by itself...for the duration of the city's construction"

(Howard, 1985)

"an area in which people share certain common facilities, necessary to domestic life"

(Mumford, 1963)

"a mundane organ of self-government"

(Jacobs, 1961)

"a group of living cells, which constitutes a unit of habitation of suitable size"

(CIAM, 1933)

"the very local unit, within which people are personally acquainted with each other by reason of residential proximity"

(Lynch, 1981)

"an enclave of people providing a social and physical element intermediate between the individual and his family and the larger heterogeneous group"

(Rapport, 1977)

Robert E, Park in 1915 represented neighbourhoods as localities with sentiments, traditions and a history of their own. Local interests and associations develop local sensibilities which make residents the basis of participation in the elections, and thus neighbourhoods become the basis of political control. A neighbourhood exists without any formal organisation (Park, 1915). Any town is made up of several neighbourhoods.

The conceptualisation of neighbourhood has been extensively used both in policy-making and research. In policy-making, neighbourhoods act as perfect laboratory for testing and executing various policies. In research, it serves as a spatial unit which helps in understanding inequalities at spatial levels. Neighbourhood concept has been dynamic, and it has changed over time. Different branches of knowledge have offered different perspectives on how the neighbourhood concept is originated.

1.1.1 Neighbourhood as a Planning Unit

In the discipline of planning, idea of a neighbourhood has been believed to be emerged from "Garden city" moment of Ebenezer Howard during the 19th century.

The neighbourhood concept as a planning unit was first used in the 1920s. Regarding this, two separate original ideas were presented in the year 1929. One idea was of the "Neighbourhoods" given by Clarence Stein and Henry Wright while the second idea was of the "Neighbourhood Unit" given by Clarence Perry.

1.1.1.1 "Neighbourhood Unit" by Clarence Perry (1929)

The idea behind individual neighbourhood was to put together a sense of belongingness among its inhabitants and development of environment friendly practices.

Earlier people were concerned about major urban problems in the industrialising cities like traffic congestion, crowded residential and working conditions, houses without open spaces, problems caused by vehicles, etc.

Perry saw traffic problem as deadly problem as it restricted the safe movement of people especially kids to nearby playgrounds and other facilities. In fact, he developed his neighbourhood unit idea as a planning tool to guide the distribution and arrangement of playgrounds in the city.

He saw traffic as a major problem as in early 20th-century modem tools modern tools to manage traffic problems like zebra crossing, traffic signals and road signs were not abundant and the road death rate was much more than one child a day (Perry, 1998).

Perry developed his neighbourhood unit concept as a solution to contemporary urban problems. Although the idea of neighbourhood unit appeared in 1923 at a joint meeting of "The National Community Centre Association" and "The American Sociological Society" in Washington DC, neighbourhood unit gained popularity as a planning tool only after publication of Clarence Perry's paper in "Regional Plan of New York and its Environs" in 1929. His work was titled as "The Neighborhood Unit, a Scheme for Arrangement for the Family-Life Community" (Perry, 1929).

He provided a concrete illustrative model for ideal structure of a neighbourhood of a specific size of population. The models offered proper guidelines for distribution of residential units, neighbourhood services and businesses activities as well as arrangement of streets. The basic principles of neighbourhood as a planning unit are as follows:

- Main roads should be along the periphery of neighbourhood unit forming boundaries to it. Therefore, it should define and differentiate the neighbourhood unit with surrounding areas and also prevent the undesirable traffic in the neighbourhood unit. Therefore, main roads must define the neighbourhood rather that dividing it.
- Radius of the neighbourhood should be one fourth of a mile and in the centre of the neighbourhood there should be school. Therefore, a child will have to walk for about one fourth of a mile to school and he would not cross the main road.
- The size of the neighbourhood should be around 5000–9000 people to keep up the school.
- Local streets should be distinguished from main roads following a hierarchical structure to ensure safety of the residents especially kids. Streets should discourage unwanted outer traffic through neighbourhood.
- Shopping centres should be located near the periphery of neighbourhood so that non-local population should be restricted to periphery only should not intrude the neighbourhood unit.
- At-least 10% land area of neighbourhood should be devoted to open spaces, playgrounds and parks for kids to enjoy outdoor activities and residents to interact.

Perry's idea of neighbourhood unit was continued to be used in much modern and adopted forms to order and organise communities of an area in such ways that satisfies their "social, administrative and service requirements for satisfactory urban existence" (Banerjee and Baer, 2013).

1.1.1.2 "Neighbourhood" by Clarence Stein and Henry Wright (1929)

Before working on the neighbourhood concept, Stein worked on the Yorkshire Village Master plan in Camden, New Jersey (Patricios, 2002). The theatrical base of Yorkshire plan was later applied to his other works too particularly "Neighbourhood" concept. As Stein and Wright clearly presented their Neighbourhood design principles in their plan for Radburn city, their concept for the neighbourhood is also known as Radburn model.

The neighbourhood concept of Stein and Wright was hierarchical one starting from enclave up to neighbourhood. Then several neighbourhoods will form the city.

An enclave in neighbourhood model of Stein and Wright was a group of 20 or more houses. These houses were arranged in U form around a street known as lane, basically a cul-de-sac (dead end) street. A pedestrian street separated enclaves. Three or more enclaves in a line formed a block. The blocks were organised around a central parkway in such way so as to encircle the open spaces. The cluster of blocks formed a superblock and around four to six superblocks formed a neighbourhood. Two neighbourhoods were separated by main roads or natural features.

In neighbourhood plan of stein and Wright, roads were to be hierarchical with main roads to border and separate neighbourhoods, middle roads to encircle superblocks and local cul-de-sac streets for access to individual properties.

Stein and Wright while considering neighbourhood as self-sufficient also organised them in superimposed way for common use of amenities and facilities such as health, education and recreational facilities. They imagined three levels of hierarchy comprising neighbourhood forming towns and towns forming a region.

1.1.2 Identification of Neighbourhood Boundaries

Neighbourhood size has been defined throughout in planning history. A variety of approaches have been used to measure boundaries of the neighbourhoods. According to Clarence Perry, a neighbourhood is a part of town and its size is measured as a radius of walking distance of five minutes from the centre of the neighbourhood (around 0.65 km^2). The neighbourhood's centre provides cultural services like presence of a school. In the early 1990s, the firm of Duany Plater-Zyberk procreated Clarence Perry's model to exhibit that his model is still functional for planning of today's cities. Perry's definition of a neighbourhood's radius of five walking minutes distance is a part of the American Institute of Architects Architectural Graphics Standards. Some studies have defined neighbourhoods based on residents' addresses and by drawing a radius of 400–500 m around their houses. Conventional neighbourhoods generally have definite sizes mostly depending upon the walking distance corresponding to a radius of quarter mile.

Some important features that can be used for marking the boundary of neighbourhoods can be streets, surrounding context, natural features like parks, river or streams or manmade features like railway lines, highways, and changes in land use or character, etc. Streets demarcate clear limits that are easy to recognise and remember. Land use change is one of the most common ways to define limit of one neighbourhood and start of another neighbourhood. For example, land use change from residential to commercial or residential to industrial easily demarcates the neighbourhoods. Similarly, presence of any university, institution, hospital, etc., can influence the surrounding population and can result in certain development and changes in the neighbourhood.

Neighbourhood boundaries can be defined based on several criteria ranging from historical, administrative boundaries, based on residents' characteristics, based on residents' perception, etc. Boundaries based on different criteria could be different from each other, and for different research questions different criteria can be used. For example, when research interest is related to social interaction and relations among residents, neighbourhood boundaries based on people's perception should be used while administrative boundaries of neighbourhoods should be used when policy application is under investigation. In the same way, to examine the characteristics of chemical and physical environment, i.e. exposure to certain environmental conditions, geographic boundaries of neighbourhoods should be used (Diez Roux 2001).

The use of administrative boundaries has also been a widespread practice, mainly due to data availability and feasibility. Although the use of administrative boundaries does not exactly fit with residents' perception of their neighbourhood, it can be justified that census boundaries were originally developed to be rather homogenous in socio-economic characteristics. Generally, census or ward boundaries possess similar social and physical attributes. Some studies have used entire census tract or block groups to represent a neighbourhood (Brownson et al., 2004; Spivock et al., 2008), while others have combined various census tracts (King, 2008; Furr-Holden et al., 2008). Rauh et al. (29) have defined neighbourhood relevant to affect health of its residents as a cluster of several census area while Pearl et al. (30) have chosen administrative block group.

Large quantitative researches over a longer time span are generally forced to rely on existing administrative boundary for which official data are available. For smaller areas, defining neighbourhoods based on local historical, social, geographic and demographic knowledge could be helpful. Several other characteristics of neighbourhoods could be taken into consideration while defining neighbourhoods.

1.1.3 Characteristic Features of Individual Neighbourhoods

With increasing urbanisation, inequality in income has increased along with class segregation and a concentration of wealth and poverty giving rise to different types of neighbourhoods (Massey, 1996). It is essential to know the factors that give neighbourhoods their individual characters. These factors could be population composition (races, classes), people having their own houses or the proportion of the population consisting of nomads, gipsies, etc. Neighbourhoods can be classified based on numerous criteria. Some of them are as follows.

1.1.3.1 Neighbourhood Socio-Economic Condition

It includes classification of the neighbourhoods based on per capita income of residents, education and occupation of the head of the households, percentage of white-collar people, percentage of residents having cars, newspaper subscriptions, land values and level of overcrowding. It is important to note that all these criteria are associated with each other and income, education and occupation are the major deciding factors for the majority of other factors.

1.1.3.2 Housing and Population

It includes percentage households living on rent, percentage of houses occupied by single persons, population size and area of a neighbourhood. Percentage households living on rent and percentage of houses occupied by single persons are also associated with socio-economic condition of neighbourhoods viz. neighbourhoods with higher socio-economic status have a significant share of owned houses mostly occupied by family men.

1.1.3.3 Density of the Neighbourhood

It involves population density, residential density as well as household density of neighbourhoods. High population density in the neighbourhoods is a signature phenomenon of low socio-economic status neighbourhoods with mostly poor residents as affluent people choose to live in less dense areas with ample availability of open green spaces.

1.1.3.4 Presence or Lack of Commercial Stores

It includes the presence of pharmacies, beauty parlours, barbershops, schools, clinics and supermarkets per thousand populations in a neighbourhood. Availability or unavailability of amenities and facilities is generally an indicator of income group residing in the neighbourhood as high-income neighbourhoods are generally full-fledged with public amenities and facilities.

1.1.4 Concept of Neighbourhood in Some Major Cities of the World

There are different concepts of neighbourhoods in different parts of the world. In Asian countries like China, the term neighbourhood is used for an urban administrative unit just lower from district level. In China, the term neighbourhood and streets are used alternatively, varying from city to city. Each neighbourhood comprises 2000 to 10,000 families. Neighbourhoods are further divided into residential units or quarters comprising 100 to 600 families. However, in most of the Chinese cities, the terms neighbourhood, community, residential unit and residential quarter are used interchangeably.

In Ottoman's Turkey Neighbourhood was used as a settlement unit to maintain social order (Aru, 1996). Neighbourhood in Ottoman cities was a place comprising families praying in the same mosque, having adequate social interaction and cohesion. Due to the importance of neighbourhoods as a social unit, Middle Eastern cities and Islamic culture are known as a composition of neighbourhoods (Ergenç, 1984; Çakır, 2012). In modern societies, however, with change of residential structure in the cities, the social fabric has started disappearing and so has the initial concept of neighbourhood (Aydın and Sıramkaya, 2014).

In the United Kingdom, neighbourhood does not have any official status; however, people use it informally for their local areas. The term is often used for local organisations like neighbourhood policing, neighbourhood watch, etc. Moreover, government data for any local area is also termed as neighbourhood data.

In Canada and the United States, the term neighbourhood often enjoys official or semi-official status. Various organisations like neighbourhood association and neighbourhood watches are there to regulate various activities in the neighbourhoods. The services that come under these organisations are neighbourhood security, neighbourhood parks, regulation of lawn care and fence heights as well as organising block parties. However, in many cities, districts and wards are used as official divisions of the city and not neighbourhood boundaries. Post office areas and zip code divisions can sometimes reflect a neighbourhood in American cities.

1.1.5 Concept of Neighbourhood in Indian Cities

Neighbourhood in India is a more fluid and socially constructed concept and is not given an official status. Although role of neighbourhood in social interaction and cohesion has been understood since old times, they are mostly used as informal divisions of the city. Although, neighbourhood concept is not incorporated in urban administration in India; however, informal neighbourhoods can be seen in different parts of the country. For example "chawl" in Mumbai and also Lajpat Nagar, Gol Market and Chandni Chowk are different neighbourhoods of Delhi. In India, the term "neighbourhhod" can be used interchangeably with the term "Mohalla".

The concept of neighbourhood however has been considered in some planned cities or planned colonies of the cities. The master plan of Chandigarh city incorporated the concept of neighbourhood for creating self-contained society, away from traffic and other ill-effects of cities by following the idea of Perry (1929). Each Neighbourhood unit in Chandigarh city, termed as sector, was self-contained and self-sufficient in terms of daily needs like grocery shopping, schools, health facilities, banks, post offices, leisure and recreation (Gupta, 2020).

Other studies related to neighbourood concept in modern urban planning in India have investigated currently existing neighbourhoods in the light of sustainable neighbourhoods. Green city Nagpur has fulfilled the requirement for a healthy and sustainable neighbourhood (Narad and Gupta, 2014) while Minal residency, Bhopal does not fulfil the requirements of a neighbourhood (Prajapati and Padhya, 2021). The results show that at some planned residential areas in India, we can see the essence of initial neighbourhood units.

In sociology, various researchers believe that neighbourhoods play an important role in building social cohesion among residents therefore the neighbourhoods must be considered while framing urban policies to solve urban social problems (Jha et al. 2021).

1.2 How Neighbourhoods Affect Health

Various social and physical characteristics of neighbourhoods are generally linked with common health status, disabilities, chronic conditions, health behaviours, injuries, mental health as well as mortality and other important health indicators (Cubbin et al., 2008). Neighbourhoods can influence our health in many ways. First and perhaps most important is through the physical characteristics of neighbourhoods. Health can be adversely affected by poor air and water quality in the neighbourhood (Macintyre and Ellaway 2002). A neighbourhood can damage the health of its people by its poor water quality, air quality, faulty drainage conditions, water logging, accumulation of litter, congestion, adverse traffic conditions, unavailability of safe places for exercise, unavailability of medical and health services, etc.

Amerigo (2002) while discussing residential satisfaction has clarified that residences and neighbourhoods are usually examined into two forms: one deals with physical and service features associated with facilities and amenities and another one deals with social features associated with community bonding in the common areas of the residences as well as in the neighbourhood (Amerigo, 2002).

Neighbourhoods can affect health of its residents by its physical and social features as well as by the services or facilities it provides. To understand the neighbourhood effect more precisely, it will be helpful to understand the forms of neighbourhood environment separately. According to Catherine Cubbin et al. (2008), neighbourhood environment can be studied in three forms, i.e. neighbourhood physical environment, neighbourhood social environment and neighbourhood service environment.

1.2.1 Neighbourhood Physical Environment and Health

Physical environment of neighbourhood involves the natural environment along with the built-or manmade environment. Components of natural environment include air, water, soil, sunshine, etc., while the built environment is the environment coming out from the manmade structures including fabrics of buildings, roads, streets, urban green spaces and health, recreational and educational facilities. Physical environment of a neighbourhood can influence health in many ways. Physical features of neighbourhoods like air and water quality, inferior housing conditions like houses with lead paints, pest and insect's infections, unavailability of stores providing fresh vegetables and other food items, unavailability of places to walk/exercise like parks, playgrounds, gyms, etc., readily availability of unhealthy food stores or liquor stores and exposure to harmful traffic conditions, etc. Researches are done worldwide to examine how physical features of neighbourhoods affect health, and it has been proved that characteristics of streets, buildings and other built material influence the habit of smoking and workout and also obesity among residents (Booth et al. 2005; Sallis and Glanz 2006; Goedon-Larsen et al. 2006). Closeness to the facilities that sell fresh food items is associated with low prevalence of obesity, and similarly closeness to the facilities that do not provide fresh food items is associated with more prevalence of obesity (Morland et al. 2006) and smoking (Chuang et al. 2005) among residents. In the neighbourhoods where facilities for exercise like parks, walking trails and pedestrian-friendly street patterns are abundant, people are more physically active. Many features of the neighbourhood physical environment such as supermarkets and parks can also be taken as features of the neighbourhood service environment.

1.2.2 Neighbourhood Social Environment and Health

The Social Environment – Social environment of a neighbourhood incorporates the quality of relationship among residents of a neighbourhood like the level of trust and cooperation. Social environment of neighbourhoods can also influence health. In a neighbourhood where people are more connected and share the feeling of togetherness, there are more chances of them to work together for the betterment of neighbourhood like litter free and safe public spaces, healthy behaviour among kids and good schools, etc. (Putnam 1993: Sampson et al. 2002). Also there are more chances of them to exchange helpful knowledge and information regarding childcare, employment and other resources affecting health and to maintain social control among youth like discouraging objectionable behaviours in terms of smoking, alcohol use, littering, crime, etc. Healthy social environment in the neighbourhoods thus prevents disorder which will help attain a community with better mental health. In the neighbourhoods where people are more connected and are willing to get involved for public welfare, homicide rates are lower (Sampson et al. 1997; Morenoff et al. 2001). In contrast, neighbourhoods with less connectedness among residents and higher social disorders are associated with anxiety and depression among residents (Cultrona et al. 2000).

1.2.3 Neighbourhood Service Environment and Health

The service environment of a neighbourhood incorporates amenities and facilities associated to health whether directly or indirectly. It includes services in the neighbourhood for health, educations, jobs, grocery and recreation, etc. Neighbourhoods can also influence health by the availability and unavailability of various services and opportunities in it. Where we live determines our access to good quality schools, health facilities, municipal services, employment opportunities as well as transportation facilities which ultimately determines our health. Availability of health facilities in neighbourhood is rather directly associated with health. Educational as well as employment opportunities affect the health in indirect ways, i.e. by providing means to attain a decent living standard both in present and future. The neighbourhood that lacks in proper educational and employment opportunities creates a socially disadvantaged society which eventually possesses poor health conditions (William and Collins 2001; Pastor 2001; Fernandez and Su, 2004).

The modern urban environment is combined with industrialisation, over-crowding, waste generation and inadequate drainage system. The speedy and unplanned urbanisation, along with unsustainable style of development, is making developing cities the focal point for evolving environmental and health perils. These problems include urban poverty, traffic mortalities, air and noise pollution as well as increasing burden on municipal services. Urbanisation has also invaded open spaces of walking and recreation in the cities leading to a sedentary lifestyle and a rise in related non-communicable diseases. Various environmental problems like pollution; overcrowding and unsanitary living conditions are important pathways for transmission of infectious diseases. Many contagious diseases flourish in neighbourhoods if there is a crisis of water supply and if quality and services of drainage, sanitation and solid waste removal are inadequate.

1.2.4 How Neighbourhood Effect is Measured

Interest of the researchers regarding how neighbourhoods can affect health has increased worldwide as it is not only academically important but impor-tant for policy makers too. Neighbourhood differences are especially impor-tant in the case of increasing concentration of poverty in certain areas and sort of geographical concentration of poverty and other deprivations. Keeping track of neighbourhood effects and how they are measured could have serious policy implications for increasing health equality and reducing health dispar-ity. Generally three practical approaches have been used to measure neigh-bourhood effects on health, i.e. ecologic studies, contextual or multi-level studies as well as comparison of certain well-defined neighbourhoods (Diez Roux 2001).

1.2.4.1 Ecologic Studies

Ecologic or ecological studies are used to examine the relationship between occurrences of diseases as well as exposure to recognised or potential causes. Here, the unit under examination is a community or population. In each com-munity or population, morbidity or mortality is examined and their association is analysed with the prevalent risk factors. Generally, the information about prevalence of diseases is extracted from published sources. Since unit of analy-sis is the community, inferences about individuals cannot be drawn. Here the main aim is to examine the association between area characteristics and rates of morbidity and mortality in those areas. The area under investigation could be very large, not at all equivalent to neighbourhoods like counties, regions (Wing et al. 1992; Tyroler et al. 1993; Raleigh and Kiri 1997) or even whole countries or very small like census tracts or electoral wards (Eames et al. 1993).

The unit of analysis in ecologic studies can be electoral wards, zip codes, counties, regions or full countries. The most commonly examined area characteristics are collective socio-economic characteristics of residents of an area or level of deprivation measured through any index. These characteristics of the area have been strongly found correlated to mortality rates (Townsend et al. 1988; Wing et al. 1992; Tyroler et al. 1993). However, there is confusion that whether these area-level variables are taken as simply area-level characteristics or collective form of individual-level variables (Diez Roux 2001). Although ecological studies are very helpful in understanding health inequality over areas, they cannot clearly state that whether health differences across areas are due to peculiar characteristics of areas themselves or it is due to different characteristics of individuals living in them. Ecologic studies cannot determine whether the individual-level variables act like confounders, mediators or modifiers to the area effects. Therefore, a need was felt of multi-level study that distinguished between the area-level characteristics (Context) and individual-level characteristics (Composition).

1.2.4.2 Contextual or Multi-Level Studies

This type of studies requires datasets both of the characteristics of individuals of the area as well the characteristics of area themselves (Rauh et al. 2001; Pearl et al. 2001). By including both individual and neighbourhood-level characteristics in regression equations while considering individuals as unit of analysis, here individual-level characteristics are controlled and only neighbourhood effect is measured. This strategy can help in measuring the neighbourhood characteristics as modifiers of individual characteristics and vice-versa. Multi-level analysis is helpful in understanding both the role of inter-neighbourhood and intra-neighbourhood variability in occurrence of diseases. It is helpful in understand how much neighbourhood-level differences can be explained by individual factors as well by neighbourhood factors themselves. Studies in this approach have tried to examine the association between individual characteristics and the area characteristics. A consistency in the results of the previous studies has been found regarding an independent effect of neighbourhood environment (Anderson et al. 1997; Yen and Syme 1999; Robert 1999); however, strength of this effect over individual-level factors is not much (Yen and Syme 1999; Robert 1999).

1.2.4.3 Comparison of Certain Well-Defined Neighbourhoods

A relatively new approach in measuring neighbourhood effect on health is a comparison of certain well-defined neighbourhoods of different characteristics (Phillimore and Morris 1991; Macintyre et al. 1993, Ellaway et al. 1997). Neighbourhoods can be defined based on their local historical, geographical and sociological as well as demographic characteristics. Simultaneously, a combination of other quantitative and qualitative techniques can also be used to collect information about neighbourhood characteristics and health conditions (Macintyre et al. 1993). This method is used to examine differences between neighbourhood's characteristics in terms of resources and services they provide and to relate these differences with health outcomes. Major limitation of this method is that very small range and number of neighbourhoods can be examined at a time. This method can be best used with local definition of neighbourhood and in the direct collection of data on the features of neighbourhoods so that it can help in understanding the ways by which neighbourhood environment influences health. In this work, we would further see the use of the current method in understanding the impact of neighbourhood environment on health.

Summary

This chapter deals with different concept of neighbourhood over space and time as well as an understanding of how neighbourhoods can impact health of its residents. The chapter has been divided into two sections. The first section deals with concept of neighbourhood while the second section deals with the ways by which neighbourhoods can affect health of its residents. The chapter starts with an understanding of different definitions of neighbourhoods and further deals with identification of neighbourhood as a planning unit, identification of neighbourhood boundaries, characteristic features of individual neighbourhoods, concept of neighbourhood in some major cities of the world as well as concept of neighbourhood in Indian context. The analysis reveals that neighbourhoods have been identified since early times; however, their official recognition as a planning unit has started only after publication of the idea of "Neighbourhood Unit" by Clarence Perry and "Neighbourhood" by Stein and Wright in 1929. In the modern world, neighbourhoods have not been given official status except in the United States and Canada; however, the term is being comprehensively used for an informal division of the city and people have a certain boundary of their neighbourhood in their minds. The second section of the chapter deals with different forms of neighbourhood environment, i.e. neighbourhood physical environment, neighbourhood social environment as well as neighbourhood services environment and ways by which they can influence residents' health. Further, various methods used to measure neighbourhood impact on health have been discussed ranging from ecological studies to contextual or multi-level studies and a comparison of certain number of well-defined neighbourhoods is done.

References

Amerigo, M. (2002). "A Psychological Approach to the Study of Residential Satisfaction". Eds. J. I. Aragones, G. Francescato, & T. Carling (Eds), *Residential Environments: Choice, Satisfaction, and Behavior*. Bergin Si Garvey Publisher, Westport (YT/London), pp. 81–99.

Anderson, R. T., Sorlie, P., Backlund, E., Johnson, N., & Kaplan, G. A. (1997). Mortality effects of community socioeconomic status. *Epidemiology*, *1*, 42–47.

Aru, K.A. (1996). *Osmanlı Türk Kentlerinin Genel Karakteristikleri Üzerine Görüşler.* Tarihten Günümüze Anadolu'da Konut ve Yerleşme. Türkiye Ekonomik ve Toplumsal Tarih Vakfı, İstanbul.

Aydın, D., & Sıramkaya, S. B. (2014). "Neighborhood" concept and the analysis of differentiating sociological structure with the change of dwelling typology. *Procedia-Social and Behavioral Sciences*, *140*, 260–269.

Banerjee, T., & Baer, W. C. (2013). *Beyond the Neighborhood Unit: Residential Environments and Public Policy.* Springer Science & Business Media, California.

Booth, K. M., Pinkston, M. M., & Poston, W. S. C. (2005). Obesity and the built environment. *Journal of the American Dietetic Association*, *105*(5), 110–117.

Brownson, R. C., Chang, J. J., Eyler, A. A., Ainsworth, B. E., Kirtland, K. A., Saelens, B. E., & Sallis, J. F. (2004). Measuring the environment for friendliness toward physical activity: a comparison of the reliability of 3 questionnaires. *American Journal of Public Health*, *94*(3), 473–483.

Çakır, İ. E. (2012). XVI. Yüzyılda Ayntab'da Toplumsal Kontrol Aracı Olarak Mahalle Halkının Rolü. *Bilig, Güz*, *53*, 31–54.

Chuang, Y. C., Cubbin, C., Ahn, D., & Winkleby, M. A. (2005). Effects of neighbourhood socioeconomic status and convenience store concentration on individual level smoking. *Tobacco Control*, *14*(5), 337–337.

CIAM (1933). "The Athens Charter". In Le Corbusier (1973, 1943) *The Athens charter*. Grossman Publisher, New York.

Cubbin, C., Egerter, S., Braveman, P., & Pedregon, V. (2008). *Where We Live Matters for Our Health: Neighborhoods and Health.* Robert Wood John Foundation.

Cutrona, C. E., Russell, D. W., Hessling, R. M., Brown, P. A., & Murry, V. (2000). Direct and moderating effects of community context on the psychological well-being of African American women. *Journal of Personality and Social Psychology*, *79*(6), 1088.

Diez Roux, A. V. (2001). Investigating neighborhood and area effects on health. *American Journal of Public Health*, *91* (11), 1783–1789.

Eames, M., Ben-Shlomo, Y., & Marmot, M. G. (1993). Social deprivation and premature mortality: regional comparison across England. *British Medical Journal*, *307*(6912), 1097–1102.

Ellaway, A., Anderson, A., & Macintyre, S. (1997). Does area of residence affect body size and shape?. *International Journal of Obesity*, *21*(4), 304–308.

Ergenç, Ö. (1984). Osmanlı Şehrindeki Mahallenin İşlev ve Nitelikleri Üzerine. Osmanlı Araştırmaları IV. İstanbul. 69–78.

Fernandez, R. M., & Su, C. (2004). Space in the study of labor markets. *Annual Review of Sociology*, *30*, 545–569.

Friedmann, J. (2010). Place and place-making in cities: A global perspective. *Planning Theory & Practice*, *11*(2), 149–165. http://dx.doi.org/10.1080/14649351003759573

Furr-Holden, C. D. M., Smart, M. J., Pokorni, J. L., Ialongo, N. S., Leaf, P. J., Holder, H. D., & Anthony, J. C. (2008). The NIfETy method for environmental assessment of neighborhood-level indicators of violence, alcohol, and other drug exposure. *Prevention Science*, *9*(4), 245–255.

Gordon-Larsen, P., Nelson, M. C., Page, P., & Popkin, B. M. (2006). Inequality in the built environment underlies key health disparities in physical activity and obesity. *Pediatrics*, *117*(2), 417–424.

Gupta, K.J. (2020). Neighborhood planning in capital city of Chandigarh-an appraisal. https://www.linkedin.com/pulse/neighborhood-planning-capital-city-chandigarh-appraisal-gupta-1f retrieved on 27-12-2022.

Hallman, H. W. (1984). *Neighbourhoods: Their Place in Urban Life.* Sage Publications, Beverly Hills, CA.

Howard, E. (1985). *Garden Cities of Tomorrow.* MIT Press, London.

Jacobs, J. (1961). *The Death and Life of Great American Cities.* Vintage Books, New York.

Jha, S., Pathak, D. N., & Das, A. K. (Eds.). (2021). *Neighbourhoods in Urban India: In between Home and the City.* Bloomsbury Publishing, India.

King, D. (2008). Neighbourhood and individual factors in activity in older adults: results from the neighbourhood and senior health study. *Journal of Aging and Physical Activity, 16*(2), 144–170.

Lynch, K. (1981). *Good City Form.* MIT Press, Cambridge.

Macintyre, S. & Ellaway, A. (2002). Place effects on health: how can we conceptualise, operationalise and measure them? *Social Science & Medicine, 55*(2002), 125–139.

Macintyre, S., Maciver, S., & Sooman, A. (1993). Area, class and health: should we be focusing on places or people?. *Journal of Social Policy, 22*(2), 213–234.

Massey, D.S. (1996). The age of extremes: Concentrated affluence and poverty in the twenty-first century. *Demography, 33*, 395–412.

Morenoff, J. D., Sampson, R. J., & Raudenbush, S. W. (2001). Neighborhood inequality, collective efficacy, and the spatial dynamics of urban violence. *Criminology, 39*(3), 517–558.

Morland, K., Roux, A. V. D., & Wing, S. (2006). Supermarkets, other food stores, and obesity: the atherosclerosis risk in communities study. *American Journal of Preventive Medicine, 30*(4), 333–339.

Mumford, L. (1963). *Technics and Civilization.* Harcourt, Bruce, New York.

Mumford, Lewis (1954). The Neighbourhood and the Neighbourhood Unit'. *The Town Planning Review, 24*(4), 256–270.

Narad, A.V. & Gupta, P.V. (2014). Role of sustainable neighbourhood in urban built environment. *IOSR Journal of Mechanical and Civil Engineering (IOSR-JMCE),* 27–31.

Park, R. E. (1915). The city: Suggestions for the investigation of human behavior in the city environment. *American Journal of Sociology, 20*(5), 577–612.

Pastor, M. (2001). Geography and opportunity. *America Becoming: Racial Trends and Their Consequences, 1,* 435–468.

Patricios, N. N. (2002). Urban design principles of the original neighbourhood concepts. *Urban Morphology, 6*(1), 21–36.

Pearl, M., Braveman, P., & Abrams, B. (2001). The relationship of neighborhood socioeconomic characteristics to birthweight among 5 ethnic groups in California. *American Journal of Public Health, 91*(11), 1808–1814.

Perry, C. (1929). *The Neighbourhood Unit: From the Regional Survey of New York and Its Environs: Volume VII: Neighbourhood and Community Planning.* Routledge.

Perry, C. (1998). *The Neighbourhood Unit (1929).* Reprinted Routledge/Thoemmes, London, pp. 25–44.

Phillimore, P. R., & Morris, D. (1991). Discrepant legacies: premature mortality in two industrial towns. *Social Science & Medicine, 33*(2), 139–152.

Prajapati, V., & Padhya, H. (2021). Smart neighbourhood planning in India. *International Journal of Research and Engineering, 9*(2), 22–25.

Putnam, R. (1993). The prosperous community: Social capital and public life. *The American Prospect*, *13*(4), 35–42.

Raleigh, V. S., & Kiri, V. A. (1997). Life expectancy in England: variations and trends by gender, health authority, and level of deprivation. *Journal of Epidemiology & Community Health*, *51*(6), 649–658.

Rapport, A. (1977). *Human Aspects of Urban form*, Pergamon Press, New York.

Rauh, V. A., Andrews, H. F., & Garfinkel, R. S. (2001). The contribution of maternal age to racial disparities in birthweight: a multilevel perspective. *American Journal of Public Health*, *91*(11), 1815–1824.

Robert, S. A. (1999). Socioeconomic position and health: the independent contribution of community socioeconomic context. *Annual Review of Sociology*, *25*, 489–516.

Rohe, W. (2009). From local to global: one hundred years of neighborhood planning. *Journal of the American Planning Association*, *75*(2), 209–230. http://dx.doi.org/10.1080/01944360902751077

Sallis, J. F., & Glanz, K. (2006). The role of built environments in physical activity, eating, and obesity in childhood. *The Future of Children*, *16*, 89–108.

Sampson, R. J., Morenoff, J. D., & Gannon-Rowley, T. (2002). Assessing "neighborhood effects": Social processes and new directions in research. *Annual Review of Sociology*, *28*, 443–478.

Sampson, R. J., Raudenbush, S. W., & Earls, F. (1997). Neighborhoods and violent crime: A multilevel study of collective efficacy. *Science*, *277*(5328), 918–924.

Smith, M. E. (2010). The archaeological study of neighborhoods and districts in ancient cities. *Journal of Anthropological Archaeology*, *29*(2), 137–154. http://dx.doi.org/10.1016/j.jaa.2010.01.00

Spivock, M., Gauvin, L., Riva, M., & Brodeur, J. M. (2008). Promoting active living among people with physical disabilities: evidence for neighborhood-level buoys. *American Journal of Preventive Medicine*, *34*(4), 291–298.

Townsend, P., Phillimore, P., & Beattie, A. (1988). *Health and Deprivation: Inequality and the North*. Routledge.

Tyroler, H. A., Wing, S., & Knowles, M. G. (1993). Increasing inequality in coronary heart disease mortality in relation to educational achievement: profile of places of residence, United States, 1962 to 1987. *Ann Epidemiol*, *3*(Suppl.), S51–S54.

Warren, D. (1981). *Helping Networks*. Notre Dame University Press, South Bend, IN.

Whittick, A. (Ed.) (1974). *Encyclopedia of Urban Planning*, McGraw-Hill Book Company, USA, pp. 714–715.

Williams, D. R., & Collins, C. (2001). Racial residential segregation: a fundamental cause of racial disparities in health. *Public Health Reports*, *116*(5), 404.

Wing, S., Barnett, E., Casper, M., & Tyroler, H. A. (1992). Geographic and socioeconomic variation in the onset of decline of coronary heart disease mortality in white women. *American Journal of Public Health*, *82*(2), 204–209.

Yen, J. H., & Syme, S. L. (1999). The social environment and health: a discussion of the epidemiologic literature. *Annual Review of Public Health*, *20*, 287.

2 The Study Area
Azamgarh City

The physical setting or natural environment of any area undeniably affects the living conditions, food habits, social, cultural and economic activities. So before the geographical analysis of any problem, it is essential to know the physical and cultural characteristics of that region. In the present study focusing on neighbourhood environment and health, Azamgarh city has been selected as the study area. Therefore, background knowledge of physical and demographic setting of the city will be helpful in understanding neighbourhood environmental conditions in the city. This chapter is in continuation of the first chapter. In the first chapter, the concept of neighbourhood over space and time and how neighbourhood affects health have been discussed. While going further and directly onto the case study, it will be beneficial to understand the historical, geographical and demographic setting of the study area on which the study is conducted. The current chapter has been divided into two sections. The first section deals with geographical and other characteristics of study area Azamgarh city, while the second section deals with identification and mapping of different neighbourhoods in Azamgarh city. The data for the current chapter has been obtained from various published sources like gazettes, official magazines as well as newspapers and personal observations.

2.1 Azamgarh City: Some Insights

Azamgarh city (26.068° N latitudes to 83.184° E longitudes) is a medium-sized city situated in the fertile land of middle Ganga Plain in north India (Figure 2.1). From the historical, political, administrative as well as cultural point of view, Azamgarh is an important city in the eastern part of Uttar Pradesh (UP). It is surrounded by Mau and Ghazipur in the east, Sultanpur and Ambedkar Nagar in the west, Gorakpur in the north and Jaunpur in the south. Situated on the loop line of the North-Eastern Railway, it is well connected by good motorable roads with important towns of UP, namely Varanasi (95 km), Gorakhpur (100 km), Allahabad (162 km) and Lucknow (271 km). The first three cities form a right triangle which bears the situation of Azamgarh on its perpendicular arm. National Highway-233 passes along the city. Azamgarh city is the administrative headquarters of Azamgarh Division,

DOI: 10.4324/9781003442486-3

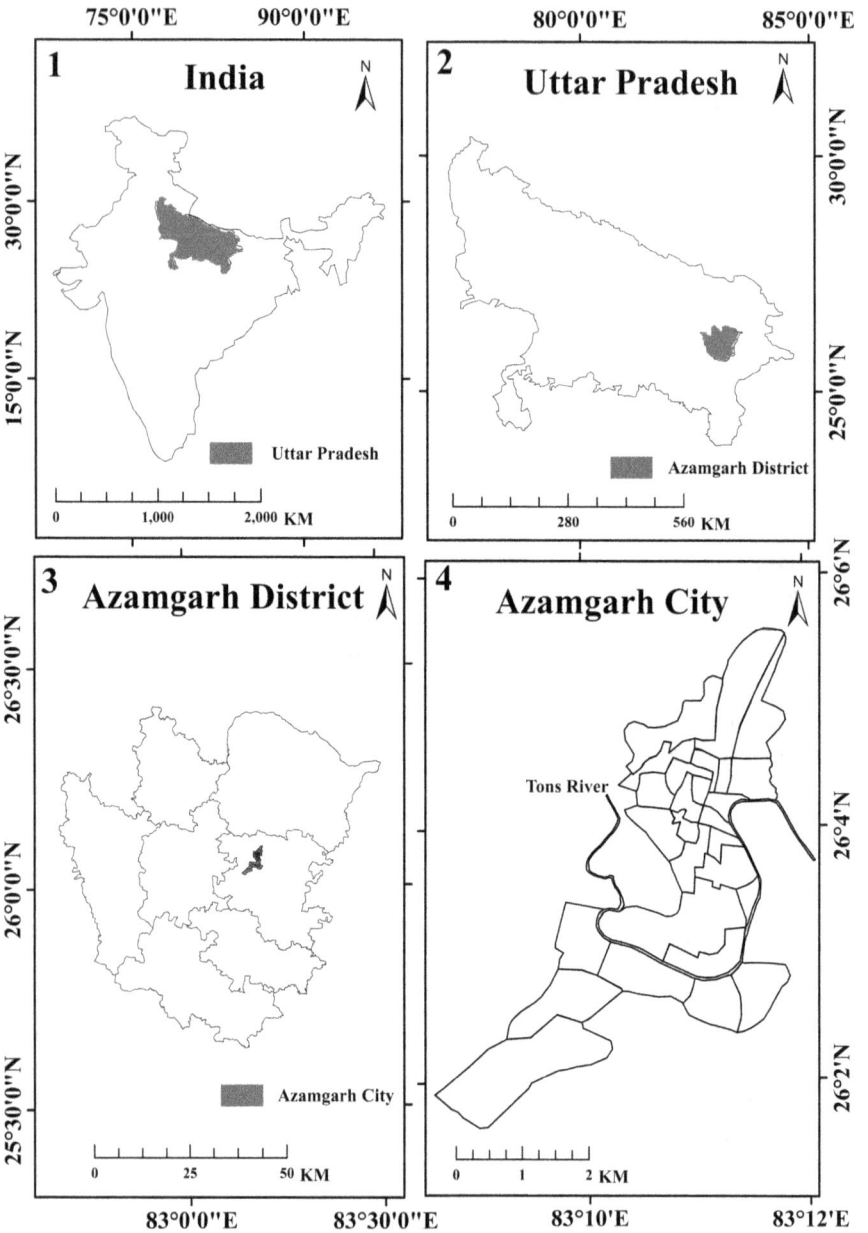

Figure 2.1 Azamgarh City: Location Map.

Source: (Authors).

covering districts namely Azamgarh, Mau and Balia. The city comprises an area of 12.71km^2 (Municipal Office, Azamgarh, 2011) nearly half is used for residential purposes and rest for commercial, industrial, transport, public utility, administrative, recreational and parks and open spaces. There are 25 wards 16294 households in the city (Census of India, 2011).

2.1.1 Origin and Evolution

Azamgarh like many other cities may be characterised as "collection of period pieces". The town originated from a group of villages which gave way to a fort town. The history of the city may be classified in three phases.

2.1.1.1 The Medieval Period

There are no antiquarian to establish the exact dates of the origin of city but it certainly had its beginning in the medieval period. It originated from two villages, namely, Ailval and Phulwaria, which were situated on the *bangar* lands along what is now the road from Gorakhpur to Allahabad. The name of the former village is still borne by mohalla of Azamgarh, while the later name changed to Siuli and later on to Reshad Nagar which is now situated in Ghulami Ka Pura ward. The site of these two villages yielded place to a fort built by Azam Khan in 1965 on the left bank of the Tones. Later the town expanded by merging within itself four neighbouring villages, namely, Maria, Arazi Bhagat, Hirapatti and KandarAzamatpur.

Azam Khan, after whom the town is named, was the son of Vikramajit, a Gautam Rajput who had embraced the faith of Islam. He selected for his fort an elevated site between the two villages which have been mentioned above. The empty areas between the two villages were settled but there remain, even to this day, a gap in settlement in the vicinity of Dharmu Nala. The town during the period of Azam Khan (1665–1680) consisted of the present mohallas of Ailval, Seetaram, Paharpur and Kot.

The nucleus of town was present Kot Chowk. The physical expansion of the town was restricted on the north, north-east and east by natural barriers such as Dharmu Nala and the jungles. The town, therefore, expanded to the west, occupying much of the upland between Dharmu Nala on the northern and eastern sides and river Tons on the southern and south-western sides. Beyond the uplands, the slope of the land becomes gradually steeper but these areas were settled during the next phase of historical development of the city.

It was during the period of Mahabat Khan (1680–1730) that the town developed considerably towards the west and south-west, covering the present localities of Anant Ram, Gurutola and Farashtola, all of them situated along the old course of Tons which facilitated the establishment of a number of bathing ghats and temples on the old bank of the river, for example Hanuman Gharhi, Gurughat and Ganesh Temple. The localities mentioned above lay close to Tons and were highly vulnerable to seasonal floods.

Iradat Khan (1731–1756), a local Raja, appears to have done much for the development of the city, but there was little expansion of the town in this period. The Nawab of Oudh, whose rule started in 1761, did a great deal towards the development of the city. New mohallas and localities were founded, for example, Asifganj, which is named after Nawab Asifuddaula and Chowk which is the present nucleus and the main shopping centre of the city.

2.1.1.2 The British Period

As the British came to power, they made Azamgarh town the headquarters of the district in 1832. Administrative buildings were in the south of the city. The area between these buildings and the town was utilised for the construction of the district jail, municipal hall, bank and education centre. Moreover, the new localities such as Kaleenganj, Matbarganj, Civil Lines, Pandey Bazar and Mukeriganj were founded. The town was provided with facilities such as educational institutions, medical centres, railways, post offices and a protective embankment.

2.1.1.3 The Modern Period

In the post-independence period, the town was benefitted much by the extension of embankment, roadways and urban amenities such as banks, schools, electrification and water supply. New localities are coming up, for example, Belaisa and Railway Station Complex, Sidhari and Harra Ki Chungi. It is clear that town is expanding towards north and north-west, the areas which are safe from the danger of floods.

2.1.2 Physical Setting of Azamgarh City

2.1.2.1 Site and Situation

The city stands on a meander loop of the Tons which surrounds the city completely on three sides. The lands adjoining the river are low-lying and contain a number of depressions, most of which are natural features. The surface of the upland areas is generally level.

The whole township may be divided into two units: (i) The upland areas, which provided the earliest site of the town and now include the mohallas of Kot, Baz Bahadur, Jalandhari, Paharpur, Takia and Katra. From these upland areas, the land gradually slopes down on all sides except in north up to Dharmu Nala, and (ii) the low-lying areas which are protected by the embankment include the localities of Asifganj, Matbarganj and Seetaram in the south.

2.1.2.2 Drainage

Azamgarh city is surrounded by the river Tons on three sides and by the seasonal Dharmu Nala on the north and north-eastern sides. Tons river is a tributary of Ganga, having its origin in Kaimur ranges of Madhya Pradesh, and it is popularly known as Tamsa River. Tons has a narrow course, therefore there are frequent floods which cause substantial damage in the area surrounding its course. Consequently, land up to 500m along the river is demarcated as flood prone and mostly used for agricultural purposes during non-flooding seasons. In today's time, a decrease is recorded in the water level of river.

Tons river has a great impact on the development and residential pattern of the city. Previously, areas only north of the Tons River were considered part of city while in southern part rural character prevailed. Gradually with the construction of bridge on Tons river, its southern counterparts started to develop and villages mingled in the city. At present in the northern part of city, old and congested character can be seen while in southern part two types of features can be spotted. In the later mingled villages still some rural character can be seen while in newly developed colonies good residential character can be seen. Newly developed, far north, areas of the city also exhibit proper residential structure.

2.1.2.3 Floods and the Changing Course of the Tons River

It may be noted that although the Tons is a small river, it seasonally brings down a large volume of water and breaks through the embankment in almost every monsoon season. It is notorious for its changing course. It is recorded that at one time it flowed very close to the town but it changed its course and thus enlarged its meander by shifting westwards and also southwards from its original course. The abandoned course was gradually and largely filled up, but it is traceable even today. The abandoned course still forms low-lying areas with a few hollows. During the rainy season the whole area becomes water logged. The stagnant waters in early winter render it unsuitable for agriculture and also for permanent human settlements because of the flood remains.

There are no records of floods which occurred in the medieval times, but one can envisage that the river surrounded the city giving it the look of an island. Systematic records of floods are available for the years 1838, 1871, 1894, 1915, 1955, 1971 and 1976 which caused great loss of life and property. Later on frequency of the flood in Tons was reduced. Last recorded flood in the river was in 2005.

It was during the flood of 1894 that the necessity of protection was keenly felt and after two years the work started on the construction of an embankment which ran along the river (which is now the abandoned course), took an easterly course, turned near the Jail and extended up to Kot Fort. It was repaired and its height was doubled in 1976.

2.1.2.4 Topography

According to its geomorphology, Azamgarh is a part of Indo-Gangetic Plains, one of the most fertile river plains in the world. The average elevation of district is 64 m. The land of Azamgarh is flat plain without any undulation or hillocks. The only up and downs in the land can be seen along the banks of rivers and streams that flow through it (Ashraf, 2009).

2.1.2.5 Soil

Azamgarh possesses one of the most fertile alluvial soil which can be geologically divided into the new alluviam (khadar) and older alluviam (bangar). The khadar land can be found in the immediate strips along the river streams, where these are rejuvenated every year. The soil of the district is fertile and is highly cultivated. The major crops produced are rice, sugarcane and wheat. Other important crops of the region are maze, gram and mustard. Mango and guava are some popular fruits in the district. The bangar soils found in the district are loamy in character; however, sometimes they attain sandy character near the rivers. In the narrow depressions of rivers, some patches of clay and *usar* can also be seen (Ashraf, 2009).

2.1.2.6 Climate

The climate of Azamgarh is humid subtropical climate which is also known as Cwa type of climate according to Koppen's climatic classification scheme. There is a significant difference in the temperature recorded in summers and winters. Summer season is longer, extremely hot and extend from April to October. South-West monsoons begin around the starting of June and last up to September. Winters are cold with occurrence of Fog as a common phenomenon.

2.1.2.6.1 TEMPERATURE

The temperature range in Azamgarh in summers is 22–46°. Diurnal range of temperature in winters is quite high with comparatively warmer days and colder nights. Temperature in winters (December–February) sometimes fell as low as 5°C mainly due to onset of cold waves from Himalayas (Table 2.1).

2.1.2.6.2 RAINFALL

Azamgarh receives an average yearly rainfall of 110 cm. Rainfall in Azamgarh city takes place from South-West monsoon as well as western disturbances. However 88% rainfall occurs from southern west monsoon during rainy season. Western disturbances are responsible for some rain in winter season too, which is beneficial for Rabi crops (Table 2.1).

2.1.2.6.3 WINDS

Loo is the most prominent wind blowing in summers in the region. Another significant feature is mostly the onset of dust storms in the evening, at the end

Table 2.1 Average Climatic Conditions in Azamgarh City

Month	Average high °C	Average low °C	Rainfall (mm)
Jan	19	8	19.3
Feb	24	12	13.5
Mar	31	17	10.4
Apr	37	22	5.4
May	38	25	9
Jun	36	27	100
Jul	32	26	320.6
Aug	31	26	260.4
Sep	31	24	231.6
Oct	31	21	38.3
Nov	27	15	12.9
Dec	22	11	4
Year	29.9	19.5	85.45

Source: Seasonal Weather Averages, Weather Underground.

of hot days followed by a light showering of rain. These storms are locally known as "*andhis*".

2.1.3 Demographic Setting

Azamgarh city municipality comprises 25 wards. City has a total population of 110,983. Male population of the city is 57,878 and female population is 53,105 (Census of India, 2011). According to Azamgarh Nagar Palika Parishad (NPP), about 12.03 % population is below 6 years, i.e. 13,352. Azamgarh city has female sex ratio of 918 which is higher than UP, i.e. 912. Sex ratio is however lower than national average, i.e. 943. Child sex ratio, i.e. number of female per thousand male within the age group 0–6 years, in the city is 848 against the state average of 902. Azamgarh city has an average literacy rate of 75.51 %, close to the national average, i.e. 74.37% and more than state average, i.e. 67.68% (Census of India, 2011). The total number of households in Azamgarh municipal council is 16,294 which are covered under supply of essential services like water and sewerage.

2.1.3.1 Population Growth

Population growth of Azamgarh city fluctuated from the year of 1911 to 2011 due to various reasons. Table 2.2 shows that the population of city in 1911 was 10,834 Population of the city has increased with an average decadal growth rate of 29.90%. The city was enjoying the highest growth rate from 1971 to 1981, i.e. 62.40% while the lowest growth rate was recorded from 1941 to 1951, i.e. 9.57%. From the year 2001 to 2011, decadal population growth was 18.66%. For the same period, decadal population growth was 20.09% for UP while it was 17.64% for India (Table 2.2). It is expected that the population of city will increase rapidly due to the migration and natural growth.

Table 2.2 Population Growth in Azamgarh City (1911–2011)

Year	Total population	Decadal population growth rate
1911	10834	
1921	14778	+36.50
1931	18046	+22.03
1941	24307	+34.69
1951	26632	+09.57
1961	32391	+21.62
1971	40963	+26.46
1981	66532	+62.40
1991	78567	+18.10
2001	93521	+19.03
2011	110983	+18.66

Source: Census of India (1971, 1981, 1991, 2001 and 2011).

Table 2.3 Literacy Rate and Sex Ratio in Azamgarh City (1991–2011)

Year	Literacy	Sex ratio
1991	61.82	851
2001	70.68	887
2011	75.51	918

Source: Census of India (1991, 2001 & 2011).

2.1.3.2 Literacy Level and Sex Ratio

Literacy is defined as the ability of reading and writing of any person (census of India, 2011). Literacy can be a measure of development and modernisation of the society. Table 2.3 depicts that literacy rate of literacy rate in the city was 61.82 which increased to 70.68 in 2001. Current literacy rate in Azamgarh City is 75.51%. At the same time literacy rate of UP is 67.5%. Sex ratio is defined as the number of females per thousand male. It is a very important indicator for the development. Sex ratio in the city has increased from 851 in 1991 to 887 in 2001 and 918 in 2011. Sex ratio in the city is higher than state average, i.e. 912 but lower than national average, i.e. 940. Low sex ratio in the city can be explained by large outmigration of youths from the district to larger cities of the country, i.e. Mumbai, Delhi, Hyderabad as well as overseas (Table 2.3).**

2.1.3.3 Occupational Structure

Work participation rate is defined as the participation of total workers out of total population (Census of India, 2011). It is very important variable of economic development, and it reflects the employment and unemployment condition of any place. Table 2.4 shows the work participation rate of the city from 1991 to 2001 and from 2001 to 2011. Agricultural workers in city have decreased from 8.45% to 3.92% in 2001 and further 2.80% in 2011. Percentage in the

Table 2.4 Occupational Structure in Azamgarh City (1991–2011)

Year	Workforce (Percentage)	Primary sector (Percentage)	Secondary sector (Percentage)	Tertiary sector (Percentage)
1991	23.74	8.45	10.78	80.77
2001	21.07	3.92	10.81	85.27
2011	21.93	2.80	6.39	90.81

Source: Census of India (1991, 2001 & 2011).

secondary sector has increased slightly from 1991 to 2001, i.e. from 10.78% to 10.81%; however, further decrease was recorded, i.e. 6.39% in 2011. This phenomenon represents pathetic industrial/manufacturing structure in the city. Proportion in the tertiary sector has increased from 80.77% in 1991 to 90.81% in 2011.

2.1.4 *Land-Use Pattern*

Land use is the result of natural and socio-economic factors of any region. It is very important to know the data of land use for sustainable management of resources and urban planning. Lulc map of the city has been prepared by using Sentinel-2A satellite data with 10 m resolution. The map suggests that about 39.83% area of the city is occupied by built-up structures. Open-green spaces cover 35.38% area of the city while tree cover occupies 21.50% area of the city. Water bodies occupy 1.90% area of the city while 1.39% area is devoted to agricultural activities (Table 2.5).**

Table 2.5 shows the classification of land uses in Azamgarh city and it is evident that out of total area, higher percentage of area is covered by residential land use, 74.73% of total built-up area. After residential land use, community services cover large area of Azamgarh city, i.e. 17.39%. Office uses cover 4.79% of the built-up area followed by commercial activities, i.e. 2.54% (Table 2.6). Least proportion (0.33%) of transportation activities has been recorded closely followed by industrial activity (0.22%).

Table 2.5 Land-Use Land-Cover in Azamgarh City

Azamgarh city; Land-use land-cover

Land-use type	Area in km²	Percentage
Built-up area	5.02	39.83
open spaces	4.46	35.38
Tree cover	2.71	21.50
water body	0.24	1.90
Agriculture	0.18	1.39
Total		100.00

Source: Sentinel 2A (10 m resolution, 2017).

Table 2.6 Land-use Categories in Azamgarh City

Serial Number	Land-Uses	Category	Percentage
1	Residential	Housing	74.73
2	Commercial	Market Street	1.14
		General Businesses	0.75
		Godown	0.65
3	Industrial	Light Industries	0.33
4	Office Uses	State Offices	4.79
5	Community Services	Health Services	1.49
		Educational Services	4.58
		Police Stations	5.42
		Fire stations	0.06
		Post Offices	0.07
		Cemetery	0.25
		Electricity Houses	4.69
		Parks	0.83
6	Transportation	Bus Station	0.22
Total			100.00

Source: Azamgarh city Master Plan 2011–31.

Azamgarh city is much smaller comparing to other giant cities of India. For example, the larger cities of India like Delhi. Mumbai, Chennai and Kolkata have population ranging from four to twelve millions (Mumbai-12,442,373, Delhi- 11,034,555, Chennai-4,646,732, Kolkata- 4,496,694, Census of India, 2011), while Azamgarh city has a population of 0.11 million only (110,983). In larger cities of India, population is mainly due to in-migration of people from rural areas or smaller cities and in Azamgarh city also trend of in-migration from surrounding villages has been increasing. However, being smaller in size, it does not attract population with the same force as larger cities do. Industrial development is totally lacking in the city and it has a service economy base. Azamgarh city, being headquarters of Azamgarh Division has administration as the main occupation along with educational as well as health services. Literacy rate in Azamgarh city is lower (75.51 %) comparing to larger cities of India (Delhi-86.21%, Mumbai-89.91%, Chennai-90.18% and Kolkata-86.31%). Azamgarh city does not have any University or airport. Its situation in eastern part of UP, makes it lagging behind in terms of urbanisation and industrialisation, as western part of UP is much urbanised due to its proximity to New Delhi and developed states of Haryana and Punjab and development of Gurugram, Delhi, Meerut Industrial region. Per capita income and quality of life is quite low as compared to developed countries. However, when it comes to environmental problems, no city in India is untouched. Also in Indian cities, we are still facing local problems related to water and sanitation while cities in the developed world are facing global problems related to climate change and global warming etc. It is due to prevalence of environmental issues in Azamgarh city, which has led its selection for the current study.

2.2 Identification and Mapping of Different Neighbourhoods in Azamgarh City

Azamgarh city has been chosen for present analysis because smaller cities like Azamgarh are on the way of becoming urban adversity. Persistent urbanisation and lack of investment in urban infrastructure development have made disastrous impacts. Attention should be given to smaller cities like Azamgarh, which are no longer small but are fast developing into big problem cities. Provision of community services is disappointing in the city with respect to garbage collection services, supply of drinking water, drainage and sanitation etc. With increasing population over the years, the city has evolved into a crowded space with poor environmental infrastructure leading to deterioration in residents' health.

2.2.1 Criteria for Identification of Neighbourhood

In Azamgarh City, different neighbourhoods have been identified based on three major criteria.

2.2.1.1 Income-Wise Dominance in the Wards

Income is the most important and perhaps the most accepted criterion to identify different kinds of neighbourhoods in any city as almost all the other characteristics of the neighbourhood like housing characteristics, percentage of renters, the presence or lack of community services etc. are dependent on what income group of people reside in the majority in any neighbourhood. In Azamgarh city, neighbourhoods are categorised into high-income neighbourhoods with the majority of residents having total monthly income above 25,000, medium-income neighbourhoods between 10,000 and 25,000 and low-income neighbourhoods below 10,000. A neighbourhood is considered low-income when more than 30% of families of the neighbourhood belong to the low-income category and vice-versa (Lemstra et al., 2006).

2.2.1.2 Population Density of the Ward

The concept of urban density was first introduced in the Garden City movement in England. Planners back then observed that places with too many people, houses and workplaces along with less air, light and open spaces recorded high social deprivation, worsening health and crime (Radberg, 1990). Population density can be defined as the number of people living in per square kilometre area. The population density of an area is one of the most important determining factors to differentiate neighbourhoods, as high population density may lead to environmental pollution and other ecological issues and vice versa. The number of people living in a particular radius decides the availability of various community services in the neighbourhood. Neighbourhoods in Azamgarh city are categorised into high-density neighbourhoods (above 20,000 persons per km²), medium density neighbourhoods (10,000–20,000 persons per km²) and low-density neighbourhoods (below 10,000 persons per km²).

2.2.1.3 Household Density of the Wards

Household density is also an important criterion. Percentage of housing units per single area decides the ratio of open space to the available land of a neighbourhood, proper ventilation to the streets and houses, and availability of various community services at the neighbourhood level. Neighbourhoods in Azamgarh city are categorised into high-density neighbourhoods (above 2700 households per km²), medium density neighbourhoods (1400–2700 households per km²) and low-density neighbourhoods (below 1400 households per km²) Distribution and Mapping of Different Neighbourhoods in Azamgarh City.

Based on the above criteria, seven different neighbourhoods have been identified in Azamgarh city, grouping all 25 wards (Figures 2.2 and 2.3).

Seven neighbourhoods of Azamgarh city are as follows.

2.2.2.1   High-Income High-Density Neighbourhood (HI/HD)
2.2.2.2   High-Income Medium-Density Neighbourhood (HI/MD)
2.2.2.3   High-Income Low-Density Neighbourhood (HI/LD)
2.2.2.4   Medium-Income High-Density Neighbourhoods (MI/HD)
2.2.2.5   Medium-Income Low-Density Neighbourhood (MI/LD)
2.2.2.6   Low-Income High-Density Neighbourhood (LI/HD)
2.2.2.7   Low-Income Medium-Density Neighbourhood (LI/MD)

2.2.1.4 High-Income High-Density Neighbourhood

This neighbourhood comprises only one ward, i.e. Asifganj. It is located in the central part of the city and is highly congested due to high residential density. The main market of the city, i.e. Takiya, is located in it, resulting in massive traffic congestion on the streets. Quality of life is, however, decent in this neighbourhood as old influential people reside in it.

2.2.1.5 High-Income Medium-Density Neighbourhood

This neighbourhood comprises three wards namely Sidhari East, Arazibagh and Matbarganj. Sidhari East and Arazibagh wards are inhabited mainly by migrants from surrounding villages of Azamgarh district. However, in Matbarganj, mostly old residents of the city reside. Good quality of life prevails in this neighbourhood encompassing downtown of the city with the presence of Chowk market in it.

2.2.1.6 High-Income Low-Density Neighbourhood

Civil Lines, Raidopur, Madya, Sidhari West, Heerapatti and Mukeriganj are the six wards that constitute this neighbourhood. Civil Lines, Raidopur and

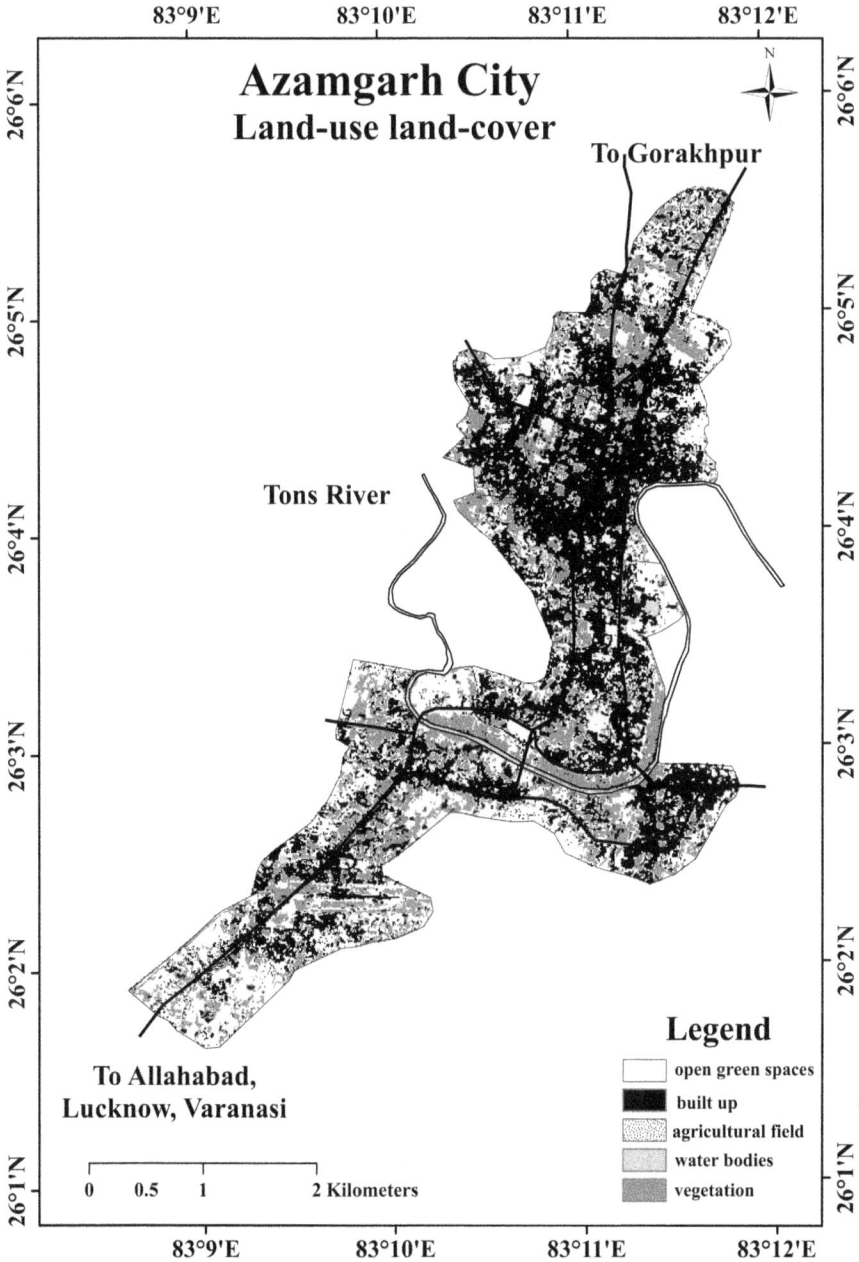

Figure 2.2 Azamgarh City: Land-Use Land-Cover.

Source: Sentinel 2A (10 m resolution, 2017).

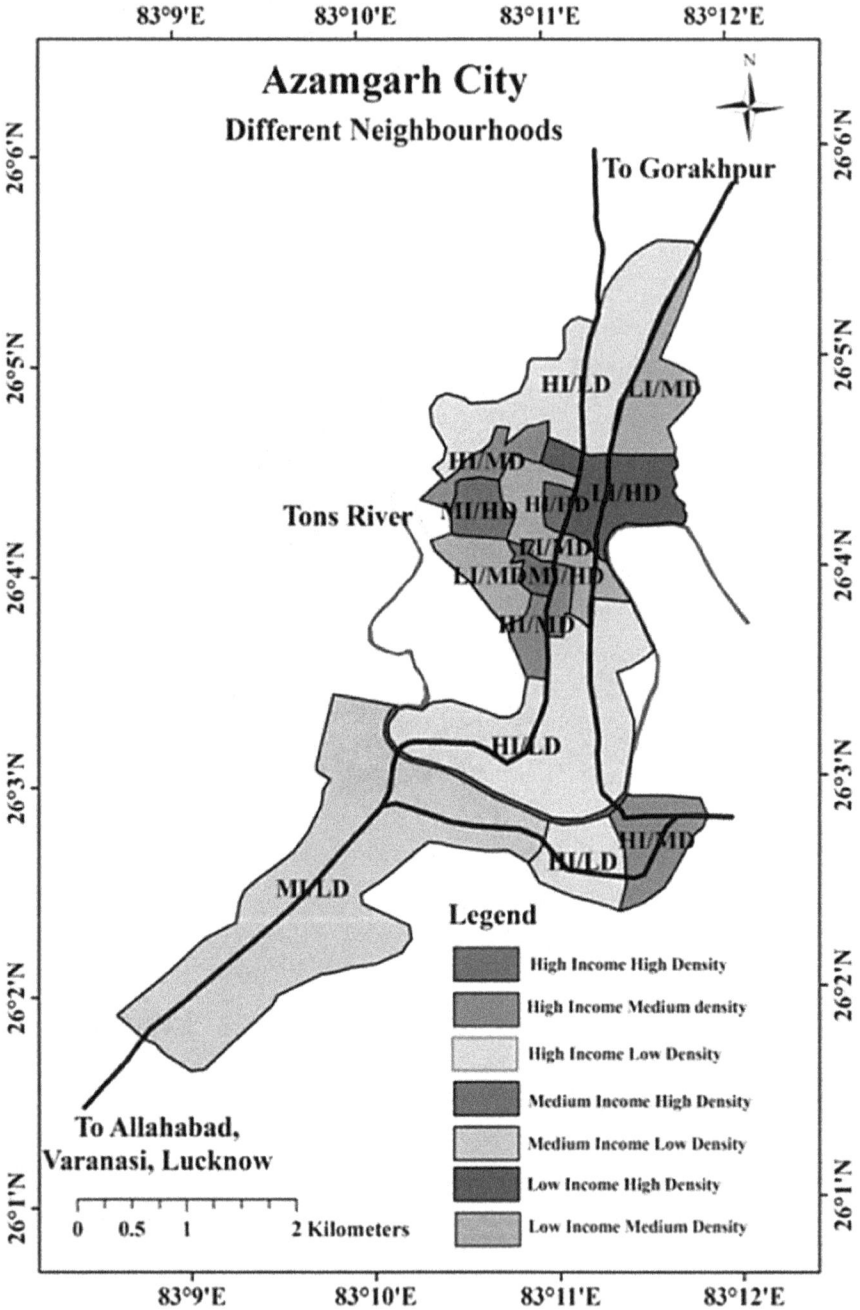

Figure 2.3 Azamgarh City: Neighbourhood Map.

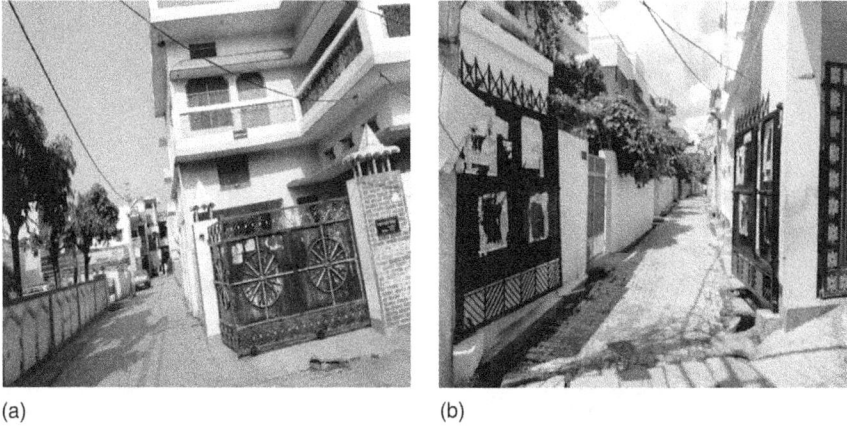

(a)   (b)

Figure 2.4 (a, b) High-Income Neighbourhoods of Azamgarh City.

Sidhari west are mostly devoted to administrative activities with civil court, D.M. office and municipal office in it resulting in low population density. Mainly officers and Govt. officials reside in these wards. The largest colony in Raidopur ward is Officers Colony, meant for various officers posted in the city. Madya, Mukeriganj and Heerapatti are other wards comprising Teachers Colony and Officers Colony. New residential units are a characteristic feature of this neighbourhood with quality of life being far better (Figure 2.4).

2.2.1.7 Medium-Income High-Density Neighbourhoods

Situated in the heart of the city this neighbourhood includes two wards namely Badarka and Katra. Both of these wards are highly congested, comprising of mostly old residential units; however, some modern houses can also be sighted in Badarka ward. Friends Colony in Badarka is a new extension of the ward and exhibit far better residential structure and quality of life. On average, a mixed type of population resides in this neighbourhood with average to low quality of life (Figure 2.5).

2.2.1.8 Medium-Income Low-Density Neighbourhood

This neighbourhood forms the southern extension of the city, in the south of river Tons, comprising wards namely Narauli, Harbanshpur and Sarfuddinpur. Sarfuddinpur and parts of Harbanshpur were previously villages; therefore, a rural character can be seen in these wards with patches of agricultural fields. Scheduled caste, as well as other backward caste, is primary population composition of this area. A fair to medium quality of life prevails in this neighbourhood.

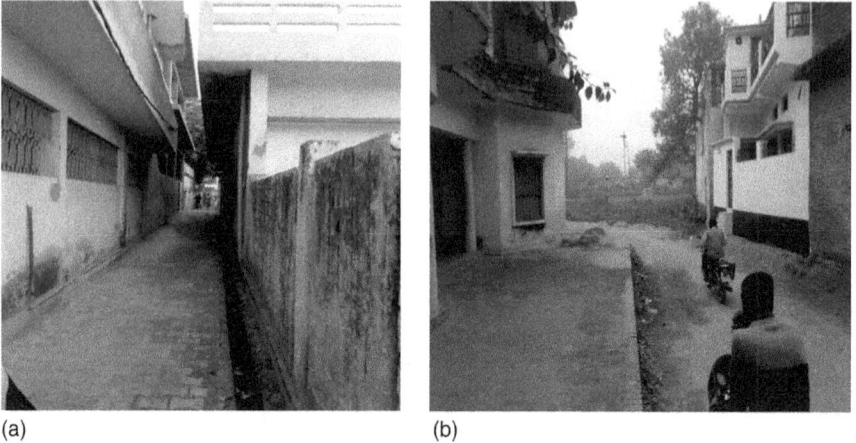

(a)   (b)

Figure 2.5 (a, b) Medium-Income Neighbourhoods of Azamgarh City.

2.2.1.9 *Low-Income High-Density Neighbourhood*

Situated along the river Tons, this neighbourhood saw the inception of the city. In the name of the fort of its founder Azam khan in this area, a colony is named as QilaMohalla. Mainly four wards Bazbahadur, Seetaram, Jalandhari and Paharpur comprise this neighbourhood. It is characterised by congested residential pattern and medium to low quality of life.

2.2.1.10 *Low-Income Medium-Density Neighbourhood*

This neighbourhood encompasses six wards namely Pandey Bazaar, Sadavarti, Ailval, Farashtola, Gurutola and Ghulamikapura. Mainly schedule caste and other backward caste people live in these wards. However, some colonies in Ghulamikapura ward, like Rahmat Nagar colony and AwasVikas colony are in relatively better condition (Figure 2.6).

2.3 Summary

This chapter deals with details about study area Azamgarh city. This chapter has been divided into two sections. The first section deals with geographical and other characteristics of study area Azamgarh city, while the second section deals with identification and mapping of different neighbourhoods in Azamgarh city. In the first section, origin and evolution in medieval, British and modern period; physical setting in terms of terms of site and situation, drainage, soil, climate; demographic setting in terms of population growth, literacy level and sex ratio, occupational structure as well land use pattern in the city are discussed in detail. In the second section, first of all criteria selected for identification of different neighbourhoods like income-wise dominance,

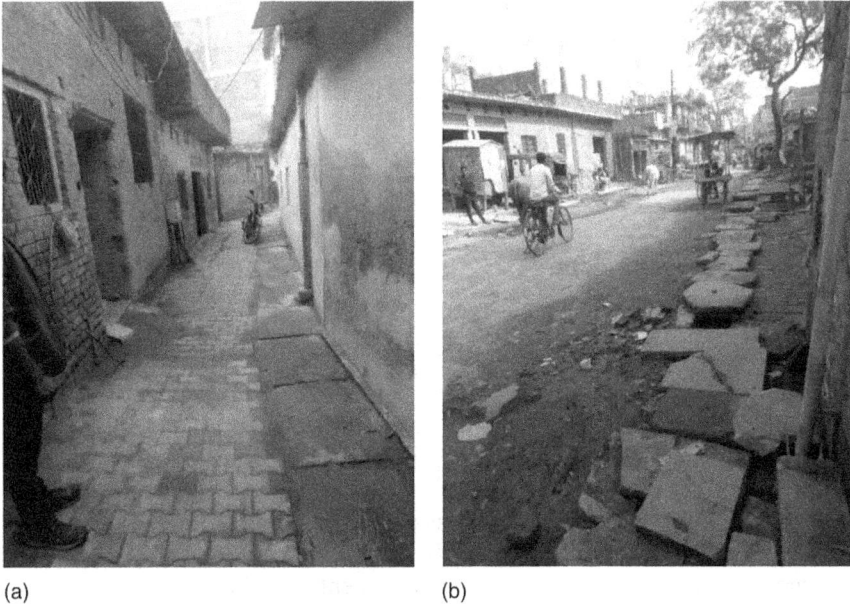

(a)   (b)

Figure 2.6 (a, b) Low-Income Neighbourhoods of Azamgarh City.

population density as well as household density are discussed. Further each neighbourhood of the city, along with its picture is discussed in detail.

References

Ashraf, M. (2009). Impact of irrigation facilities in agricultural development in Azamgarh district (Doctoral thesis, Aligarh Muslim University, Aligarh), http://hdl.handle.net/10603/55439

Azamgarh city Master Plan (2011–31), Azamgarh Development Authority, Azamgarh.

Census of India. (1991). *Primary Census Abstract.* Office of the Registrar General & Census Commissioner, India.

Census of India. (2001). *Primary Census Abstract.* Office of the Registrar General & Census Commissioner, India.

Census of India. (2011). *Primary Census Abstract.* Office of the Registrar General & Census Commissioner, India.

Lemstra, M., Neudorf, C., & Opondo, J. (2006). Health disparity by neighbourhood income. *Canadian Journal of Public Health/Revue Canadienne de Sante'ePublique, 97,* 435–439.

Municipal Office, Azamgarh City. (2011).

Radberg, J. (1990). Doktrinochtathetisvensktstadsbyggande, 1875–1975.

"Seasonal Weather Averages" Weather Underground. (2010), December. Retrieved 22 December 2010, temperature data from Weather Underground.

Sentinel 2A. (2017), 10 m resolution.

3 An Overview of Neighbourhood Environmental Characteristics in Azamgarh City

"Environment refers to the sum total of conditions which surrounds man at a given point of space of time" (Park, 1980); and neighbourhood, in its purest definition, is the vicinity in which people live. Neighbourhood Environment thus refers to the environment around the house, the locality in which people live. The immediate social and physical environment around the house is termed as neighbourhood environment. Significant components of the neighbourhood environment are physical environment, social environment and service environment. According to Amerigo (2002), neighbourhoods are typically studied from two perspectives, one on physical characteristics relating to facilities and amenities and the other focusing on aspects relating to social networks established in the neighbourhoods. Catherine Cubbin et al. (2008) divided the neighbourhood environment in the following three forms.

- **The Physical Environment** – Physical environment of neighbourhood involves the natural environment along with the built-or manmade environment. Components of natural environment include air, water, soil, sunshine, etc. while the built environment is the environment coming out from the manmade structures including fabrics of buildings, roads, streets, urban green spaces and health, recreational and educational facilities (Health Canada, 2002).
- **The Social Environment** – It includes the quality of relationship such as trust, connectedness and cooperation among residents.
- **The Service Environment** – The service environment of a neighbourhood incorporates amenities and facilities associated to health whether directly or indirectly. It includes services in the neighbourhood for health, educations, jobs, grocery and recreation, etc.

3.1 Neighbourhood Physical Environment

The physical environment includes the natural environment as well as the built environment, i.e. environment resulting from the anthropogenic constructions. The built environment encompasses the fabrics of buildings, infrastructure and

DOI: 10.4324/9781003442486-4

open urban spaces (Cubbin, 2008). The physical environment in which people live has a significant impact on their access to resources and services (Kwon et al. 2019). In the present work, the physical environment is concerned with the built environment in the city and not the natural environment, i.e. climate, weather, soil, etc. as the natural environment is homogenous in the entire city.

The physical environment is an essential component of the neighbourhood environment but has received least research-based studies so far.

The physical environment in Azamgarh city has been measured with the help of an in-depth survey of 7 neighbourhoods and 1629 households. Information was collected from these neighbourhoods with the help of a questionnaire (Appendix-I), interview and observation as well as secondary data from satellite sensors and various government offices. Following variables were selected to study the neighbourhood physical environment in Azamgarh City:

3.1.1   Residential Density
3.1.2   Built-Up Density
3.1.3   Open Spaces/Parks/Playground

3.1.1 Residential Density

Residential density or housing density is a quantitative measure of the intensity by which any land is occupied either by population or development works. Residential or housing density can be defined as the number of residential dwellings per unit area of land. It is measured in India as number of houses per square kilometre of area. Residential density is a vital component of land use in any area, as distribution of population has important repercussions on the availability of basic amenities and facilities such as transport, utilities and social infrastructure. Percentage of housing per unit area decides ratio of open space to all the available land of a neighbourhood and proper ventilation to the streets and houses. With the increasing pressure on the land, not only the number of dwellings grew, but houses are also becoming smaller and thus resulting in less room per person in the houses. Housing density exhibits the pressure of households on the existing available services and utilities, i.e. drinking water, sanitation, parks and open green spaces. Housing density in the neighbourhood leads to neighbourhood overcrowding, and it is equally important as housing overcrowding. Neighbourhood overcrowding can contribute to the deterioration of the neighbourhood environment in many ways such as traffic congestion, worsening of air quality, potential reduction of outdoor spaces, noise problem and lack of privacy. The higher the housing density of a neighbourhood, the poorer will be the quality of the urban environment (Mishra, 2001). The housing density is measured as one of the important indicators to influence its resident's health status and is responsible for the rapid and continued spread of airborne diseases.

Housing or residential density in Azamgarh city is measured with the help of census data as the number of dwellings per square kilometres. The average

Table 3.1 Neighbourhood-Wise Residential Density in Azamgarh City

Neighbourhoods	Residential Density (Per Square Km)	Density Range
MI/LD	677	Below 1500
HI/LD	976	Below 1500
HI/MD	1955	1500–3000
LI/MD	1997	1500–3000
LI/HD	3125	Above 3000
MI/HD	3369	Above 3000
HI/HD	4689	Above 3000

Source: Census of India, 2011.

household density of the city is 1282 houses per square km land. Out of seven neighbourhoods in the city two neighbourhoods come under the category of below 1500, two in 1500–3000 and three neighbourhoods have household densities more than 3000 houses per km square.

A perusal of the Table 3.1 shows that housing density is the highest in HI/HD neighbourhood, i.e. 4689 houses per square kilometre followed by MI/HD (3369) and LI/HD (3125), respectively. These neighbourhoods comprise of wards namely Asifganj, Badarka, Katra, Paharpur, Bazbahadur, Seetaram and Jalandhari. These wards are localised in the central old part of the city and represent typical downtown characteristics of Indian cities with mixed land use and high household density. LI/MD and HI/MD neighbourhoods have household densities of 1997 and 1955, respectively, consisting of wards namely Farashtola, Gurutola, Pandeybazaar, Sadavarti, Ailval, Arazibagh, Matbarganj, Ghulami Ka Pura and Sidhari East. These neighbourhoods are situated surrounding the central high-density neighbourhoods; however, two wards Sidhari East and Ghulami Ka Pura are found in the outer part of the city as these wards are mostly inhabited by migrants and continue to attract population from outside the city. MI/LD and HI/LD neighbourhoods form the outer limit of the city, both in the north and south including wards like Heerapatti, Mukeriganj, Madya, Civil Lines, Raidopur, Sarfuddinpur, Narauli and Harbanshpur representing newly formed regions of the city mainly developed for administrative and commercial purposes, resulting in low residential density. Wards like Sarfuddinpur and parts of Harbanshpur, which formerly came under villages, have newly been included in the city boundary and naturally, have low household density now.

3.1.2 Built-Up Density

Built-up density is the percentage share of built-up area with its total area of a particular spatial unit. Built-up density is calculated by dividing the built-up area of a spatial unit by its total area and then multiplied by 100. Areas characterised by buildings, tar, asphalt and concrete as well as systematic street patterns are defined as built-up area. Classes of the built-up area include residential, commercial, industrial, communications, transportations, utilities and others; while non-built-up classes include parks/gardens and playgrounds, vacant lands, agricultural lands, plantation/orchards, forest, barren, marshy area and water bodies. With the increasing population, the demand of people for shelter is rising, consequently increasing pressure on lands. Built-up areas consisting of homes, shops and offices are essential for living and working of people, but they are using more and more urban spaces, resulting in low open green spaces and rise in residential densities. Built-up density is directly related to residential density – the higher the residential density, the lower the environmental quality (Mishra, 2001). With the increasing built-up density, environmental threats such as air and noise pollution are likely to increase, as the development of roads and transportation causes most of these issues. Higher built-up densities are responsible for damaging open green spaces in the cities, as well as the quality of life of people in overcrowded residential neighbourhoods. The environmental problems that can result from the high built-up densities are noise and air pollution, crowding on streets and public services, and lack of open green spaces (Kimhi, 2005).

Built-up area in Azamgarh city is calculated with the help of satellite data of the year 2017. Sentinel imagery of 10 m resolution has been used to identify different land use classes in the city. Total built-up area in Azamgarh city is 5.02 km², representing 39.83% area of the city.

Neighbourhood-wise analysis revealed that density of built-up area is highest in HI/HD neighbourhood, i.e. 82.50% followed by MI/HD (77.39%) and LI/HD (66.64%), respectively (Table 3.2 and Figure 3.1). These neighbourhoods include wards, namely Asifganj, Bazbahadur, Jalandhari, Paharpur, Seetaram, Badarka and Katra, developed in the first stage of city growth, with the highest density of population, representing the core area of the city. These neighbourhoods mainly comprise residential areas of the city; however, commercial as well as transportation are other common land uses. Built-up density is the lowest in MI/LD neighbourhood covering wards Sarfuddinpur, Harbanshpur and Narauli. Presence of Tons river, around three sides of the city, has great impact on growth and development of the city and areas south of the river are not as developed as the northern counterparts. Sarfuddinpur

Table 3.2 Neighbourhood-Wise Built-Up Density in Azamgarh City

Neighbourhoods	Built-Up Density (Percentages)
HI/HD	82.50
HI/MD	50.25
HI/LD	37.28
MI/HD	77.39
MI/LD	25.87
LI/HD	66.64
LI/MD	47.10

Source: Sentinel 2A Satellite Sensor (10 m), 2017.

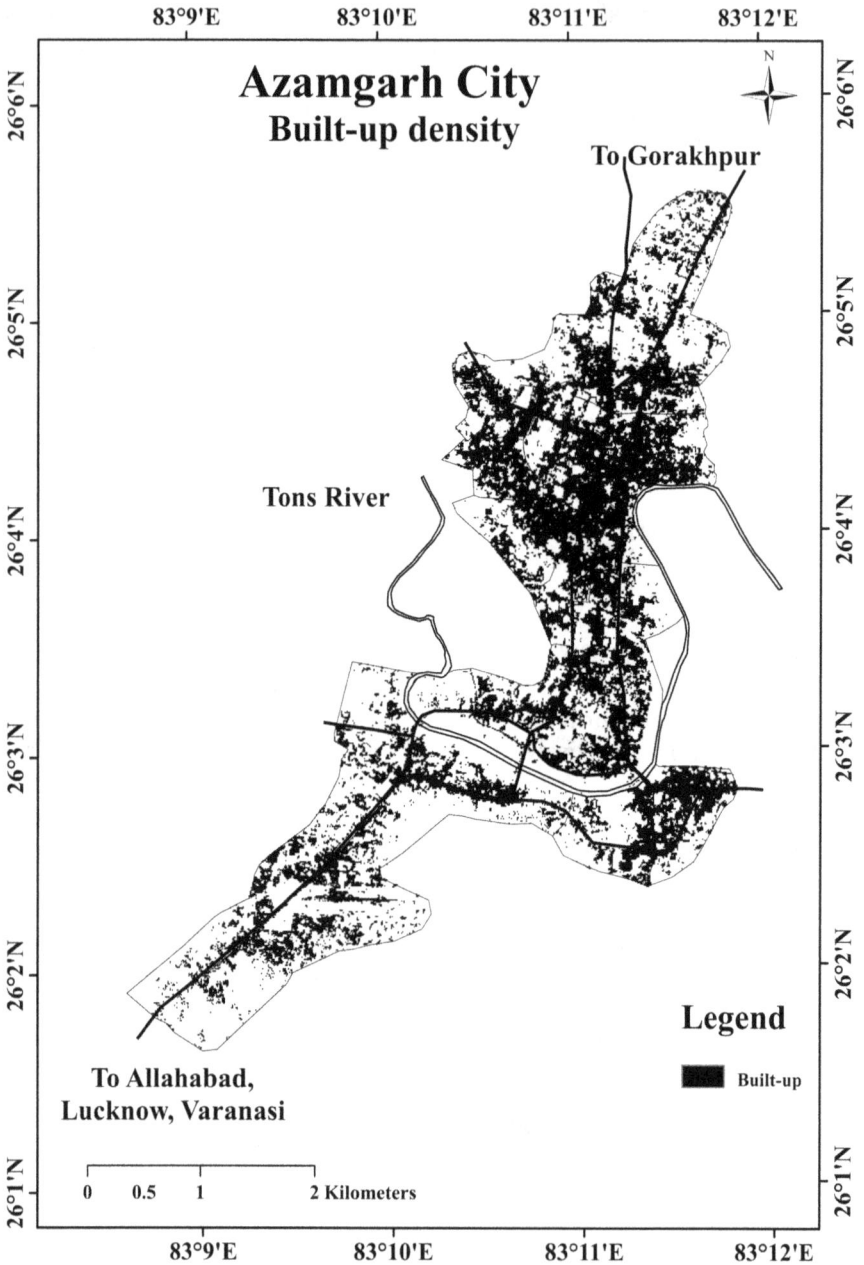

Figure 3.1 Azamgarh City: Built-Up Density in Different Neighbourhoods.

Source: Sentinel 2A Satellite Sensor (10 m), 2017.

and parts of Harbanshpur (south of river Tons), which were previously villages and were later incorporated into the municipal boundary, still show fairly rural character with low built-up area and larger open spaces. The density of population is also low in these areas. Commercial and Transportation land use are significant features of these neighbourhoods.

3.1.3 Open Spaces/Parks/Playgrounds

Urban green space is another crucial aspect for neighbourhood environment assessment as it provides pollution-free environment in the city. Urban green spaces include parks, gardens and recreational venues, informal green spaces like riverfronts and indigenous vegetation types, etc. Green space in urban areas offers a sense of better place for living as it makes available a place of recreation for all groups of society. Open green spaces provide clean air to the residents by acting as urban lungs; absorbing pollutants and releasing oxygen. It has also been proved that green spaces help individuals to recover from physical and mental traumas (Gupta et al., 2012). Green spaces are a necessary infrastructure of a city, making significant contributions to the city, aesthetically and ecologically, as well as to the public health and quality of life (Low et al., 2007). The more the area of open and green spaces in the city, the better is the quality of the environment (Rahman et al., 2011).

Azamgarh City has a fair 35.38% area, devoted to open green spaces, however, the situation is far from satisfactory, while analysing this data neighbourhood-wise (Table 3.3). Percentage of green space is the lowest in HI/HD neighbourhood (8.85%), followed by MI/HD neighbourhood (11.96%). These neighbourhoods are located in the old, congested part of the city packed with concrete structures with barely any open space (Figure 3.2). However, the percentage of open green spaces in MI/LD neighbourhood is 43.8%, followed by HI/LD (35.5) and LI/MD (32.11)%, respectively. These neighbourhoods are basically situated along the river and a wide belt along both sides of the river is declared as flood-prone area, used for cultivation in dry seasons that is why green spaces show high proportion in these neighbourhoods.

Table 3.3 Neighbourhood-Wise Open Green Spaces in Azamgarh City

Neighbourhoods	Open Green Spaces (Percentage)	Open Space Per Capita (in m^2)
HI/HD	8.85	2.41
HI/MD	28.97	19.4
HI/LD	35.5	29.44
MI/HD	11.96	6.375
MI/LD	43.8	124.28
LI/HD	24.79	9.92
LI/MD	32.11	6.69

Source: Sentinel 2A Satellite Sensor (10 m), 2017.

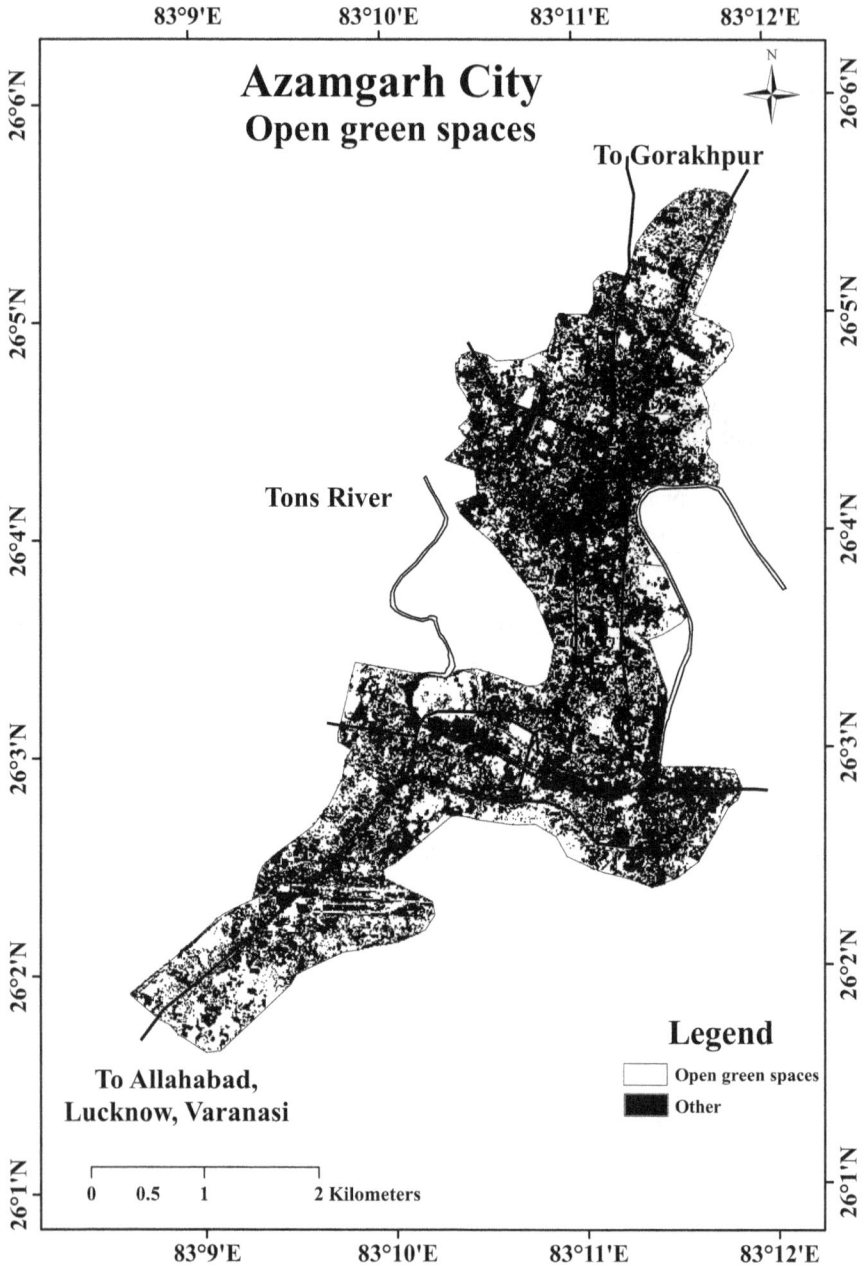

Figure 3.2 Azamgarh City: Open Green Spaces in Different Neighbourhoods.

Source: Sentinel 2A Satellite Sensor (10 m), 2017.

Table 3.4 Neighbourhood-Wise Parks and Playgrounds in Azamgarh City

Neighbourhoods	Parks/playgrounds (Numbers)	
	Parks	Playgrounds
HI/HD	0	0
HI/MD	0	1
HI/LD	5	0
MI/HD	0	0
MI/LD	0	0
LI/HD	0	1
LI/MD	1	2
Total	6	4

Source: Municipal Office, Azamgarh City, 2017.

World Health Organisation has suggested to ensure a minimum availability of at least 9 m^2 green open space per each city resident (Singh et al., 2010). Vienna, world's most livable city, provides as high as 120 m^2 open green space per capita, followed by Stockholm (87.5) and Amsterdam (45.5), respectively. Azamgarh City has succeeded to provide 40.18 m^2 green space per capita; however, this data is highly misleading, as when we see neighbourhood-wise per capita green space availability, a considerable variation is found in this regard. Per capita green space availability is the highest in MI/LD neighbourhood, i.e. 124.28 m^2 and is the lowest in HI/HD, i.e. 2.41 m^2 only, followed by MI/HD 6.35, LI/MD 6.69 and LI/HD 9.92 m^2. Green spaces in one's neighbourhood are essential for healthy life; however, a thorough analysis of open green spaces in the city does not show a good picture (Table 3.3).

There are total six parks in Azamgarh city, out of which five parks can be found in the HI/LD neighbourhood and only one in LI/MD neighbourhood (Table 3.4). These six parks are Kunwar Singh Park and Mehta Park in Civil Lines, Thandi Sadak Park in Madya, Kashi Ram Awas Park in Raidopur, Hariaudhnagar Park in Heerapatti and Awas Vikas Colony Park in Ghulami Ka Pura. Presence of parks in the neighbourhood is a major place of recreation as it encourages residents for walking, jogging as well as other physical activities. Data shows that mostly medium- and low-income neighbourhoods are devoid of park facility around their houses. Parks are even absent in medium- and high-density counterparts of high-income neighbourhoods. There are four official playgrounds in the city, one in HI/MD neighbourhood as Sukhdev Pahalwan Stadium, one in LI/HD and two in LI/MD neighbourhood.

3.2 Neighbourhood Service Environment/Infrastructure/Access to Amenities

Service environment of a neighbourhood includes resources found in it for health care, education, employment, recreation, transportation and other services directly or indirectly tied with health (Cubbin et al., 2008). Improvement in neighbourhood physical, social and service environment has been considered as an important approach to elevate community health. Potential health impacts of such initiatives have also been recognised by the U.S. Public Health Service Task Force on Community Preventive Services and other teams of experts. Municipal bodies in India are accountable to provide public health services to the residents in the form of water supply, sewage and sanitation as well as eradication of communicable diseases. Residents suffer if the water supply in their neighbourhood is erratic, drains are open and unclean, streets are littered with solid waste and there is darkness in their neighbourhoods at night. Neighbourhoods can influence the health of their residents by the availability of various services, opportunities, facilities and amenities in it. One's access to quality of community services, healthcare services, recreational services, educational and employment opportunities, transportation and other public services, greatly depends upon how near or far these are located. Although health effect of various neighbourhood characteristics is generally small in comparison to individual factors, but most studies have found these factors significant in explaining differences in health outcomes and health-related behaviours (Pearce et al.,2006). Quality of healthcare influences health in direct ways while educational and employment opportunities as well as other public services influence health in indirect ways like by providing the means to attain a good standard of living presently or in the near future. Easier and direct access to places of shopping, exercise, work, meeting neighbours, having health check-up, etc., leads to good health not only by lowering time and cost of access but also by freeing resources for other uses. It also affects lifestyle (Knox, 1982). It has been observed that characteristics of physical, social and service environment generally overlap like access to supermarkets represent both service and physical environment. Many other characteristics of physical environment like parks, transportation and connectivity can be taken as characteristics of the service environment. Condition of streets, drains, availability of water supply and street lighting represent both physical and service environment.

Service environment in Azamgarh is assessed under the following heads:

3.2.1   Water Supply
3.2.2   Solid Waste Management
3.2.3   Waste Water Management
3.2.4   Roads (Connectivity and Accessibility)
3.2.5   Safety/Street lighting
3.2.6   Health Facilities
3.2.7   Educational Facilities
3.2.8   Recreational Facilities
3.2.9   Religious Facilities
3.2.10 Markets
3.2.11 Shopping Malls
3.2.12 Impact of Amenities and Facilities on Well-Being

Data has revealed a distinct geographical variation in access to various amenities and facilities in different neighbourhoods of Azamgarh city including various municipal services like water supply, sanitation, etc., educational opportunities, health services, recreational facilities and public transport choices.

3.2.1 Water Supply

Proper supply of safe water is important for public health, either to be used for drinking purposes, domestic uses, food production or recreational purposes. Appropriate supply of water, sanitation and good management of water resources can increase the country's economic growth besides causing poverty reduction.

As per the data of 2015, 88% of the total Indian population had access to improved water sources, which is 96% in urban areas and 85% in rural areas (WHO and UNICEF, 2017). Under the Indian constitution water supply and sanitation is a state responsibility and in urban areas, states delegate this responsibility to municipalities, known as urban local bodies. Therefore water supply in Azamgarh city is managed by Azamgarh municipal council. Groundwater is the primary source of water supply in the city which is drawn with the help of motor pumps, collected in 6 water tanks and supplied in the entire city through a network of pipelines. Out of the six water tanks, two are located in Pandeybazar ward, two in Civil Lines ward, one in Matbarganj and one in Sidhari ward. As far as the capacity of the tanks is concerned, three tanks have water holding capacity of 350 KL, two have 1000 KL and one tank has 2100 KL capacity of water with the total amount of water supplied in the city being 135 LPCD. An estimated 15 million litre of water is supplied daily. In addition to these, there are total 1285 public hand pumps and 36 government water taps in the city. There are 15460 households enrolled by the water tax department to whom water is supplied, representing 94% households of the city and about 837 households officially do not have access to municipality water while the number of households not getting official water supply is much higher at the ground level.

Household survey as shown in Table 3.5 revealed that out of the total, 92.80% households have water connection inside their premises while 7.20% households have to fetch water from outside their premises. Sources of water supply inside the premises include private piped water connections, submersible borings and hand pumps. Data revealed that about half of the households have their own submersible borings and other half have piped connections inside houses. The main source of water supply outside the premises is roadside public hand pump providing water to 6.26% of the total households while only 0.67 households take water from roadside water pipes installed by the municipality. Neighbourhood-wise analysis of data revealed that 19.39% of LI/HD, 15.08% of LI/MD, 13.33% of MI/LD and 2.53% households of HI/LD neighbourhoods do not have water supply facility inside their houses.

Table 3.5 Neighbourhood-Wise Sources of Water Supply (in Percentages) in Azamgarh City

Neighbour-hoods	Source of Water Supply		If Inside the Premises			If Outside the Premises	
	Inside the Premises	Outside the Premises	Hand pump	Piped Connection	Boring	Roadside Handpump	Roadside Pipe
HI/HD	100.00	0.00	6.25	51.25	42.50	0.00	0.00
HI/MD	100.00	0.00	3.25	45.65	51.10	0.00	0.00
HI/LD	97.47	2.53	19.88	20.82	56.77	0.67	0.00
MI/HD	100.00	0.00	1.00	56.94	42.06	0.00	0.00
MI/LD	86.67	13.33	9.75	36.42	40.50	11.67	1.67
LI/HD	80.61	19.39	1.96	37.83	40.82	16.39	3.00
LI/MD	84.84	15.08	3.57	47.12	34.81	15.08	0.00
Total	92.80	7.19	6.52	42.29	44.08	6.26	0.67

Source: Based on Field Survey, 2016–2017.

Furthermore, of the households having water inside their houses, half of them have their own boring systems to fetch water. In the wards like Ailval and Narauli, water supply pipes do not reach to each and every house and residents are forced to have their own water supply system i.e. either hand pump or submersible. Since both are low-income wards, it was a great expense for the residents to have their private water connection. Water also does not reach to *Harijan basti* in Raidopur ward and Pura Jodhi in Heerapatti ward. Since these are high-income areas, majority of the households have their own boring system but it is the poor population that suffers and is dependent on public hand pumps or forced to have their own boring systems.

3.2.2 Solid Waste Management

Municipal solid waste is the unwanted and unusable solid materials generated by living communities in residential, commercial or industrial areas (Syed, 2006). Composition of solid waste comprises of degradable materials like paper, clothing, food and vegetables, moderately degradable materials like cardboard and wood and non-degradable materials like leather, plastic, rubber, metal, glass and electronic waste (Jha et al., 2011). In India, the total waste generated in urban areas per day is 188,500 tonnes or 68.8 million tonnes per year at the rate of 0.5 kg of waste generated per capita per day. For urban areas of Uttar Pradesh, this data is 15,500 MT per day (Government of India, 2018). The total solid waste generated in Azamgarh city is 5.99 metric tonnes or 5999 kg per day. Per capita waste generation in the city thus can be estimated as 0.05 kg per head per day. Major sources of solid waste generation in the city are households, commercial and industrial establishments, hospitals, slaughterhouses, road sweeping, drain cleaning and construction and demolition sites. However, the major share of solid waste is generated by households in Azamgarh city. For proper solid waste management, there are three main steps involved. These are collection and segregation, transportation and disposal. Azamgarh municipal council is responsible for collection, transportation and disposal of solid waste generated within the city.

3.2.2.1 Collection of Waste

The first major step in the management of solid waste is the collection of waste. Collection of solid waste involves door to door collection or collection from dust bins or well-defined collection points. However, during the field survey, it was observed that door to door collection is not very efficient in the city and sanitation workers collect waste of only those households from the door, which have paid them extra for this service. Provision of dustbins around the houses to dump household waste is also lacking as during field survey, majority of the households claimed that no dustbins are provided by the municipality. Thus residents in the city are left with no choice but to drop the household waste in roadside collection points from where waste is lifted by sanitation workers. Total 173 sanitation workers have been appointed by municipality which means on an average, one sweeper has to collect waste from 94 houses other than the waste generated by commercial and industrial sites, hospitals, hotels, restaurants and construction and demolition sites.

However, field survey has revealed that not all the parts of the city are covered by municipal waste collection services and around 20% households dispose their waste at other than the municipal collection points (Table 3.6) of which 8.61% households throw their waste in open fields, 1.72% dump it in adjacent water bodies, 6.26% in their backyards and 2.89% households burn their household waste. Neighbourhood that is least covered by municipal services is MI/LD neighbourhood where wards Sarfuddinpur and Harbanshpur are new extensions of the city. This could be due to its distance from the city centre, that's why municipal services are not efficient in this part and residents either throw their garbage in open fields or backyards or burn it. In wards like Civil Lines, Paharpur and Farashtola, households themselves clean their neighbourhood through sweeping the roads and streets. Around 80% household waste is collected by sanitation workers of which 14.35% waste is collected directly from the houses of residents, for which they pay some extra money to sanitation workers and around 65% residents drop their garbage to the roadside collection points from where sanitation workers collect them.

3.2.2.2 Transportation of Waste

Another major step in solid waste management is the transportation of waste-to-waste disposal points. For collection and transportation of waste 90 handcarts and various other vehicles are used. Other vehicles include eight tractors, five Tata motors, three dumpers and four JCB machines. Total 173 sanitation

Table 3.6 Neighbourhood-Wise Collection and Disposal Practices of Household Waste (in Percentages) in Azamgarh City

Neighbour hoods	Disposal/Collection of Household Waste			If collected by Municipality		Other (Disposal to)			
	By Municipality	Households Themselves	Other	Roadside Collection Points	Household Collection System	Open Field	Water Body	Back Yard	Burn
HI/HD	95	0	5	64	31	5	0	0	0
HI/MD	73.78	0	26.22	55.78	18	4.29	0	14.41	7.52
HI/LD	78.61	3.7	17.69	58.98	23.33	12	2.22	3.47	0
MI/HD	94	0	6	82.4	11.6	6	0	0	0
MI/LD	47.81	0.86	51.33	45.31	2.5	19.47	8.35	10.8	12.71
LI/HD	82.46	2.89	14.65	77.46	5	7.07	0.5	7.08	0
LI/MD	81.37	3.1	15.53	72.32	9.05	6.47	1	8.06	0
Total	79.01	1.5	19.49	65.18	14.35	8.61	1.72	6.26	2.89

Source: Based on Field Survey, 2016–2017.

workers have been employed by municipality of which 116 are on permanent job while 57% work on ad hoc basis.

3.2.2.3 Disposal of Waste

The most common methods used for disposal of solid waste in most countries of the world are open dumping, landfill, composting, recycling and reuse. Mostly in underdeveloped countries, the popular method is open dumping where solid waste is dumped in the open grounds, far from the settlements and left to decay and decompose. In Azamgarh city too, open dumping method is used as means for disposal of waste material and after sometime when huge heaps of garbage are created, it is burnt down by the municipality. For waste disposal, earlier the location called "Bandha" near the river Tons was used, but was criticised on the ground that it was located inside the city and residents suffer from a number of environmental problems due to dumping and burning of waste in the city. Therefore new dumping site was proposed by the municipality, which is located in village Manjhgawan, Tehsil Sadar, Pragna Nizamabad Azamgarh. The total area of the dumping site is 17,494.56 m², and now it has started being used as a dumping site for Azamgarh municipality. However, disposal at inner-city dumping site has still not stopped completely.

3.2.3 Waste Water Management

Drainage is natural or artificial removal of household wastewater as well as storm water (rainwater) from an area. Drainage systems are built to make sure that household wastewater, sewage and storm water is tidily transported to disposal points, thus keeping the environs well drained, free of waste and clean. Components of a sound drainage system incorporate closed drainage channels having piped drains, clean drainage pipes and conduits.

Azamgarh city generates 17.3 MLD (million litres per day) sewage water per day which can be estimated as 134 LPCD (litre per capita per day). Municipal Office and District Urban Development Authority (DUDA) in Azamgarh city are responsible for designing, planning and implementation of wastewater and sewage management. India's big cities have proper sewage systems, combined with underground pipes, pumping stations and well-equipped treatment plants. However, these systems are quite expensive to build and operate. Thus, smaller cities like Azamgarh do not have this facility. Drainage system of Azamgarh city includes small, medium- and large-sized drains and wastewater disposing sites. There is no provision of sewage treatment in the city and waste water is directly disposed into the water bodies. Two main wastewater disposal sites of the city are Tons river flowing in the middle of the city and Dharmu Nala, which surrounds the city from the north east side. Water from the nalas is pumped into the river with the help of pumping sets. However, at different places, the capacity of pumping stations is not enough to discharge all the water into the river and in rainy season it results in flooding on the roads and surrounding areas.

Total length of drainage network in the city is 12275 m including 35 big nalas. Wastewater after being discharged from houses with the help of small drains, goes to big nalas and then is disposed in other nalas and ultimately into the Tons river.

Households in general, generate two types of wastewater, one is grey water that comes from the kitchen, washing clothes, bathroom and from other activities and the other one is black water that comes from flush toilets and is totally contaminated with bodily excreta. The grey water is meant to go to drains while black water to the sewer lines but in most of the times black water gets mixed with grey water outside the houses and turns out to be disposed in the city drains and ultimately in surrounding water bodies. There is no separate sewer line in Azamgarh city, and both grey as well as black water after leaving the houses get mixed up in the drains and flow together to the dumping sites. Underground sewer line is still under construction in the city and is not being used till date.

Wastewater that is not being treated and disposed directly to the surrounding water bodies results not only in water pollution leading mainly to eutrophication but also produces breeding grounds for various insects leading to the occurrence of various types of water as well as vector-borne diseases.

Neighbourhood survey has revealed the state of the drainage system in Azamgarh city (Table 3.7). A perusal of the Table shows that about 10.53% households do not have drainage system around their houses and this percentage is highest as 22.16 in LI/MD neighbourhood, 20.75% in LI/HD density neighbourhood, 11.30% in MI/LD neighbourhood and 10.75% in MI/HD neighbourhood. In LI/MD neighbourhood, houses in Farashtola are situated along the river, and they dispose of their wastewater directly into the river while in Sadavarti, majority of the households dispose of their wastewater in a pond located in the middle of the ward. Households that neither have proper drainage network nor water bodies near their houses let the wastewater flow in

Table 3.7 Neighbourhood-Wise Drainage Condition and Disposal of Wastewater (in Percentages) in Azamgarh City

Neighbourhoods	Drainage Around Houses		If Exists		If Not exists (Wastewater goes to)	
	Exists	Not Exists	Closed	Open	Water Body	Around Houses/Kachcha Drains
HI/HD	99.13	0.87	90.00	10.00	0.87	0.00
HI/MD	97.40	2.60	66.45	34.44	1.60	1.00
HI/LD	94.70	5.30	57.78	42.22	2.47	2.83
MI/HD	89.25	10.75	55.00	45.00	3.22	7.53
MI/LD	88.70	11.3	70.00	30.00	6.70	4.60
LI/HD	79.25	20.75	37.00	63.00	11.22	9.53
LI/MD	77.84	22.16	31.00	69.00	9.56	12.6
Total	89.47	10.53	58.05	41.95	5.09	5.44

Source: Based on Field Survey, 2016–2017.

nearby fields or *kachcha nalis* that further join the main drains of the city. A bitter phenomenon that was observed during the field survey was that proper drainage system was not provided to *Prajapati colony* in Arazibagh, *Harijan basti* in Sidhari East, *Mallah basti* in Madya, *Harijan basti* in Raidopur and *Qasaibada* in Paharpur. Although these wards come under the high-income counterparts of the city, but in the shadow zone of beautiful houses, there are several *Harijan, Prajapati* and *Mallahbastis* and situation in these *bastis* show a very different picture than the rest of the neighbourhood. In those areas, where drainage does not exist, wastewater from houses either goes to water bodies in informal *kachcha* drains or flows around the houses (Table 3.7).

However, the situation of the existing drainage is also far from satisfactory as only 58.05% drains around the houses were reported closed while 41.95% households reported the presence of open drains in the neighbourhoods. Neighbourhoods with the highest percentage of open drains were LI/HD, LI/MD and MI/HD, where the problem of open drains was mainly prominent in Katra, Paharpur, Bazbahadur, Gurutola, Pandeybazar and Seetaram wards.

Ill maintained drainage systems and poor wastewater management practices could adversely affect the environment in many ways like leading to water-logged sites and deteriorating the health of the nearby residents due to increase in unsanitary conditions and water as well as vector-borne diseases.

3.2.4 Roads (Connectivity and Accessibility)

Roads are the chief infrastructure of a city as they are meant to connect far off locations creating a network of places. A well-ordered network of roads is required to access various services and facilities from all corners of the city. Quality of the roads as well as road density represents the spatial efficacy of the city's built-up environment. The analysis here is concerned with internal

Table 3.8 Neighbourhood-Wise Quality of Roads (in Percentages) in Azamgarh City

Neighbourhoods	Quality of Roads					
	Road Type			Width of Roads		
	Kachcha	Pucca	Both	Good	Reasonable	Poor
				(>15 feet)	(7–15 feet)	(>7 feet)
HI/HD	0	100	0	0	20	80
HI/MD	0	100	0	0	45	54.99
HI/LD	3.33	91.67	5	18.33	65.84	15.83
MI/HD	0	100	0	0	0	100
MI/LD	1	71.67	18.33	38.89	49.44	11.67
LI/HD	0	72.91	27.09	0	55	45
LI/MD	4.17	95.83	0	10.84	55.83	33.33
Total	2.5	90.3	7.2	9.72	41.59	48.68

Source: Based on Field Survey, 2016–2017.

roads of the city connecting houses and other services. To assess the quality of roads, surveyed residents were asked questions regarding type and width of roads.

Major findings of the field survey are shown in the Table 3.8. The table reveals that 90% residents reported pucca roads, 7.20% both types of roads and 2.50% reported the presence of *kachcha* roads in their neighbourhoods. *Kachcha* roads in their neighbourhoods were reported by 10% households from MI/LD, 4.17% from LI/MD and 3.33% households from HI/LD neighbourhoods while 27.09% from LI/HD and 18.33% from MI/LD reported both *kachcha* and *pucca* roads in their neighbourhoods. *Kachcha* roads become a menace in the rainy season due to formation of puddles and affecting accessibility and connectivity of a neighbourhood. The Table reveals how roads show a bit satisfying picture in high-income neighbourhoods, and *kachcha* and mixed type of roads can still be seen in low- and medium-income neighbourhoods. The width of the roads also plays a vital role in the overall quality of the roads in a city.

Congested street pattern not only leads to high residential density but also influences the overall quality of the life of residents. Congested or narrow streets result in packed residential areas as well as the spread of contagious diseases in the community. Wide streets let the fresh air pass from all the houses and also give an impression of a decent living space. An analysis of width of roads in Azamgarh city shows that about 48.68% residents reported narrow or congested streets around their houses and this was 100% in MI/HD, 80% in HI/HD, 54.99% in HI/MD and 45% in LI/HD neighbourhood. Data shows that the width of the streets is far from satisfactory in the central part of the city where all high- and medium-density neighbourhoods are located. Width of streets is reasonable to good in low-density counterparts of the city which mainly constitute the newly developed northern and southern extension of the city.

Another aspect of connectivity is road density of an area. Road density is calculated by dividing total length of the roads to the total area of a particular spatial unit. Higher road density represents higher connectivity. Since majority of the facilities and amenities like hospitals, schools, etc. are located along major roads in the city, their neighbourhoods possessing higher density of roads show better connectivity towards the facilities. A perusal of the Figure 3.3 shows that road density is higher in the central and Civil Lnes part of the city. Neighbourhoods that represent higher road density are HI/HD and LI/HD, HI/MD and LI/HD while low road density is recorded in the neighbourhoods MI/HD and MI/LD neighbourhoods.

Connectivity by road as well as proper means of transport is another major requirement of an area. Azamgarh city is connected with other cities through roads and railway. There is one railway station, one bus station and three auto stands in Azamgarh city. The railway station is located in Sarfuddinpur ward and the bus station in Civil Lines ward while out of three auto stands; Narauli auto stand is located in the Narauli ward, Bilaria Ki Chungi in Heerapatti and Harra Ki Chungi in Mukeriganj ward. National and state highways connect the city to Gorakhpur, Allahabad, Varanasi and Lucknow, while internal roads that are managed by municipality connect different parts of the city. As far as means of connectivity within the city is concerned, public transport facilities like buses and trains are provided only to connect outer regions but in the city, important means of transport are private autos, e-rickshaws and manual rickshaws. On the major roads of the city, autos can be spotted but in the neighbourhood narrow lanes only manual rickshaws can ply. E-rickshaw is the new introduction in the region and has gained popularity in quite less time. Manual rickshaws and e- rickshaws can be boarded from small streets of each neighbourhood and on the major roads one can easily find autos.

3.2.5 Safety/Street lighting

Street lighting offers many vital benefits. Not only it enhances security in the neighbourhoods but also increases the quality of life by lengthening bright hours so that various activities can occur. Many urban groups believe that extra lighting can help prevent crime and create a pleasant environment in the neighbourhood. Safety of pedestrians, drivers and riders can also be improved by street lighting. The distribution of light on various buildings can increase the perception of safety in the neighbourhoods. Often it is seen that the areas with less lighting are more crime-prone than those of well-lit ones.

Street lighting is vital to community's health, and several researches have found that improved street lighting, either by increasing number of lights or brighter lights, reduces crime rate by significant percentages (Farrington et al., 2002). Other studies have also confirmed that lighting improvement can reduce crime and improve safety. Improved street lighting in the neighbourhoods can

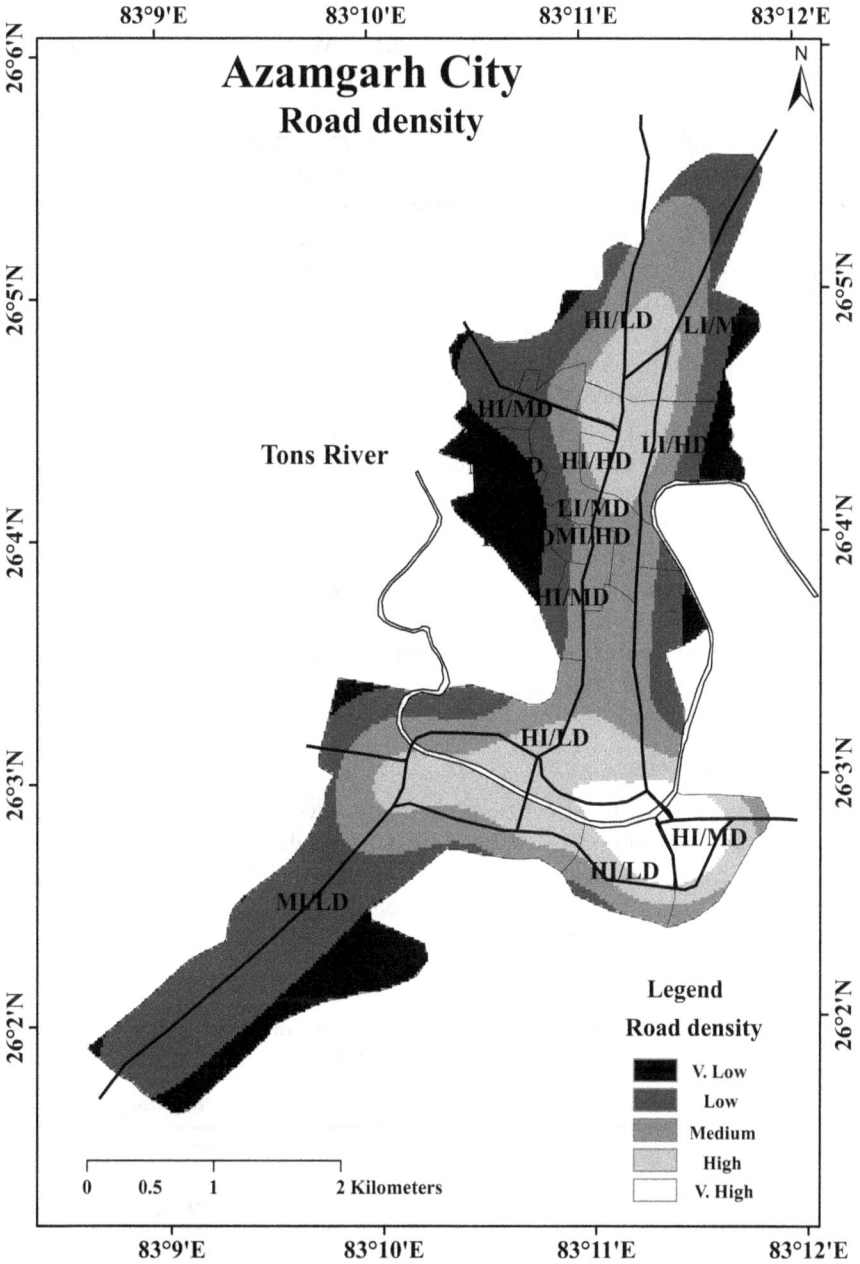

Figure 3.3 Azamgarh City: Road Density.

Source: Google Earth, 2019.

make communities feel safe. It reduces road accidents, allows safer movement of vehicles and helps in smooth traffic flow. Moreover, many communities believe that street lighting is a means to fight crimes in their neighbourhoods. Street lighting thus leads to a more active, healthy and enhanced neighbourhood. Street lighting system in Indian cities is managed by local urban bodies, i.e. municipalities and it is an indicator of an agreeable municipal keep up. Availability of street lighting in Azamgarh city is represented by the fact that there were 3603 street lights in the city until May 2018. On an average 4.5 households or 31 people are served by a single street light.

As far as the distribution of street lighting in the city is concerned, Table 3.9 shows that about 75% people reported availability of street lighting in their neighbourhoods, but it is not uniform throughout the city. While in HI/HD neighbourhood presence of street lighting was reported by 100% residents, this was 73.33 and 83 in HI/MD and HI/LD neighbourhoods respectively. Map shows that these are mainly high-income neighbourhoods where more than 80% households reported street lighting while remaining parts of the city comes under the category of 60–70 and 70–80% of street lighting. The lowest percentage was recorded from MI/LD neighbourhood, i.e. 60 %. Reason for less illumination in this neighbourhood could be its distance from the city centre as well as its socio-economic status. However low-income neighbourhoods closer to the city centre are well lit at night but not as illuminated as high-income counterparts of the city.

3.2.6 Health Facilities

Urban environment can affect health in many ways and out of them, access to health care is very important. A person's health is directly related to the availability and quality of healthcare services in their neighbourhood. A number of previous studies have verified the potential health impacts of healthcare services.

Table 3.9 Neighbourhood-Wise Availability of Street lighting (in Percentages) in Azamgarh City

Neighbourhoods	Street lighting
HI/HD	100.00
HI/MD	73.33
HI/LD	83.00
MI/HD	67.50
MI/LD	60.00
LI/HD	72.50
LI/MD	69.44
Total	75.11

Source: Based on Field Survey, 2016–2017.

Data revealed that there are 6 government and 93 private health services in the city including hospitals, nursing homes, primary health centres and small clinics. Out of the government facilities, there is one divisional district hospital, one district women hospital, one urban health post, one medical care unit, one PHC (primary health centre) and one TB (tuberculosis) clinic in the city (CMO Office, 2016–2017). Government services are located in HI/LD, LI/MD, MI/HD and HI/MD neighbourhoods mainly in Mukeriganj, Matbarganj, Ghulami Ka Pura, Ailval and Badarka. Although private health facilities are well distributed in the entire city, but a large concentration of hospitals can be seen in Arazibagh, Mukeriganj and Heerapatti wards of the city covering HI/LD and HI/MD neighbourhoods. Hospitals and nursing homes are also concentrated along the major roads in Madya and Narauli ward while clinics are almost equally distributed and are accessible in all parts of the city. From Table 3.10, it can be seen that there are total 38 major registered hospitals and nursing homes and 55 clinics in the city. Out of this, 16 major hospitals are located in HI/LD, 9 in HI/MD and 7 in MI/LD neighbourhood with 74, 37 and 29 doctors and 193, 87 and 78 hospital beds, respectively. The analysis reveals a significant concentration of hospital and nursing homes in high- and medium-income neighbourhoods.

3.2.7 Educational Facilities

In Azamgarh city, total one twenty-four schools and three degree colleges are located including 31 government schools and 93 private schools (Table 3.11). Government primary schools are well distributed and can be found in almost every neighbourhood of the city. Same is the case for private schools; however, a significant concentration of private schools in HI/LD, MI/LD and LI/HD

Table 3.10 Neighbourhood-Wise Distribution of Health Facilities (in Numbers) in Azamgarh City

Neighbour hoods	Government Services	If Yes		Private Services	If Yes		No. of Doctors	No. of Hospital Beds
		Health Centres	Hospital/ Nursing Homes		Clinics	Hospitals and Nursing Homes		
HI/HD	0	0	0	5	5	0	6	7
HI/MD	1	0	1	15	9	9	37	87
HI/LD	2	1	1	32	13	16	74	193
MI/HD	1	1	0	4	4	0	6	8
MI/LD	0	0	0	15	8	7	29	78
LI/HD	0	0	0	10	7	3	21	39
LI/MD	2	2	0	12	9	3	24	62
Total	6	4	2	93	55	38	197	474

Source: CMO Office, Azamgarh, 2016–2017.

Table 3.11 Neighbourhood-Wise Distribution of Educational Facilities (in Numbers) in Azamgarh City

Neighbourhoods	Government Schools	Private Schools	Degree Colleges
HI/HD	0	0	0
HI/MD	7	10	0
HI/LD	6	36	1
MI/HD	3	5	1
MI/LD	3	18	0
LI/HD	2	9	1
LI/MD	10	15	0
Total	31	93	3

Source: Basic Shiksha Adhikari, Azamgarh, 2016–2017.

neighbourhoods can be seen (Figure 3.4). Important schools in Azamgarh city are Children Senior Secondary School, St. Xavier's School, SKP Inter College, Shibli Nursery School and College, Pratibha Niketan School, Wesley Inter College, Krishna Inter College, etc. However, some most prestigious schools are also located outside the city boundary like Jyoti Niketan School, G.D. Global School, Azamgarh Public School, Central Public Schools, etc. From the field survey, it was found that children from all parts of the city were going to some most prestigious schools and location of schools in a different neighbourhood or outside the city did not matter. Almost all the big schools provide transport facility to the students and parents are also mainly focused to send their children in good schools no matter how far the schools are located. However, for elementary levels like nursery and kindergarten children go to nearby schools but after that, they are transferred to other schools. It is also an important point to note that these are mainly affluent parents that send their children to good schools, may be far from their houses, while children from low- and medium-income households go to neighbouring schools. Degree colleges that are located in the city are Shibli National PG College, DAV PG College and Shri Agrasen Mahila Snatkottar Mahavidyalay. Other educational and training institutions are ITI, Polytechnic College and Management College.

3.2.8 Recreational Facilities

Recreational facility refers to parks, clubs, swimming pools for water sports, tennis courts, health clubs or gyms developed for the common amusement of residents in an urban area. Recreational activities can greatly improve physical as well as mental health. Residents who take part in activities like walking, jogging or have gym membership generally maintain low body fat, lower blood pressure and cholesterol level. Recreational activities also help manage stress and mental wellness, vital for overall physical health. Recreational activities help in improving the quality of life too, as people who participate in recreational activities are more likely to feel satisfied with their lives. One of the

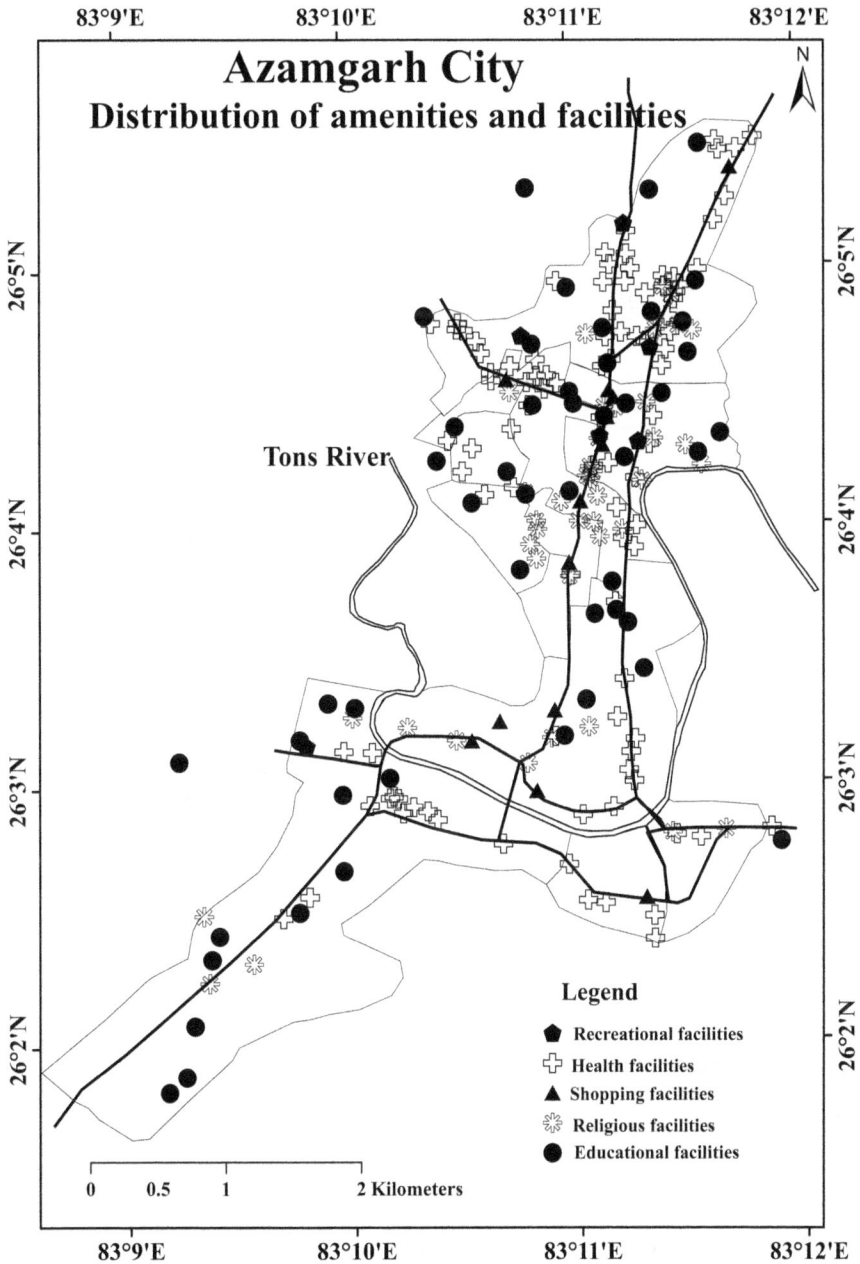

Figure 3.4 Azamgarh City: Distribution of Amenities and Densities.

Source: (i) CMO Office, Azamgarh, 2016–2017 (ii) Google Maps, 2019 (i) Basic Shiksha Adhikari, Azamgarh (2016–2017).

Table 3.12 Neighbourhood-Wise Distribution of Recreational Facilities (in Numbers) in Azamgarh City

Neighbourhoods	Recreational Facilities				
	Parks	Gyms	Cinema Halls	Restaurants	Libraries
HI/HD	0	0	0	3	0
HI/MD	0	0	1	4	0
HI/LD	5	3	2	11	1
MI/HD	0	0	0	3	0
MI/LD	0	1	0	4	0
LI/HD	0	2	0	3	1
LI/MD	1	0	0	2	0
Total	6	6	3	28	2

Source: (i) Municipal Office, Azamgarh and Field Survey, 2016–2017 (ii) Google Maps, 2019.

crucial components of people's comfort is the availability of recreational opportunity. Presence of parks in different neighbourhoods enhances well-being not only of the residents but of the city as well (Bakar et al., 2016). Recreational facilities in Azamgarh city include parks, gyms, libraries, cinema halls and restaurants (Table 3.12).

There are total six parks in Azamgarh city out of which five are located in HI/LD neighbourhood in the wards namely Civil Lines, Madya, Heerapatti, Raidopur while one is located in LI/MD neighbourhood, in the ward Ghulami Ka Pura. Presence of parks in the neighbourhood is a major place of recreation as it encourages residents for walking, jogging as well as other physical activities. Data shows that mostly medium- and low-income neighbourhoods are devoid of park facility around their houses. Parks are even absent in medium- and high-density counterparts of high-income neighbourhoods. As far as accessibility of gyms is concerned, out of total six gyms located in Azamgarh city, three can be found in HI/LD neighbourhood in Mukeriganj and Heerapatti, two in LI/HD neighbourhood in Paharpur and one in MI/LD neighbourhood in Harbanshpur ward of the city. There are three cinema halls in Azamgarh city namely Vishal Theatre in Sidhari West, Murli DDplex in Mukeriganj, both in HI/LD neighbourhood, and one is Suraj Talkies in Matbarganj in HI/MD neighbourhood. Thus it can be seen that all the three Cinema halls are located in high-income counterparts of the city.

There are two Public libraries in Azamgarh city, namely Mahapandit Rahul Sankrityayan Library located in Civil Lines and Darul Musannifeen Shibli Academy located near Shibli College in Paharpur. These libraries cover HI/LD and LI/HD neighbourhoods of the city. Another important source of recreation in the city is restaurants where residents go to spend some quality time. Significant concentration of restaurants can be seen in Civil Lines area or the main markets along Gorakhpur Allahabad Highway. However, some newly opened restaurants can also be seen in Narauli, Arazibagh, Heerapatti and Sidhari in the commercial areas (Figure 3.4).

3.2.9 Religious Facilities

Importance of religious sites in the neighbourhood needs no explanation as people generally prefer to live in the neighbourhoods that provide places of worship to the residents. Hindus prefer to visit a temple daily, weekly, or on festivals, while Muslims visit mosques for prayer, five times a day or at least once in a week and it is mandatory for Christians to attend Church at every Sunday. Therefore the presence of these sites in the neighbourhood not only save time, energy and travelling cost of the residents but also enhances overall well-being. Population composition of Azamgarh city shows that Hinduism is the major religion with 70.22% followers. Around 29.06% of residents follow Islam, 0.34% Christianity, 0.18% Buddhism and 0.01% follow Jainism (Census of India, 2011).

Since in Azamgarh city, a majority of Hindus and Muslims, in comparison to other religions, is observed, the same phenomenon was seen regarding the distribution of religious sites. Temples and Mosques are well distributed throughout the city and can be found in almost every neighbourhood. However, a significant concentration of both temples and mosques can be seen in central and most congested parts of the city due to high density of the area (Figure 3.4). Significant temples of Azamgarh city include Bhanwarnath Temple, Panchdev Temple, Shiv Mandir, Krishna Temple, Durga Temple Kali Mata Temple, Mahavir Temple, etc. Some important Mosques of the city include Jama Masjid Azamgarh, Tedhiya Masjid, Sidhari Masjid, Masjid Usman Ghani, Rahmat Nagar Mosque, etc. Only two churches are there in the city namely Holy Trinity Church and Masihi Prarthana Bhavan located in Civil Lines and Harbanshpur, respectively.

3.2.10 Markets

While small grocery shops can be found around houses in all the neighbourhoods, not all the essential goods can be accessed in each neighbourhood. Markets are the places where all everyday essentials, comfort goods and luxury goods can be bought. In other words, a market is a place from where we purchase food, clothing, footwear, home appliances, and stationery and housekeeping items. Large markets are located in some particular locations, not equally accessible from all the corners of the city. There are two major markets in Azamgarh city namely Chowk market and Takiya market, along Allahabad-Gorakhpur highway passing in the mid of the city and located in the wards of Matbarganj, Sadavarti, Asifganj and Paharpur (Table 3.13 and Figure 3.4).

Markets include shops of food grains, electricity, stationery, gold and silver, provisional stores, clothing and service shops. Markets show a mixed type of function and specialised markets lack in the city. From the map it is apparent that markets are located in the north-central parts of the city well accessible from other parts except Heerapatti and Ghulami Ka Pura wards. Some shops can also be seen along the roads in Sarfuddinpur and Harbanshpur wards, but not much developed like the markets of the city.

Table 3.13 Distributions of Markets in Azamgarh City

Neighbourhoods	Presence of Market	Name of the Market	Ward Name
HI/HD	Yes	Takiya	Asifganj
HI/MD	Yes	Chowk	Matbarganj
HI/LD	No	–	–
MI/HD	No	–	–
MI/LD	No	–	–
LI/HD	Yes	Takiya	Paharpur
LI/MD	Yes	Chowk	Sadavarti

Source: (i) Municipal Office, Azamgarh City (ii) Based on Field Survey, 2016–2017.

3.2.11 Shopping Malls

A shopping mall is a latest, basically North American term for a shopping centre that has many shops. Malls are big multi-storeyed, air-conditioned structures with shops on different floors selling both branded and non-branded items. Malls sell not only clothing, footwear, home appliances, stationery and housekeeping items but also fresh fruits, vegetables as well as dairy products. Therefore the presence of shopping malls in the neighbourhoods is highly appreciated by residents as they can buy all the essential goods under a single roof. Malls also sell goods from different prestigious brands that are not generally available in local markets. Malls in Azamgarh city are mainly located in the major markets along the Allahabad Gorakhpur highway. There are total 16 shopping malls in Azamgarh city, out of which nine are located in HI/LD, three in HI/MD, two in LI/MD, one in HI/HD, and one in LI/HD neighbourhoods (Table 3.14). Malls of HI/LD were V. Mart, Grihpurti Mall, Vishal Mega mart (Civil Lines), Family Bazar, Vinayak Tower (Madya), V2 Mart, One city Mall, Style up (Mukeriganj) and JK the Mall (Sidhari West). In HI/MD, these were India-2 Mart, Sanskaar (Matbarganj) and M Mart, Kolkata Bazar (Arazibagh). V. Mart in Asifganj, Royal Shopping Mall, City Life Mall (Paharpur) and Sunbeam (Sadavarti) were other malls.

A considerable concentration of malls can be seen in high-income counterparts of the city and practically no shopping mall is located in MI/LD and MI/HD neighbourhood (Table 3.14 and Figure 3.4). However MI/HD neighbourhood has the advantage of its location in the central part of the city, and shopping malls are not very far from its wards like Badarka and Katra, but the situation is notably worse for MI/LD neighbourhood covering wards like Sarfuddinpur, Harbanshpur and Narauli, in the south of river Tons.

3.2.11.1 Impact of Amenities and Facilities on Well-Being

Many aspects of urban life can be favourable to human well-being, in terms of access to education, healthcare facilities, social support, physical security as well as material resources (Butterworth, 2000). Researches in the field of environmental psychology as well as in urban planning have also shown that

Table 3.14 Neighbourhood-Wise Distribution of Shopping Malls (in Numbers) in Azamgarh City

Neighbourhoods	Number of Malls	Name of the Malls (Wards)
HI/HD	1	V. Mart (Asifganj)
HI/MD	3	India-2 Mart, Sanskaar (Matbarganj), M Mart, Kolkata Bazar (Arazibagh)
HI/LD	9	V. Mart, Grihpurti Mall, Vishal Mega mart (Civil Lines), Family Bazar, Vinayak Tower (Madya), V2 Mart, One city Mall, Style up (Mukeriganj), JK the Mall (Sidhari West)
MI/HD	0	–
MI/LD	0	–
LI/HD	2	Royal Shopping Mall, City Life Mall (Paharpur)
LI/MD	1	Sunbeam (Sadavarti)
Total	16	

Source: (i) Municipal Office, Azamgarh City, 2016–2017. (ii) Based on Field Survey, 2016–2017 (iii) Google Maps, 2019.

physical surrounding and well-being are affected by one another (Lee and Maheswaran, 2011). It has been found that individual well-being is significantly affected by the physical, social and service environment in which the individuals live. In a given location, an individual's well-being can be affected by educational and employment opportunities, prices of goods and services as well as presence and quality of place-specific amenities and facilities (Winters and Lee, 2017). Urban planners and city development authorities have also recognised the impact of amenities and facilities.

Field survey has revealed that about 81.95% residents have admitted that availability of health facilities, schools, markets, shopping malls, recreational as well as religious sites in the neighbourhoods leave a positive impact on them and they would prefer to live in the neighbourhoods laced with proper facilities in it. This percentage is 83.23 in HI/LD, 89.98 in HI/HD, 89.64 in LI/MD, 85.79 in MI/HD, 84.56 in LI/HD, 83.44 in HI/MD and 79.85 in MI/LD neighbourhood (Table 3.15).

3.3 Social Environment

The physical and the social environments are not independent of each other. Environment of any place is the result of continuous interaction between natural and human-made components, social practices, and the relation between individuals and groups (Syme, 1992). Social environment of a neighbourhood includes the quality of relationship such as trust, connectedness and cooperation among residents. A society is a network of social relationships which provides a set of values and norms which helps in keeping harmonious relationship

Table 3.15 Neighbourhood-Wise Impact of Amenities and Facilities on the Well-Being (in Percentages) in Azamgarh City

Neighbourhoods	Positive Impact of Neighbourhood Amenities on Well-Being*		
	Yes	No	Can't say
HI/HD	83.23	6.75	10.02
HI/MD	83.44	10.56	6.00
HI/LD	88.25	7.44	4.31
MI/HD	79.79	7.63	12.58
MI/LD	79.85	11.13	9.02
LI/HD	80.56	4.39	15.05
LI/MD	78.50	8.25	13.25
Total	81.95	8.02	10.03

Source: Based on Field Survey, 2016–2017.
* Based on resident's perception.

among members of the society and offers them full opportunity for development and privilege of a decent life. A socially healthy neighbourhood is formed by strong social relationships among residents, together with the level of mutual trust and sense of connectedness among neighbours. Inhabitants of a close-knit neighbourhood are more likely to work together for the welfare of the neighbourhood like cleaner and safer public places, exchanging information regarding neighbourhood resources and maintain informal social controls like discouraging wrongdoings or other unwanted actions such as smoking or drinking among adolescents, etc. Neighbourhoods in which residents show mutual trust and are willing to interfere for public welfare has been associated with lesser homicide rates. On the other hand, less closely-knit neighbourhoods have been linked with anxiety and depression (Cubbin, 2008).

Social Environment in different neighbourhoods of Azamgarh city was measured by the degree of neighbours visiting each other, willing to help each other and finding them trustworthy. Five-point Likert scale was used to record the responses of the residents regarding their social environment. Table 3.16 and revealed that out of the total, about 70% residents agree that they visit each other out of which 7.94% opted 'strongly agree' while 61.26 did agree. Neighbourhood data revealed that 'strongly agree' responses were recorded only from HI/LD and MI/LD neighbourhoods while 'agree' response was given by almost 60–70% residents of all the neighbourhoods. Total 9.30% residents were 'neither agree nor disagree' while 21.51% responded 'disagree' about visiting their neighbours. This percentage was highest in MI/HD neighbourhood, i.e. 40% followed by HI/HD, i.e. 33.33 and HI/MD, i.e. 26.67%. When the question came of neighbours willing to help each other, again about 70% residents chose 'agree' to this however proportion of 'strong agree' declined this time as only 4.76% residents opted for this (Table 3.17). 'Neither agree nor disagree' responses followed the same pattern as in case of neighbours visiting each other. Neighbourhood-wise response also did not deviate.

Table 3.16 Neighbourhood Social Cohesion and Connectedness (Visit Each-Other) (in Percentages) in Azamgarh City

Neighbourhoods	Visit Each Other				
	Strongly Agree	Agree	Neither Agree nor Disagree	Disagree	Strongly Disagree
HI/HD	0.00	66.66	0.00	33.33	0.00
HI/MD	0.00	73.33	0.00	26.67	0.00
HI/LD	33.33	31.95	29.17	5.56	0.00
MI/HD	0.00	60.00	0.00	40.00	0.00
MI/LD	22.22	54.45	6.67	16.67	0.00
LI/HD	0.00	70.42	21.25	8.33	0.00
LI/MD	0.00	72.00	8.00	20.00	0.00
Total	7.94	61.26	9.30	21.51	0.00

Source: Based on Field Survey, 2016–2017.

Table 3.17 Neighbourhood Social Cohesion and Connectedness (Willing to Help Each Other) (in Percentages) in Azamgarh City

Neighbourhoods	Willing to Help Each Other				
	Strongly Agree	Agree	Neither Agree nor Disagree	Disagree	Strongly Disagree
HI/HD	0.00	66.66	0.00	33.33	0.00
HI/MD	0.00	65.00	0.00	35.00	0.00
HI/LD	33.33	31.95	29.17	5.56	0.00
MI/HD	0.00	60.00	0.00	40.00	0.00
MI/LD	0.00	76.67	6.67	16.67	0.00
LI/HD	0.00	70.42	21.25	8.33	0.00
LI/MD	0.00	72.00	8.00	20.00	0.00
Total	4.76	63.24	9.30	22.70	0.00

Source: Based on Field Survey, 2016–2017.

Another variable to determine social capital was whether residents find their neighbours trustworthy or not (Table 3.18). It was found that all the questions like visiting each other, willing to help each other and find neighbours trustworthy were responded with the same pattern indicating that all three questions were just modified form of each other like in a neighbourhood where residents visit each other; they help as well as trust each other and vice-versa.

Another important finding of the study was that people's perception of their neighbourhoods was much different than the predefined neighbourhoods, and it was much smaller than census boundaries. Perception of the neighbourhoods was the smallest in case of newly developed residential areas where mostly migrants had settled from different parts of the city as well as from outside the city and most significant in case of old low-income residential areas where people have lived for generations. The social environment was found good in well-developed colonies like Hariaudhnagar and Officers

Table 3.18 Neighbourhood Social Cohesion and Connectedness (Trustworthy) (in Percentages) in Azamgarh City

Neighbourhoods	Trustworthy				
	Strongly Agree	Agree	Neither Agree nor Disagree	Disagree	Strongly Disagree
HI/HD	0.00	66.66	0.00	33.33	0.00
HI/MD	0.00	65.00	0.00	35.00	0.00
HI/LD	33.33	31.95	29.17	5.56	0.00
MI/HD	0.00	60.00	0.00	40.00	0.00
MI/LD	0.00	76.67	6.67	16.67	0.00
LI/HD	0.00	70.42	21.25	8.33	0.00
LI/MD	0.00	72.00	8.00	20.00	0.00
Total	4.76	63.24	9.30	22.70	0.00

Source: Based on Field Survey, 2016–2017.

Colony in which similar type of people live while in mixed type of areas it was not much satisfactory. Practically no interaction was found among the main areas of the wards and *Harijan, Prajapati and Mallah bastis*, and residents of these *bastis* were totally segregated from the mainstream population. Overall social environment in Azamgarh city was found satisfactory as people live a social life in their well-defined limits and about 70% of them reported well of their neighbours.

3.4 Summary

In this chapter, a full general overview of neighbourhood environment in Azamgarh city is provided. Neighbourhood environment of Azamgarh city is studied primarily into three parts, i.e. physical, social and service environment. The physical environment of the neighbourhoods includes residential density, built-up area and open spaces. Service environment includes supply of various municipal services such as street lighting, solid waste management, wastewater management and water supply conditions and other amenities and facilities like education and health facilities in different neighbourhoods while social environment includes social relation among residents of the neighbourhood. This chapter is based on information collected during the field survey from different neighbourhoods of Azamgarh city as well as a lot of secondary sources like satellite data and municipal as well as other offices in Azamgarh city.

An analysis of neighbourhood physical environment in the city revealed that residential density and proportion of built-up area is the highest in the old central part of the city consisting of wards Bazbahadur, Paharpur, Seetaram, Jalandhari, Gurutola and Sadavarti while proportion of open spaces was good in other wards like Civil Lines, Sidhari, Mukeriganj, Heerapatti, Narauli, Harbanshpur and Sarfuddinpur. Most of the parks are located in the high-income parts of the city like Civil Lines, Madya, Heerapatti and Raidopur.

A study of service environment in Azamgarh city revealed that High-income neighbourhoods are well lit at night. It was found that water supply pipelines of the city do not cover all the houses of the city and 7.19% of residents still do not have water facility inside their houses. Out of the total household waste generated in the city only about 80% waste is collected by the municipality while rest of the 20% is either collected by households themselves or deposited to open fields, backyards, water bodies or burnt. An investigation of drainage system in the city revealed that about 90% have reported the presence of drainage facility in their neighbourhood out of which 32.29% reported presence of open drains, while rest 10% residents reported disposal of wastewater in *kachcha nalis* along the roads, in the fields and water bodies. There are 6 government and 93 private hospitals, nursing and clinics. Arazibagh, Heerapatti and Mekeriganj are the hospital hubs of the city. There are 31 government, 93 private schools and 3 degree colleges in the city and schools outside the city are also quite popular among residents. Market is developed along the Gorakhpur Allahabad highway and comes in the wards of Civil Lines, Matbarganj, Sadavarti, Asifganj and Paharpur. Shopping malls can also be spotted on the same road in the main market; however, a significant concentration of malls can be found in high-income neighbourhoods of the city like in Civil Lines, Madya, Mukeriganj and Arazibagh. As far as availability of the recreational site is concerned there are 6 parks, 6 gyms, 3 cinema halls and 2 libraries in Azamgarh city which is inadequate for the population. Restaurants can also be spotted in the city with a major concentration along Allahabad Gorakhpur highway and in Civil Lines and other commercial areas. However, distribution of religious sites is somewhat satisfactory as temples and mosques can be accessed from almost all the parts of the city, but the case is a bit different for church, as there are only two churches in the city which can be justified on the basis that only 0.34% population of the city practices Christianity. Autos, E-rickshaw and manual rickshaws are popular means of transportation in the city to connect different neighbourhoods as well as amenities and facilities in the city.

Neighbourhood social environment in Azamgarh city is measured by the degree of trust and connectedness among neighbours. It was found that overall social environment in the city was good, as about 70% residents showed connectedness with their neighbours but a big social gap between the majority population and other marginalised communities like schedule caste was found.

References

Amerigo, M. (2002). "A Psychological Approach to the Study of Residential Satisfaction". Eds. Aragones, J. I., Francescato, G., & Carling, T. *Residential Environments: Choice, Satisfaction, and Behavior*. Bergin Si Garvey Publisher, Wesport (YT/ London), pp. 81–99.

Bakar, N. A., Malek, N. A., & Mansor, M. (2016). Access to Parks and Recreational Opportunities in Urban Low-Income Neighbourhood. *Procedia-Social and Behavioral Sciences, 234*, 299–308.

Butterworth, I. (2000). The relationship between the built environment and wellbeing: a literature review. Prepared for the Victorian Health Promotion Foundation.

Census of India. (2011).

Cubbin, C., Egerter, S., Braveman, P., & Pedregon, V. (2008). *Where We Live Matters for Our Health: Neighborhoods and Health*. Robert Wood John Foundation, New Jersey.

Farrington, D.P., & Welsh, B. (2002). *Effects of Improved Street Lighting on Crime: A Systematic Review*. Home Office Research, London, United Kingdom, p. 39.

Government of India. (2018). Ministry of New and Renewable Energy LokSabha Unstarred Question No. 2974.

Gupta, K., Kumar, P., Pathan, S. K., & Sharma, K. P. (2012). Urban Neighborhood Green Index–A measure of green spaces in urban areas. *Landscape and Urban Planning*, *105*(3), 325–335.

Health Canada. (2002). *Natural and Built Environments*. Division of Childhood and Adolescence, Health Canada, Ottawa.

Jha, A. K., Singh, S. K., Singh, G. P., & Gupta, P. K. (2011). Sustainable municipal solid waste management in low income group of cities: a review. *Tropical Ecology*, *52*(1), 123–131.

Kimhi. (2005). "Urban Environmental Quality," The Centre for Environmental Policy Studies Series #12, the Jerusale Institute for Israel Studies, Jerusalem. http://www.jiis.org.il

Knox, P. L. (1982). "Residential Structure, Facility Location and Patterns of Accessibility." Eds., Cox, K. R., & Johnston, R. J. *Conflict, Politics and the Urban Scene*. St. Martin's Press, New York, pp. 62–87.

Kwon, M., Pickett, A. C., Lee, Y., & Lee, S. (2019). Neighborhood physical environments0.1 recreational wellbeing, and psychological health. *Applied Research in Quality of Life*, *14*, 1–19.

Lee, A. C., & Maheswaran, R. (2011). The health benefits of urban green spaces: a review of the evidence. *Journal of Public Health*, *33*(2), 212–222.

Low, N., Gleeson, B., Green, R. and Radovic, D. (2007). *The Green City; Sustainable Homes, Sustainable Suburbs*. Routledge, London.

Mishra, B., Singh, R. B., & Anupama, M., (2001). "Delhi Metropolis: Housing and Quality of Life". Ed. Mishra, R.P. *Million Cities of India*, Vol. 1, Vikas Publising, New Delhi, pp. 196–228.

Park, C.C. (1980). *Ecology and Environmental Management, a Geographical Perspective*. West-view Press, Boulder, Colorado.

Pearce, J., Witten, K., & Bartie, P. (2006). Neighbourhoods and health: a GIS approach to measuring community resource accessibility. *Journal of Epidemiology & Community Health*, *60*(5), 389–395.

Rahman, A., Kumar, Y., Fazal, S., & Bhaskaran, S. (2011). Urbanisation and quality of urban environment using remote sensing and GIS techniques in East Delhi-India. *Journal of Geographic Information System*, *3*(1), 62–84.

Singh, A.S., Pandey, D.N., & Chaudhry, P. (2010). *Urban Forests and Open Green Spaces: Jaipur, Rajasthan*. Rajasthan State Pollution Control Board, Jaipur.

Syed, S. (2006). Solid and liquid waste management. *The Emirates Journal for Engineering Research*, *11*(2), 19–36.

Syme, S.L. (1992). "Social Determinants of Disease". Ed. Last, J.M., & Wallace, R.B. *Public Health and Preventative Medicine*, Appleton & Lange, Norwalk, CT, pp. 953–970.

WHO and UNICEF. (2017). *Progress on Drinking Water, Sanitation and Hygiene: 2017 Update and SDG Baselines.* World Health Organization (WHO) and the United Nations Children's Fund (UNICEF), Geneva.

Winters, J. V., & Li, Y. (2017). Urbanisation, natural amenities and subjective well-being: evidence from US counties. *Urban Studies, 54*(8), 1956–1973.

4   Understanding Neighbourhood Environmental Problems in Azamgarh City

The term neighbourhood has been used to refer to an individual's immediate residential environment, possessing both physical and social characteristics (Diez-Roux, 1998). Thus the neighbourhood environmental problems are those problems that people face in and around their houses. Researches on neighbourhood effects have contributed a lot while examining health differences among populations (Pickett and Pearl, 2001). It has been estimated that the environment is responsible for as much as 24% of the global burden of diseases. A noteworthy proportion of the overall environmental diseases burden can be credited to comparatively few dimensions of risk. These involve irregular supply and poor quality of water, inadequate sanitation, poor ambient and indoor air quality, toxic materials and global environmental change. In some cases, simple preventive measures can reduce the risk of diseases. Serious environmental problems in poor neighbourhoods often create health hazards. Insufficient water supply, improper sanitation, heaps of waste and smoky cooking fuels are all linked with urban poverty and inadequate environmental services.

Environmental problems that are found in the immediate housing environment have immediate and threatening effects on the health of the residents. Though these problems are not long term, as compared to global environmental challenges, they do induce unanticipated threat to the environmental basis for human survival. Many cities are presently burdened by infectious diseases namely typhoid, malaria, diarrhoea etc. supported by poor living conditions. These are the result and a combined interaction of social determinants of health, including insufficient infrastructure and services that mainly impact the health of the poor and slum inhabitants (WHO, 2010).

In the previous chapter, general overview of neighbourhood environment in Azamgarh city was discussed. Three significant forms of neighbourhood environment like physical, social and service environment were examined. It has been observed that residential density and proportion of built-up area is the highest in the old central part of the city. Most of the parks are located in the high-income parts of the city, and all the houses of the city are not covered by water supply pipelines. Out of the total household waste generated in the city,

DOI: 10.4324/9781003442486-5

about 80% waste is collected by the municipality. The drainage system in the city revealed that about 90% reported presence of drainage while rest 10% residents reported disposal of wastewater in *kachchanalis* along the roads, in the fields and water bodies. A study of service environment in Azamgarh city revealed that there are 6 government and 93 private hospitals, nursing homes and clinics, 31 government schools, 93 private schools and 3 degree colleges in the city. A significant concentration of shopping malls can be found in high-income neighbourhoods of the city like in Civil Lines, Madya, Mukeriganj and Arazibagh. As far as availability of recreational site is concerned, there are 6 parks, 6 gyms, 3 cinema halls and 2 libraries in Azamgarh city which is unsatisfactory pertaining to the size of the total population. Autos, e-rickshaw and manual rickshaws are major means of transportation in the city to connect to the different neighbourhoods as well as amenities and facilities in the city. Overall social environment in the city was pleasant as about 70% residents showed connectedness with their neighbours, but a big connection gap between the majority population and other marginalised communities like schedule caste was found.

This chapter is in continuation of the previous chapter. It examines the neighbourhood environmental problems that are responsible for the regional differences in physical, social and service environment, ultimately leading to various problems. This chapter presents an overview of the significant neighbourhood environmental problems of Azamgarh city. The city and household survey helped in identifying several acute problems which they face in their day-to-day life.

This chapter has been divided into two sections. In the first section, an attempt has been made to understand what actually neighbourhood problems are. In the second section, an identification of major neighbourhood problems in Azamgarh city is made, and further, the identified neighbourhood environmental problems of the city are discussed comprehensively under three major categories i.e. neighbourhood physical environmental problems, neighbourhood service environmental problems as well as neighbourhood social environmental problems.

4.1 Understanding Neighbourhood Environmental Problems

There is now widespread agreement that neighbourhood environmental problems are important but there is little coherence in identifying critical problems. The confusion is what environmental problems mean in a neighbourhood context.

The neighbourhood environmental problems deal with development issues in broader terms. Defining environmental problems as "the degradation of air, water and land" will be too narrow in neighbourhood context as it will isolate various environmental health problems predominantly suffered by socio-economically poor people. Thus it is suggested that neighbourhood environmental problems are deadly for the physical as well as social environment, including a biased distribution of amenities and facilities which create neighbourhood service environment.

Accordingly, these problems are region-specific. Based on the definition above for neighbourhood environmental problems, here in this chapter, neighbourhood problems identified for the study area include:

- Localised neighbourhood environmental problems (Physical and human-induced problems), i.e. inadequate water supply, sanitation, waste collection, substandard housing etc.
- City regional neighbourhood environmental problems (overcrowding, Air and noise pollution, waste management, river pollution, etc.)
- Neighbourhood problems that are termed as social problems like residential segregation, neighbourhood disorder etc.

Environmental management is understood as a technical process which involves discussions, conflicts, debates, certain compromises and decision making. Generally, true information can help to motivate policy makers, reformers and various government officials to make appropriate decision and also provide the right motivation. Similarly wrong and inadequate ground information can result in a fallacious and inoperative decision. Moreover, incompetently conceived problems are easily disregarded and accordingly planning funds and resources may be directed to in trivial problems. Thus the most consequent problems remain least vocal and highlighted which leads to ignorance of most needy segment of the population in policy-making.

In underdeveloped urban areas, several acute problems arise surrounding people's home, frequently creating environmental and health risks. Inadequate water supply, smoky air (due to cooking fuels and industries), spillover solid and liquid waste, pest and insect infestation are related to socio-economic backwardness and insufficient environmental services. Thus, the health of the vulnerable section of the population (women, small children, elderly) spending much time close to their home environment are directly and indirectly threatened by these problems.

Accordingly, neighbourhood associated environmental problems can play a vital pathway in environmental improvements. It can contribute to helping policy makers, officials and decision-makers to determine their way ahead with the problems. For example, in those areas where water supply drains, electricity and waste collection services are unreachable grandeur, it is of immense importance that priority setting must be highlighted and informed to the government officials. So that cost of devoting resources should be processed to needy segments in order to deal with human sufferings.

Facts and figures are critical at the city level for successful planning and essential improvements in household and neighbourhood environment. Understanding neighbourhood environmental problems is not only the need for household and community but is also crucial for inclusive development of the cities.

4.2 Identification of Major Neighbourhood Environmental Problems in Azamgarh City

People are not aware of the fact that it is the immediate housing environment which exercises the greatest and produces the most immediate impact on their health and well-being (Rahman, 1998). An overcrowded neighbourhood with congested streets, inadequate water supply and quality, weak drainage system, waterlogging conditions, litter on the streets and with several environmental hazards like air and noise pollution has direct and indirect adverse impacts on the health of its residents. Most of the environmental disease burden includes few risk factors like unsafe water and sanitation, indoor smoke from solid fuels, toxic exposures and global environmental change as well as haphazard patterns of development that adds to air pollution, traffic issues and other forms of urban environmental deterioration. Environmental hazards and related diseases kill millions worldwide every year (WHO, 2004). Many cities are presently burdened by infectious diseases namely typhoid, malaria, diarrhoea, etc., supported by poor living conditions.

Based on an in-depth survey of different neighbourhoods, interviews and observations a wide range of urgent neighbourhood environmental problems that were reported from almost all the residents of the city, were selected for analysis. These problems include

- Neighbourhood physical environmental problems like neighbourhood over-crowding, narrow or congested streets, substandard housing and slums, air and noise pollution, water quality problem etc.
- Neighbourhood service environmental problems like insufficient water supply, improper drainage, waterlogging, accumulation of solid waste and unequal distribution of amenities and facilities.
- Neighbourhood social environmental problems like residential segregation and neighbourhood disorder.

4.2.1 *Neighbourhood Physical Environmental Problems*

Neighbourhood physical environmental problems can also be understood as neighbourhood built environmental problems. These are the problems that people face due to human-made structures in their neighbourhoods ranging from residential houses, commercial buildings, patterns of roads and streets as well as the presence or absence of parks etc. Neighbourhood physical problems identified in the city include neighbourhood overcrowding, narrow or congested streets, substandard housing and slums, air and noise pollution as well as water quality problem.

4.2.1.1 *Neighbourhood Overcrowding*

"Crowding refers to people's psychological response to density; that is, to their feeling of being crowded, having a lack of privacy or an increase in unwanted interactions or psychological distress" (Gove et al., 1979; Crothers et al., 1993; Jazwinski, 1998). Overcrowding can never be measured quantitatively, and it should not be confused with density. Crowding is concerned with people's perceptions towards residential density and built-up area, i.e. their sense of being crowded, issues of breach in privacy or lack of privacy or a rise in unwanted interaction (Gray, 2001). Therefore for research purpose, crowding has been measured with people's perception of overcrowding in their neighbourhood related to high population and household density, narrow lanes and lack of public spaces etc. However, based on the fact that its people's perception, that is more important, it cannot be discarded that overcrowding is directly related to density. Various urban sociologists and psychologists have done researches on the impact of neighbourhood overcrowding. It is mostly the unplanned areas that face the problem of overcrowding. Planners of the Garden City movement observed that places with too many people, houses and workplaces, along with less air, light and open spaces recorded high social deprivation, worsening health and crime (Radberg, 1988). At the household level, overcrowding is generally measured by persons per room, persons per bedroom or persons per unit square foot (Blake et al., 2007).

However at neighbourhood level, percentage of residential units per unit area is responsible for proportion of open space in a neighbourhood and ventilation in the streets and buildings. Overcrowding at the community level can be hypothesised as pressure on local infrastructure and resources. Neighbourhood overcrowding affects all the residents as it increases the number of people using public amenities and occupying public places. Housing density in the neighbourhood leads to neighbourhood overcrowding and it is equally vital as housing overcrowding. Neighbourhood overcrowding can contribute to the deterioration of the neighbourhood environment in several ways such as traffic congestion, worsening air quality, potential reduction of outdoor spaces, noise problem and lack of privacy. The higher the housing density of a neighbourhood, the poorer the quality of urban environment (Mishra, 2001). Since overcrowding is linked with rapid spread of infectious diseases and increased violent behaviour (Gray, 2001), it can severely affect city life.

Perception of residents regarding the sense of overcrowding in their neighbourhoods has been shown in Table 4.1. The Table reveals that of the total sampled households, 59.44% households of Azamgarh city have reported a sense of overcrowding in their neighbourhoods. Overcrowding was reported the highest in MI/HD, LI/HD and HI/HD neighbourhoods, i.e. 95%, 77.60% and 66.66%, respectively, and it was least in MI/LD, i.e. 18.33% followed by HI/LD, i.e. 34.17%. A perusal of the Table shows that in MI/HD neighbourhood overcrowding is high, i.e. 95% and in the same neighbourhood residential density, i.e. 3369 houses per sq. km and built-up density, i.e. 77.39% are also high. The lowest overcrowding was reported from MI/LD neighbourhood, i.e. 18.33% and in the same neighbourhood residential density is as low as 677 houses per sq. km and built-up density is only 25.87% of the total area (Tables 4.1 and 3.2).

Table 4.1 Neighbourhood-Wise Overcrowding
(in Percentages) in Azamgarh City

Neighbourhoods	Overcrowding*
MI/HD	95
LI/HD	77.6
HI/HD	66.66
LI/MD	64.33
HI/MD	60
HI/LD	34.17
MI/LD	18.33
Total	59.44

Source: Based on Field Survey, 2016–2017.
* Based on resident's Perception.

Therefore, it can be said that perception of neighbourhood overcrowding is highly dependent on residential density and built-up area as neighbourhoods in which overcrowding was reported the highest are the same neighbourhoods with the highest residential density and built-up area in the central part of the city covering wards Badarka, Katra, Bazbahadur, Paharpur, Gurutola, Jalandhari and Asifganj. Least overcrowding was reported in Sarfuddinpur, Harbanshpur, Narauli, Civil Lines, Madya, Heerapatti, Mukeriganj and Raidopur, etc. These wards constitute southern as well as northern extension of the city with low built-up area and low residential density. The analysis, therefore, could conclude that although overcrowding is a subjective concept, it is directly affected by the density of an area.

4.2.1.2 Narrow Streets

Width of the streets plays an important role in the quality as well as the appearance of neighbourhood environment. Congested street pattern not only leads to high residential density but influence the overall quality of life of the residents. Congested or narrow street results in packed residential areas as well as transfer of contagious diseases in the community. Wide streets let the fresh air and sunlight pass from all the houses and also give an impression of an enjoyable living space. Narrow streets also can also contribute to the deterioration of the neighbourhood environment in several ways such as traffic congestion, worsening air quality, potential reduction of outdoor spaces, noise problem and lack of privacy. High population density and unplanned growth are the main reasons behind congested street pattern in the city. Residents generally built their houses on their own, without any monitoring by the city authority. Therefore to make their houses spacious, they even occupy streets making the roads narrower.

For the analysis, streets are divided into three categories based on their width, i.e. good (>15 feet), average (7–15 feet) and narrow or congested (<7 feet). Narrow streets are those streets from which passage of four-wheeler

Table 4.2 Neighbourhood-Wise Narrow Streets
(in Percentages) in Azamgarh City

Neighbourhoods	Narrow Streets
	(>7 feet)
HI/HD	80
HI/MD	54.99
HI/LD	15.83
MI/HD	100
MI/LD	11.67
LI/HD	45
LI/MD	33.33
Total	48.68

Source: Based on Field Survey, 2016–2017.

vehicles is difficult and only one vehicle could pass at once. An analysis of width of roads in Azamgarh city shows that about 48.68% residents reported narrow or congested streets around their houses and this was 100% in MI/HD, 80% in HI/HD, 54.99% in HI/MD and 45% in LI/HD neighbourhood covering wards namely Katra, Badarka, Asifganj, Matbarganj, Bazbahadur, Paharpur, Jalandhari and Seetaram (Table 4.2). These wards are localised in the central old part of the city and represent typical downtown characteristics of Indian cities with mixed land use and high household density. Overcrowding was also reported the highest in these neighbourhoods. In the field survey, streets were also found from which a four-wheeler vehicle could not pass. Households, mainly of medium- and low-income neighbourhoods, have reported that there were not adequate access roads for vehicle movement. Residents from these neighbourhoods usually take a walk from their houses and then board vehicles from main roads. The problem of narrow streets was least prevalent in the neighbourhoods MI/LD and HI/LD, i.e. 11.67% and 15.83%, respectively. These neighbourhoods mainly constitute the newly developed northern and southern extension of the city. Low-density, low built-up area and open spaces are essential characteristics of these neighbourhoods. Neighbourhood survey thus found that older parts of the city have narrower roads than the newly developed residential neighbourhoods.

4.2.1.3 Substandard Housing and Slums

It has been estimated that around 2.4 million or 30% of the Indian population is either houseless or live in mud or thatched houses. In case of small cites of India, like Azamgarh city, the problem is not the absence of housing facilities but the absence of adequate housing facilities. A clean, decent and safe house is the central goal of a majority of the population as it determines the quality of life of residents and generates the most enormous and direct influence on their physiological as well as psychological development (Thangval et al., 1987).

Quality of a house is an index of its resident's health and well-being. Proper housing is especially vital for women, children and elderlies as they spend most of their time inside the houses. Housing is a crucial determining factor for health, and substandard housing is a significant public health issue. Poor households living in cramped conditions may generate many urban problems as well. A large number of local users of smoky fuels may create neighbourhood air pollution problem and can even contribute to broader city problems.

Housing quality in Azamgarh city has been measured by the type of house in which residents live. If the house is made up of *kachcha* material like mud, wood, IG sheets it would be called as *kachcha* house; if it is made up of pucca material like brick, concrete, tiles it would be classified as *pucca* house and the houses made up of both *kachcha* and *pucca* materials would come in the category of *semi-pucca* houses. Type of house is also a representation of the social and economic background of the residents. Substandard houses in this discussion include houses made of *kachcha* or *semi-pucca* material. Other characteristics of houses like overcrowding, indoor air pollution, leaking roofs, poor sanitation, dampness and mould are all dependent upon the type of house. Substandard quality of housing is reported to increase the incidence of diseases. In Azamgarh city, a substantial proportion of residents live in substandard housing conditions. The household and the neighbourhood environment cannot be separated, since problem in one environment will have impact on the other such as lack of proper sanitation inside houses to remove wastewater and excreta would result in open drains in the neighbourhoods which can contaminate groundwater and also find its way into solid waste, open land, drainage ditches, etc., where pests etc. may breed and can cause severe health hazards. Solid waste may cause accumulation of water where mosquitos can breed. Thus all these problems are typically interrelated.

The generalised picture of the cities, highlights that even though high- and upper-middle-income groups have managed to live in decent houses in better neighbourhoods, the problem is still prevalent in case of poor population. They live in dilapidated houses in areas where shabbiness, congestion and lack of services are dominant problems. These areas suffer from inadequacy of essential services, amenities, facilities and face several complex environmental problems such as water, sanitation and hygiene, crowding and congestion, solid waste dumps, open drains and waterlogged areas as well as faecal matter and land contamination. It is a well-known fact now that poor quality of housing leads to health risks of the residents (Seng et al., 2018).

Table 4.3 reveals that about 20.86% of the total households have reported living in substandard houses and this percentage was the highest in LI/MD, i.e. 35.35% followed by LI/HD, i.e. 30.68, MI/LD, i.e. 26.40, MI/HD, i.e. 16.82%. Large clusters of substandard housing can be seen in harijan bastis in Farashtola, Sidhari east, Katra, Harbanshpur, Ghulami ka pura, Mukeriganj, Raidopur, Narauli, Pandeybazaar, in Prajapati colony in Arazibagh and *Mallah basti* in Madya. These *bastis* are mainly developed in the central part of the city and along the banks of river Tons. Slum like condition can be seen in

Table 4.3 Neighbourhood-Wise Substandard Housing
(in Percentages) in Azamgarh City

Neighbourhoods	Substandard Housing
HI/HD	7.77
HI/MD	15.20
HI/LD	13.80
MI/HD	16.82
MI/LD	26.40
LI/HD	30.68
LI/MD	35.35
Total	20.86

Source: Based on Field Survey, 2016–2017.

Kaleenganj in Farashtola, Kundigarh in Badarka and parts of Katra and Ghulami ka pura ward. Slums can be seen in most polluted land sites, for example around solid waste dumps, waterlogged sites, beside the open drains and sewers, etc.

4.2.1.4 Air Pollution

Air pollution refers to the presence of unwanted materials like gases, particulate matters and biological molecules in the atmosphere that unpleasantly affects well-being and health of humans and other organism on the planet (Perkins, 1974). Air pollution can cause diseases, allergies and even death of humans. According to 2014 WHO report, air pollution in 2012 has caused the death of around 7 million people worldwide.

Most common air pollutants are particulate matters, nitrogen oxide, sulphur dioxide, carbon monoxide and ozone. In the present analysis, ambient air quality has been analysed with the help of data related to particulate pollution only. Particulate matter is basically a mixture of organic and inorganic particles including dust, pollen, soot, smoke and liquid droplets. Exposure to particulate matter in the ambient air could be both short term and long term. Effects of long-term exposure to moderate concentrations are more prominent in comparison to short-term exposure to peak levels of particulate pollution. Areas near busy roads where the concentration of particulate matters are predominantly higher are referred as "hotspots". In urban areas, about 10% of the total population may be residing in these hotspots and are more exposed to particulate pollutants than the rest of the population.

For the present analysis, data for Air Pollution was obtained from the pollution report "Air Kills" by an NGO named Climate Agenda (2018). The report is an attempt from the NGO to assess the air quality of smaller cities of Uttar Pradesh where the practice of air monitoring is not taking place. The report is an endeavour to break the cliché that deteriorating air quality is a problem of major cities only and it has also tried to represent the ground phenomenon.

Particulate Matter, i.e.$PM_{2.5}$ and PM_{10} in Azamgarh city were monitored by Climate Agenda NGO at total 8 locations including five traffic intersection inside and immediate outskirts of the city, i.e. Hafizpur Chowraha, Narauli, Bhanwarnath, Sidhari Chowraha, Chowk Chowraha; one Traffic intersection cum commercial point, i.e. Paharpur which represents intersection near Takia market; one residential point, i.e. Civil Lines (Tables 4.4 and 4.5). Data was collected in December when particulate matters were at their peak in the absence of strong winds and with absolute stability in the environment.

Interpolation map of Azamgarh city for $PM_{2.5}$ and PM_{10} was constructed using this data to obtain a visual representation of pollutant level in the city. Values of $PM_{10}$and $PM_{2.5}$ for another residential point, i.e. near Belaisa were obtained by taking average of the values of remaining points. Inverse Distance Weighting (IDW) method was used to generate interpolation map of Azamgarh City for $PM_{2.5}$ and PM_{10} (Figure 4.1 and 4.2).

Table 4.4 Air Quality Monitoring Stations in Azamgarh City

Category	Monitoring Stations	Latitude	Longitude	PM2.5 ($\mu g/m^3$)	PM10 ($\mu g/m^3$)
National Ambient Air Quality Standards				60	100
Residential	Civil Lines	26.05217	83.1745	114	250
	Near Belaisa (Average)	26.02633	83.14301	245	384
Traffic Intersection	Hafizpur Chowraha	26.09411	83.1985	343	428
	Narauli	26.04747	83.17733	324	536
	Bhanwarnath	26.08894	83.16908	315	393
	Sidhari Chowraha	26.04253	83.18981	231	322
	Chowk Chowraha	26.06719	83.18361	160	293
Traffic Intersection cum Commercial	Paharpur	26.07381	83.18592	354	481
Others	Railway Station	26.03969	83.1615	146	273

Source: Report "Air Kills" Climate Agenda, 2018.

Table 4.5 Level of Air Pollution at Different Locations in Azamgarh City

Category of Area/Zone	Monitoring Stations
Residential	Civil Lines (HI/LD); Near Belaisa, Average (Outskirts)
Commercial cum Traffic Intersection	Paharpur (Takia Market Intersection) (HI/HD)
Traffic Intersections	Sidhari Chowraha (HI/LD); Chowk Chauraha (HI/MD); Narauli Railway station (MI/LD); Hafizpur Chowraha, Bhanwarnath (Outskirts)

Source: Report "Air Kills" Climate Agenda, 2018.

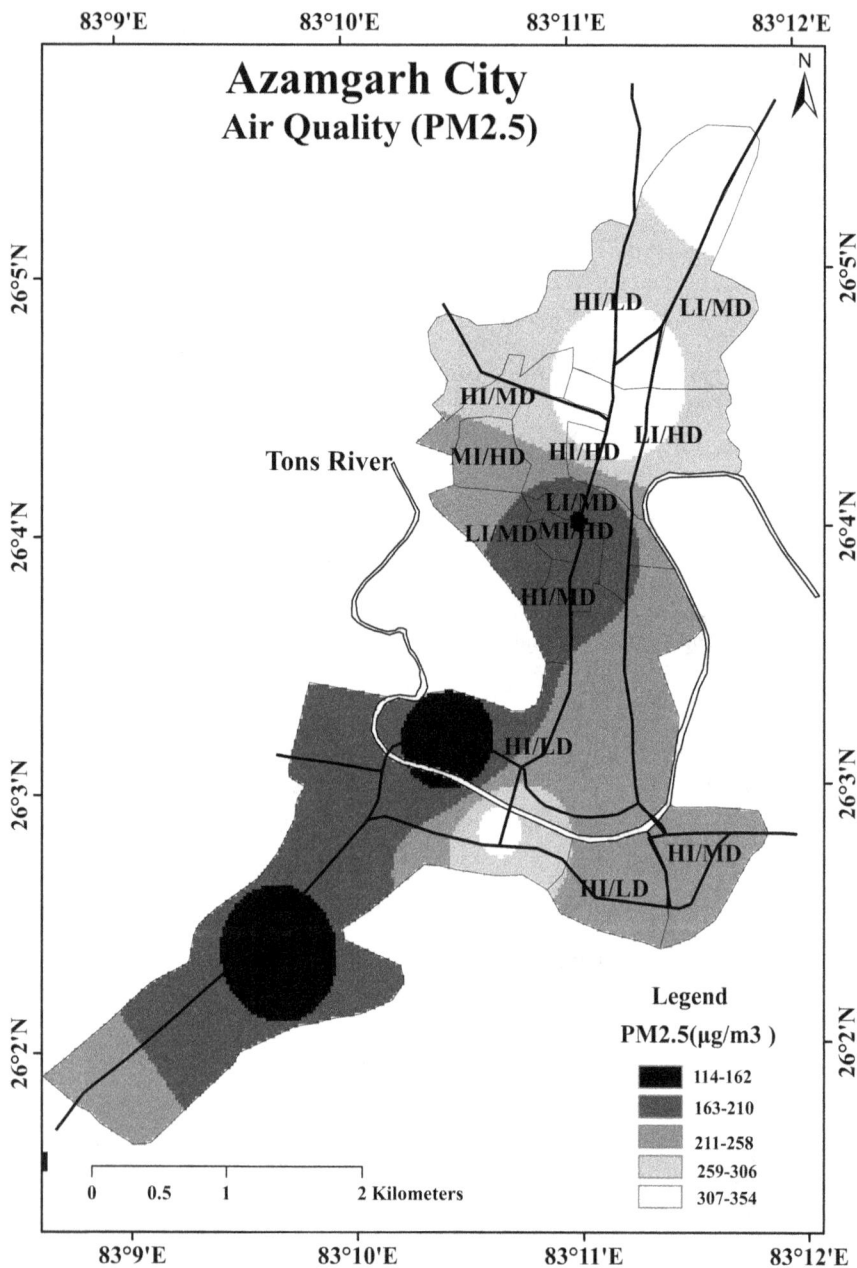

Figure 4.1 Azamgarh City: Level of PM$_{2.5}$ at Different Locations.

Source: Report "Air Kills" Climate Agenda, 2018.

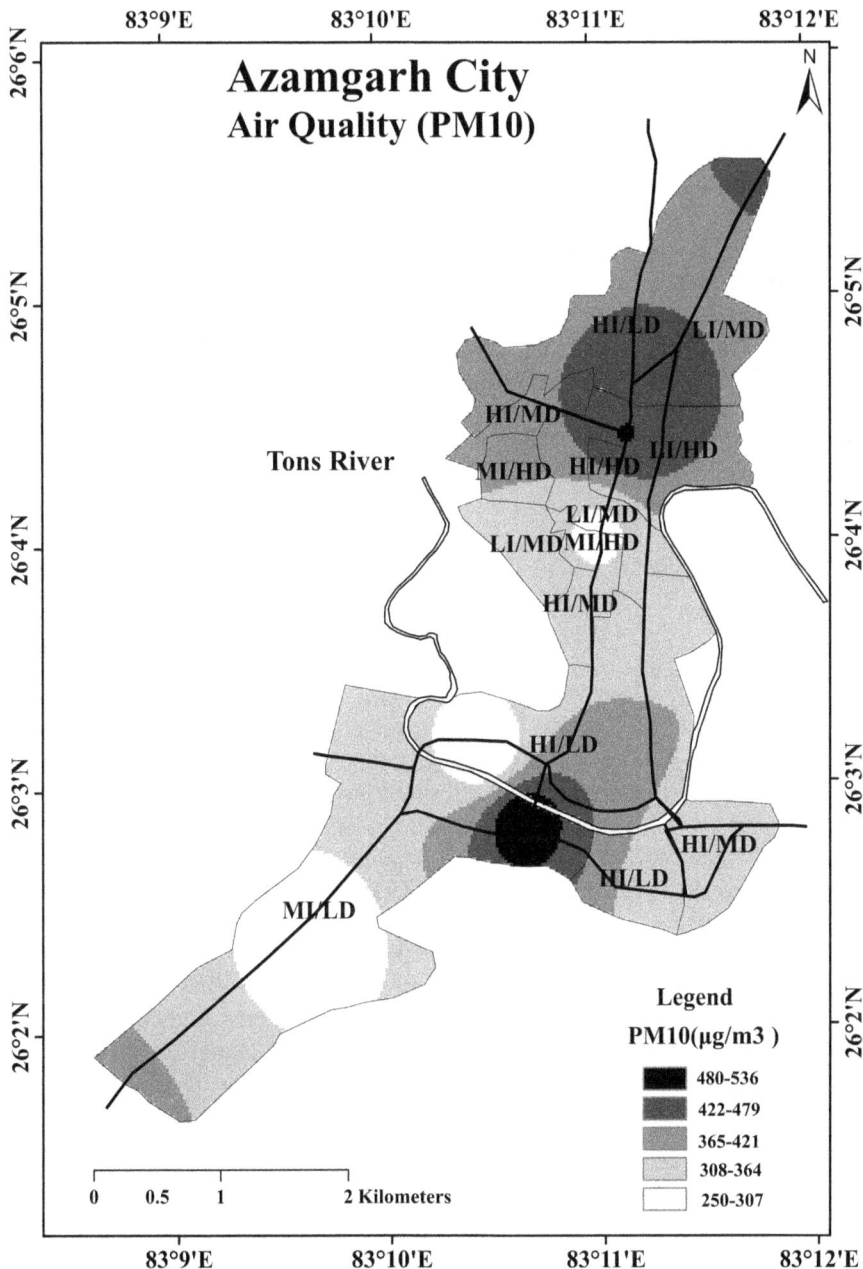

Figure 4.2 Azamgarh City: Level of PM$_{10}$ at Different Locations.

Source: Report "Air Kills" Climate Agenda, 2018.

A perusal of Table 4.5 and Figure 4.1 shows that value of $PM_{2.5}$ is higher than the National Standards (i.e. 60 μg/m³ for $PM_{2.5}$ and 100μg/m³ for PM_{10}) at all the monitored points. Minimum value of $PM_{2.5}$ was recorded as 114 at Civil Lines in HI/LD neighbourhood in a residential area which is still two times higher than the national standard. Nearby bus station and commercial activities in Civil Lines could be responsible for the elevated levels of $PM_{2.5}$. $PM_{2.5}$ was found the highest at Paharpur representing traffic intersection near Takia market in HI/HD neighbourhood where its value was recorded as high as 354 μg/m³. It was found that diesel generators are being used in the city, basically in the markets as electricity is not a 24-hour service in the city. Emission from diesel generators as well as from vehicles passing by the Allahabad Gorakhpur highway along which the market is located could be the reason behind higher level of particulate pollutants. Values are also exceptionally high at other traffic intersection points like Sidhari Chowraha, Narauli, Hafizpur Chowraha and Bhanwarnath. Year-long construction activities, which is a common phenomenon in smaller cities, and most importantly, the pool of vehicles at intersection points can attribute to elevated levels of particulate pollution.

Particulate pollution at railway station is not as high as compared to other points indicating that railway engines are not the major contributor of air pollution in the city. From the map, it is clear that value of $PM_{2.5}$ is higher than 211 in most of the city and only some parts of MI/LD, HI/LD, MI/HD and LI/MD neighbourhoods come within the range of less than 210 μg/m³.

Interpolation map of PM_{10} also shows more or less the same picture. Table 4.5 and Figure 4.2 depict that value of PM_{10} was as high as 536 which is five times higher than national standard and the lowest value recorded was 250 which is still 2.5 times higher than the national standard. The highest value was recorded at Narauli located in MI/LD neighbourhood while the lowest value was recorded in Civil Lines located in HI/LD neighbourhood. Main taxi stand of the city is located in Narauli and most of the commercial activities are also located in the region, which could be the reason behind this high value.

From the map, it is clear that about half of the city area lies in the range of more than 365 μg/m³. Vehicular emissions, dust on the bumpy roads, construction activities in the city particularly along the roads, Diesel Generators and waste burning in the city are significant sources of particulate matter concentration in Azamgarh City. Another rationale is that since the average low temperature in December falls as low as 11°C (Seasonal weather average, 2010), people burn open fire to cope from cold which also contributes to elevated particulate pollutants.

Further, an attempt was made to get the resident's response in the appraisal of air pollution in their respective neighbourhoods. Responses of the residents were in conformity with the location of their houses. Households located near the traffic intersections and markets as well as along the major roads have reported that air is not good enough in their neighbourhoods. Table 4.6 reveals that 19.31% households represented air pollution as a problem in their neighbourhoods. Neighbourhoods that have complained about major problem of air pollution are HI/HD and MI/LD and neighbourhoods with 26.33% noise

Table 4.6 Neighbourhood-Wise Air Pollution (in Percentages) in Azamgarh City (Resident's Perception)

Neighbourhoods	Air Pollution*		
	Yes	No	Can't say
HI/HD	24.48	49	26.5
HI/MD	18.68	47.86	33.5
HI/LD	17.24	52.92	29.8
MI/HD	19.68	46.85	33.5
MI/LD	26.33	54.15	19.5
LI/HD	15.5	41.29	43.2
LI/MD	13.25	38.23	48.5
Total	19.31	47.19	33.5

Source: Based on Field Survey, 2016–2017.
* Based on Resident's Perception.

pollution in MI/LD and 24.48% in HI/HD neighbourhood. The HI/HD neighbourhood is located in the downtown of the city and presence of the central market, i.e. *Takiya* and constant traffic on the major Gorakhpur Allahabad road makes it the busiest places of the city with the worst air quality. The neighbourhood MI/LD is located in the southern part of the city and includes traffic intersections, Taxi Stand as well as major roads of the city, therefore exposure to air pollution was higher in this neighbourhood. Air pollution was reported medium to low in MI/HD, HI/LD and LI/HD neighbourhoods. In Matbarganj (MI/HD neighbourhood) due to the presence of Chowk intersection, people have reported the problem of pollution, while in case of Sidhari (HI/LD neighbourhood) it is due to presence of the Sidhari intersection in it, however, the households from Mukeriganj, Farashtola that were situated on the major roads have also complained of the air quality problem (Table 4.6). It has been found that majority of the respondents of the city maintained that air pollution is not a problem in the city, however, data for particulate pollution shows a different picture. About 33.51% residents chose "can't say" for air pollution in their neighbourhood. Therefore, further researches are recommended to understand the scenario of air pollution in Azamgarh city.

4.2.1.5 Noise Pollution

Noise pollution refers to an unwanted sound or a sound which causes terrible distress on the ears. Sound is a form of energy that is transmitted by pressure variations which human ears can detect. Sound level is measured in decibel unit (dB). Noise pollution has become a major issue in urban areas as it creates discomfort, affects one's peace of mind and deteriorates people's quality of life. Noise pollution has been witnessed rising in cities as a consequence of growing population, increasing industrial and commercial activities, transportation and communication system as well as changing lifestyle of people (Hogan and Latshaw, 1973). Outdoor noise from all sources is becoming an instant cause of fatigue and health deterioration. The Noise Pollution (Regulation and Control) Rules, 2000 has provided standards in respect of noise. According to it, standard limit are: 75dB for day time and 70dB at night for industrial area, 65 dB in day 55 dB at night in commercial area and 55 dB in day and 45 dB at night in residential areas. The U.S. EPA (2005) has recognised 70 dB as a safe average for a 24-hour day (EPA, 2005). Air quality in the neighbourhood could be poor due to nearness to the sources of vehicle exhaust emissions like bus stations, airports and major roads (Perlin et al., 2001) owing to poor urban planning. These sources also contribute to substantial noise exposures, which could be associated with several adverse health effects (Stansfeld et al., 2000). Researchers have documented that environmental problems such as air and noise pollution and hazardous waste sites are not evenly distributed across all the neighbourhoods. It has been suggested that air and noise pollution is the highest in disadvantaged and racially excluded neighbourhoods (Casey et al., 2017).

Noise pollution studies are mainly of two kinds: one is continuous noise study while other is periodical noise study. For the present analysis, periodical noise measurement was chosen as it is more appropriate and less expensive. According to British Standard BS 3452:1966 "method for measurement of noise emitted by motor vehicles" the sample time should be in between 5 minutes to 55 minutes (BS 3452, 1966). For the present analysis, a sample time of 5 minutes was selected. Noise samples were collected in dB (A) scale at every 10 seconds interval (6 counts per minute) or a total of 30 reading in a sample. Average of all the readings were taken as representative of the particular area/zone. The observations were taken at a distance of 1.5 meters from the edge of roads and the right angle to the centreline of road. On the day of monitoring, weather was clear and sunny with light breeze having a speed of 1.6–3.3 m/s (Weather Online, 2019).

Precision Sound Level Meter, Model Number GM1351, which can measure noise levels within the range of 30–130 dB was used during survey. Total 16 locations, 5 residential, 2 commercial, 5 silence and 4 traffic stations were chosen to monitor (Table 4.7, and Figure 4.3). Interpolation map of Azamgarh city

Table 4.7 Location of Noise Monitoring Stations in Azamgarh City

Category of Area/Zone	Noise Monitoring Stations
Residential	Sidhari East, Millat Nagar (HI/MD); Badarka (MI/HD); Rahmat Nagar (LI/MD); Sarfuddinpur (MI/LD)
Commercial	Chowk (MI/HD); Takiya (HI/HD)
Silence	Shibli College (LI/HD); DAV College, Lifeline Hospital(HI/LD), Sadar Hospital (LI/MD); GD Global School (Outskirts)
Traffic Intersections	Hydel Intersection, Bus Station (HI/LD), Narauli, Pahalwan Sukhdev Tiraha (MI/LD)

Source: Based on Field Survey, 2019.

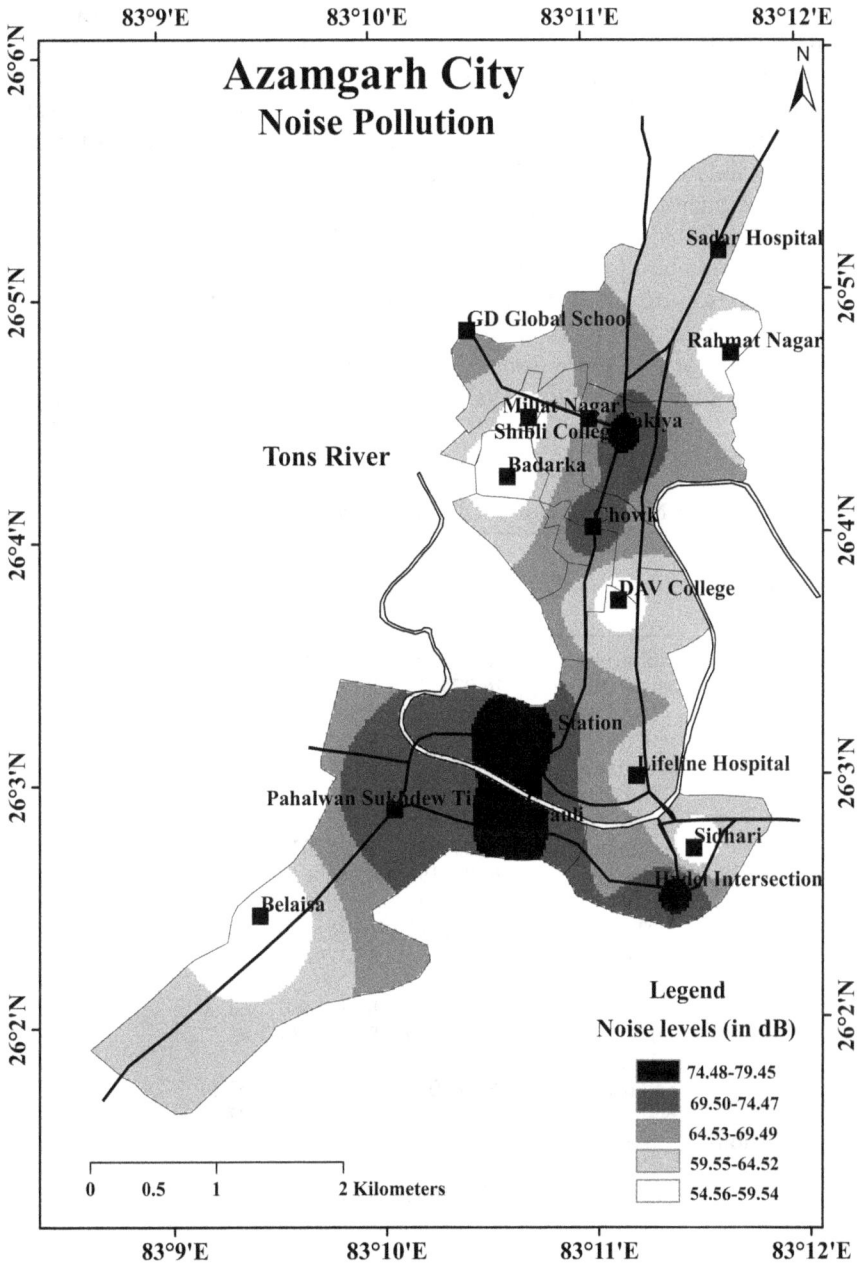

Figure 4.3 Azamgarh City: Level of Noise Pollution at Different Locations (2019).

Source: Based on Field Survey, 2019.

for noise level was constructed using the data to obtain a visual representation of noise levels in the city. IDW method was used to generate the interpolated map of noise pollution in the City.

A perusal of the Table 4.8 and Figure 4.3 reveals that noise pollution level is within the standard limits for the residential areas; however, it exceeds the pre-scribed standards at commercial and silence zones as well as traffic intersec-tions. The highest noise levels were recorded at traffic intersection points, ranging from 79.45 dB at Bus station to 71.84 dB at Pahalwan Sukhdev Tiraha against the standard limit of 65 dB.

Situation was also pathetic in case of commercial points where noise level was as high as 78 dB at Takiya and 70.15 at Chowk. The worst scenario was recorded in case of Silence Zones. Since most of the major schools, colleges and hospitals are located along the major roads in the city, not a single station

Table 4.8 Level of Noise Pollution at Different Locations in Azamgarh City

Category of Area/Zone	Locations	Latitude	Longitude	Noise Level (dB)	Ambient Noise Standards
Residential	Sidhari East	26.045000	83.191139	54.91	55
	Millat Nagar (Arazibagh)	26.074778	83.178722	57.18	
	Badarka	26.070754	83.176958	54.55	
	Rahmat Nagar (Ghulami ka pura)	26.079023	83.194701	55.9	
	Sarfuddinpur	26.040861	83.157028	55	
Commercial	Chowk	26.067191	83.183642	70.15	65
	Takiya	26.064972	83.183611	78.13	
Silence	DAV College	26.062111	83.185556	56.24	50
	GD Global School	26.080833	83.174000	68.85	
	Shibli College	26.074611	83.183460	63.56	
	Lifeline Hospital	26.050060	83.186734	62.57	
	Sadar Hospital	26.086087	83.193853	63.11	
Traffic Intersections	Naraul Taxi Stand (Narauli)	26.046694	83.177056	77.66	65*
	Bus Station (Civil Lines)	26.053000	83.177472	79.45	
	Hydel Intersection	26.042068	83.189743	77.19	
	Pahalwan Sukhdev Tiraha	26.047981	83.167728	71.84	

Source: Based on Field Survey, 2019.
* Standard, Jordanian Environmental Protection Law, 2000.

could reach up to the standard except DAV college, which was close to it. Noise level was the highest near GD Global School, i.e. 68.85 dB followed by Shibli College 53.56 dB and Sadar Hospital 63.11 dB. Noise level was 56.24 at DAV college due to its off-road location.

In residential areas, dB value was 54.55 for Badarka and 54.91 for Sidhari, and it crossed the standard limit only in case of Millat Nagar for which factors like community horns and generators were responsible.

From the interpolation map (Figure 4.3), it is clear that Traffic is a major source of noise pollution in the city. Locations like traffic intersections, commercial zones as well as places situated very close to the major roads have recorded high values for noise levels. Other sources of noise in the city include generators, construction works, railways, vendors along the roads as well as community horns.

Furthermore, an attempt was made to get the resident's response to ascertain their awareness in case of noise pollution in their respective neighbourhoods. Since the development of the city has taken place in a traditional pattern where commercial and small manufacturing activities are located along the roads and no separate commercial and industrial zones are delimited, the distance between residential and other zones is also less.

Responses of residents were in conformity with the nature of the roads along which their neighbourhoods were located. Households located along the major roads as well as markets complained of higher noise pollution. Households of the streets complained lower noise pollution and those from the bystreets reported minimum noise pollution in their respective neighbourhoods. Table 4.9 reveals that of the total sampled households, 36.31% reported noise pollution a problem in their neighbourhoods. Neighbourhoods that have complained about major problem of noise pollution are HI/HD and MI/LD, and neighbourhoods with 47.67% noise pollution in HI/HD and 43.85% in

Table 4.9 Neighbourhood-Wise Noise Pollution (in Percentages) (Resident's Perception) in Azamgarh City

Neighbourhoods	Noise Pollution*	
	Yes	No
HI/HD	47.67	52.33
HI/MD	32.22	67.78
HI/LD	35.06	64.94
MI/HD	36.65	63.35
MI/LD	43.85	56.15
LI/HD	32.5	67.5
LI/MD	26.23	73.77
Total	36.31	63.69

Source: Based on Field Survey, 2016–2017.
* Based on Resident's Perception.

MI/LD neighbourhood. The HI/HD neighbourhood is located in the downtown of the city and presence of the central market, i.e. *Takiya* and constant traffic on the major Gorakhpur Allahabad road, makes it the most busy and noisy places of the city. The neighbourhood MI/LD is located in the southern part of the city and includes Railway Station, Taxi Stand as well as major roads of the city therefore exposure to noise problem was higher in this neighbourhood. Noise pollution is medium to low in MI/HD, HI/LD and LI/HD neighbourhoods. In Matbarganj (MI/HD neighbourhood) due to the presence of Chowk market people have reported the problem of noise while in case of Civil Lines (HI/LD neighbourhood) it is due to the presence of Bus Station in it. However the households from Mukeriganj, Farashtola that were situated on the major roads have also complained of the problem.

4.2.1.6 Water Quality Problem

It is a well-known fact that human health and survival depends upon the use of uncontaminated and clean water for drinking and other purposes (Anwar and Aggarwal, 2014). In Azamgarh city, groundwater is the leading and only source for drinking water. Groundwater is the water present underneath the earth's surface in pore spaces of soil, in cavities and fissures of rocks. It is a decent source of freshwater due to its relatively low vulnerability to pollution in comparison to surface water. However, the quality of groundwater has been deteriorated due to some critical factors like increasing population, industrialisation, urbanisation, etc. (Tyagi et al., 2013). Consumption of contaminated drinking water is estimated to cause more than 5,00,000 diarrhoeal deaths each year (WHO, 2009). Contaminated water can spread diseases like diarrhoea, dysentery, cholera, typhoid and polio. Diarrhoea is the most commonly known diseases associated with contaminated water. Schistosomiasis is another acute and chronic disease caused by consumption of infested water, affecting about 240 million people a year. Therefore analysis of drinking water quality is a valuable approach to estimate the health impacts of drinking water in Azamgarh city.

Water quality of any particular area can be assessed using physical, chemical and biological parameters. Quality parameters of water involve pH, total dissolved solids, total suspended solids, dissolved oxygen, total hardness, calcium, magnesium, chlorine, chloride, fluoride, nickel, arsenic, iron, lead, coliform bacteria etc. The values of these parameters are harmful to human health if they crossed the standard defined limits (United States EPA, 2009; BIS, 2012; WHO, 2012; CPCB, 2013). Water will be called safe for drinking if it lies below the standard limits defined by various agencies like WHO, BIS (Bureau of Indian Standards) and the United States EPA (Environmental Protection Agency). Drinking water must also be aesthetically acceptable as human beings are accomplished with a sense of sight, smell and taste.

A total of nine samples were collected for physico-chemical analysis in August 2019. Out of the nine samples, two samples were taken from municipal taps (Matbarganj and Sarfuddinpur), three samples from public hand pumps

(Harbanshpur, Paharpur and Bazbahadur) and four samples from submersible pumps installed inside the houses (Arazibagh, Civil Lines, Heerapattiand Sidhari). For collecting the water sample, taps and hand pumps were operated for about 5 minutes to flush out stagnant water in it. Then the samples were collected in sterilised polythene bottles and labelled with adequate information. The samples were placed in a thermocol box and transported to Environmental Engineering Lab, Civil Engineering, Aligarh Muslim University, Aligarh. Tests were performed by the researcher, in Environmental Engineering Lab, under the guidance of lab attendant and technicians. Methods adopted for physico-chemical analysis of samples has been shown in the Table 4.10. Standard values of parameters according to BIS and WHO have been presented in Table 4.11. Concentrations of parameters in different samples of the water have been shown in Table 4.12.

Table 4.10 Standard Methods Involved for Physico-Chemical Analysis of Water

Parameters	Standard Methods
pH	pH meter
TDS	TDS meter
EC	Conductivity meter
Chloride	Argentometric titration
Alkalinity	EDTA
Total Hardness	EDTA
Ca	EDTA
Mg	EDTA
Chlorine	Starch Iodide Test
TSS	Filtering and Weighing method

Table 4.11 Standard Values for Different Parameters of Water

Parameters*	BIS		BIS Standard	WHO Standard
	Desirable Limit	Permissible Limit		
pH	6.5–8.5	6.5–8.5	6.5–8.5	6.5–8.5
TDS	500	2000	500	2000
EC	–	–	–	750
TSS	–	–	–	30**
Alkalinity	200	600	200	–
Total Hardness	200	600	200	500
Chloride	250	1000	250	200
Calcium	75	200	75	200
Magnesium	30	100	30	150
Chlorine	0.2	1	0.2	–

Source: BIS, 2012.
* unit mg/L except EC (μS/cm).
** Standard NEMA (National Environmental Management) Kenya, not available in BIS and WHO standard.

Table 4.12 Concentrations of Parameters in Different Water Samples of Azamgarh City

Samples	Sampling Point	Source of Water	pH	EC (µS/cm)	TDS (mg/L)	TSS (mg/L)	Alkalinity (mg/L)	Total Hardness (mg/L)	Ca (mg/L)	Mg (mg/L)	Chloride (mg/L)	Chlorine (mg/L)
1	Harbanshpur	Hand pump	8.31	441	239	96	184	230	148	82	16	0
2	Matbarganj	Municipal tap	7.7	1113	615	16	384	234	82	152	121	0
3	Civil Lines	Submersible pump	7.79	614	335	46	162	192	66	81	40	0
4	Bazbahadur	Hand pump	7.69	1369	792	6	500	280	120	160	190	0
5	Arazibagh	Submersible pump	7.81	400	375	36	188	184	72	112	40	0
6	Paharpur	Hand pump	7.61	1074	574	52	440	214	64	150	108	0
7	Sarfuddinpur	Municipal tap	7.91	1065	543	31	252	221	81	140	192	0
8	Heerapatti	Submersible pump	7.56	650	481	28	187	176	84	77	231	0
9	Sidhari	Submersible pump	7.38	885	354	42	132	137	62	75	248	0

Source: Calculated by Researcher in Environmental Engineering Lab, Civil Engineering, AMU, Aligarh, 2019.

Table 4.13 Relative Weights of Different Parameters

Parameters	weight (w_i)	Relative Weight (W_i)
pH	4	0.14
EC	3	0.11
TDS	4	0.14
TSS	3	0.11
Alkalinity	3	0.11
Hardness	2	0.07
Ca	2	0.07
Mg	2	0.07
Chloride	2	0.07
Chlorine	3	0.11
	$\Sigma w_i = 28$	$\Sigma W_i = 1$

Data has been analysed using the BIS standard as BIS has provided both desirable as well as permissible limits for different parameters. Parameters above the desirable limit can be tolerated up to permissible limit in the absence of an alternate source of water; however, beyond permissible limit water is not acceptable at all. In the present analysis, desirable limit provided by BIS has been taken as standard value for water parameters. However, for the parameters for which BIS did not provide any standard like EC and TSS etc., WHO and other standards are used.

pH of water refers to the concentration of hydrogen ions in it. pH ranges from 0 to 14. Water with a pH of 7 is considered neutral while it is called acidic below 7 and alkaline above 7. pH of the water should range between 6.5 and 8.5 to be acceptable for drinking. pH level below 7 makes the water acidic which can corrode distribution pipes and leach metals in water. Low pH water can cause irritation of mucous membrane, tuberculosis and other health problems in humans (Srinivas et al., 2013). Table 4.12 reveals that the pH of all the samples ranges between 7.38 and 8.31 suggesting that pH of the water in Azamgarh city is within the desirable limit.

Electrical Conductivity is the ability of water to pass an electric current and it depends upon the salt content in the water as dissolved salts and other inorganic materials. Uncontaminated water is a poor conductor of electric current rather a good insulator. Electrical Conductivity ranges between 0–800 µS/cm is good for drinking water provided there is no organic pollution and not too much of the suspended clay material. WHO has marked 750 as standard limit (Bhat and Pandit, 2014) for EC, above which water is not recommended to be consumed. A perusal of the Table reveals that out of the total 9 samples, EC is beyond the standard limit in 4 samples i.e. in Matbarganj, Bazbahadur, Paharpur and Sarfuddinpur.

The term **TDS, i.e. Total dissolved solids** refers to the inorganic salts and small amounts of organic matter present in the water. A certain level of TDS in water is essential for life. Water with deficient concentrations of TDS may be unacceptable because of its flat, insipid taste and absence of desired minerals in it.

Water with TDS less than 300 mg/litre is considered as excellent, 300–600 mg/L as good, 600–900 mg/L as fair and 900–1200 mg/L as poor. Early studies have linked concentration of TDS in water with increasing incidence of cancer, coronary heart diseases and mortality (Fawell et al., 2003). BIS has demarcated 500 mg/L as the desirable limit for drinking water. The table reveals that four samples exceeded the desirable limit of drinking water in terms of total dissolved solids and these samples are from Matbarganj, Bazbahadur, Paharpur and Sarfuddinpur.

Water hardness is defined as the sum of calcium and magnesium concentration, and it is a measure of the capacity of water to precipitate soap. Water is considered soft with a concentration of calcium carbonate below 60 mg/L, moderately hard with 60–120 mg/L, hard with 120–180 mg/L and very hard with more than 180 mg/L (McGowan, 2000). The desired limit for water hardness is 200 mg/L. The hard water is not suitable for drinking purpose and causes gastro diseases (Mohsin et al., 2013). Total hardness of the sampled water from Azamgarh city ranges from 130 to 180 with an average value of 196. It has been found that water hardness crosses the desirable limit at five stations namely Harbanshpur, Matbarganj, Bazbahadur, Paharpur and Sarfuddinpur.

Calcium and Magnesium are important determinant of water harness. Both calcium and magnesium are vital minerals and helpful to human health in numerous respects, and an inadequate intake of any of these can result in harmful health effects. Insufficient intake of calcium can lead to kidney stones, hypertension, stroke and obesity. The desirable limit of calcium in water is recommended as 75 mg/L. Calcium concentration in the water exceeds the desirable limit in five samples of water namely Harbanshpur, Matbarganj, Bazbahadur, Sarfuddinpur and Heerapatti. Magnesium deficiency has also been linked with hypertension; however, an increasing concentration of magnesium can result in diarrhoea, especially in people with low kidney function. Desirable limit of magnesium in water is 30m mg/L revealing that magnesium concentration with an average of 75 mg/l is beyond the desirable limit in all the samples.

Chlorides are inorganic minerals formed by the combination of chlorine gas and metals. Some common chlorides in the water include sodium chloride and magnesium chloride. Chlorine alone as Cl_2 in the water is poisonous; however, in a combination of metals such as sodium, it is crucial for life by providing needed salts to humans. The acceptable limit for chloride in the water is 250 mg/L and a higher concentration is linked to heart and kidney diseases (Kumar and Puri, 2012). Chloride increases the electrical conductivity of water and thus its corrosivity. The table reveals that chloride concentration is within the standard limits in all the samples. **Chlorine** alone as Cl_2 can be dangerous and can lead to vomiting, coma and even death (International Occupational Safety and Health Information Centre, 2009); however, the concentration of chlorine is found negligible in all the samples (Table 4.12).

Alkalinity in the water is primarily due to carbonate, bicarbonate and hydroxide contents. An overall surplus of alkalinity in the body can cause gastrointestinal issues and skin irritations. Higher alkalinity may lead to a metabolic *alkalosis* with the symptoms such as nausea, vomiting and muscle twitching. BIS has demarcated concentration of $CaCO_3$ 200 mg/L (alkalinity) as a desirable limit. The table reveals that most of the samples are within the desirable limit except four samples, i.e. Matbarganj, Bazbahadur, Paharpur and Sarfuddinpur.

Total Suspended Solids or TSS may include silt, decaying plants and animal substance, sewage and industrial waste. High concentration of suspended solids in the matter are generally related to elevated levels of pathogens like bacteria, germs, parasites and other microorganisms which can cause problems like nausea, twinges, diarrheal disease and headache. Neither WHO nor BIS has provided standard value of TSS in the drinking water; therefore, for the present analysis, the standard provided by NEMA (National Environmental Management Authority) Kenya has been used. NEMA has suggested 30 mg/L of suspended solids as standard limit for drinking water which suggests that out of the total 9 samples, only two samples lie within the standard limits, i.e. Matbarganj and Bazbahadur while total remaining samples have shown more suspended solids in the water which could be harmful to people consuming it.

To get a comprehensive picture of the overall quality of groundwater in the city, the Water Quality Index (WQI) is calculated. WQI can reduce the bulk of information into a single value to express the data into a logical and straightforward form (Semiromi et al., 2011). WQI provides a single number that presents overall water quality at a particular location and time, based on numerous water quality parameters.

The relative weights of parameters for WQI calculation are given in Table 4.13. The WQI values are classified into five categories, ranging from excellent water quality to water unsuitable for drinking. For WQI <50, water will be excellent, 50–100 good, 100–200 poor, 200–300 very poor and for WQI >300 water will be unsuitable for drinking.

The computed WQI values and water type of the different samples are presented in Table 4.14. Interpolation map of Azamgarh city for water quality index is constructed using the data to obtain a visual representation of water quality in the city. Inverse Distance Weighing (IDW) method is used to create an interpolation map of WQI for the City (Figure 4.4).

Table 4.14 Water Quality Index for Different Samples in Azamgarh City

Samples	Name	WQI Value	WQI Category
1	Harbanshpur	124	Poor
2	Matbarganj	129	Poor
3	Civil Lines	95	Good
4	Bazbahadur	147	Poor
5	Arazibagh	97	Good
6	Paharpur	143	Poor
7	Sarfuddinpur	125	Poor
8	Heerapatti	98	Good
9	Sidhari	97	Good
Average		117	Poor

Source: Calculated by Researcher in Environmental Engineering Lab, Civil Engineering, AMU, Aligarh, 2019.

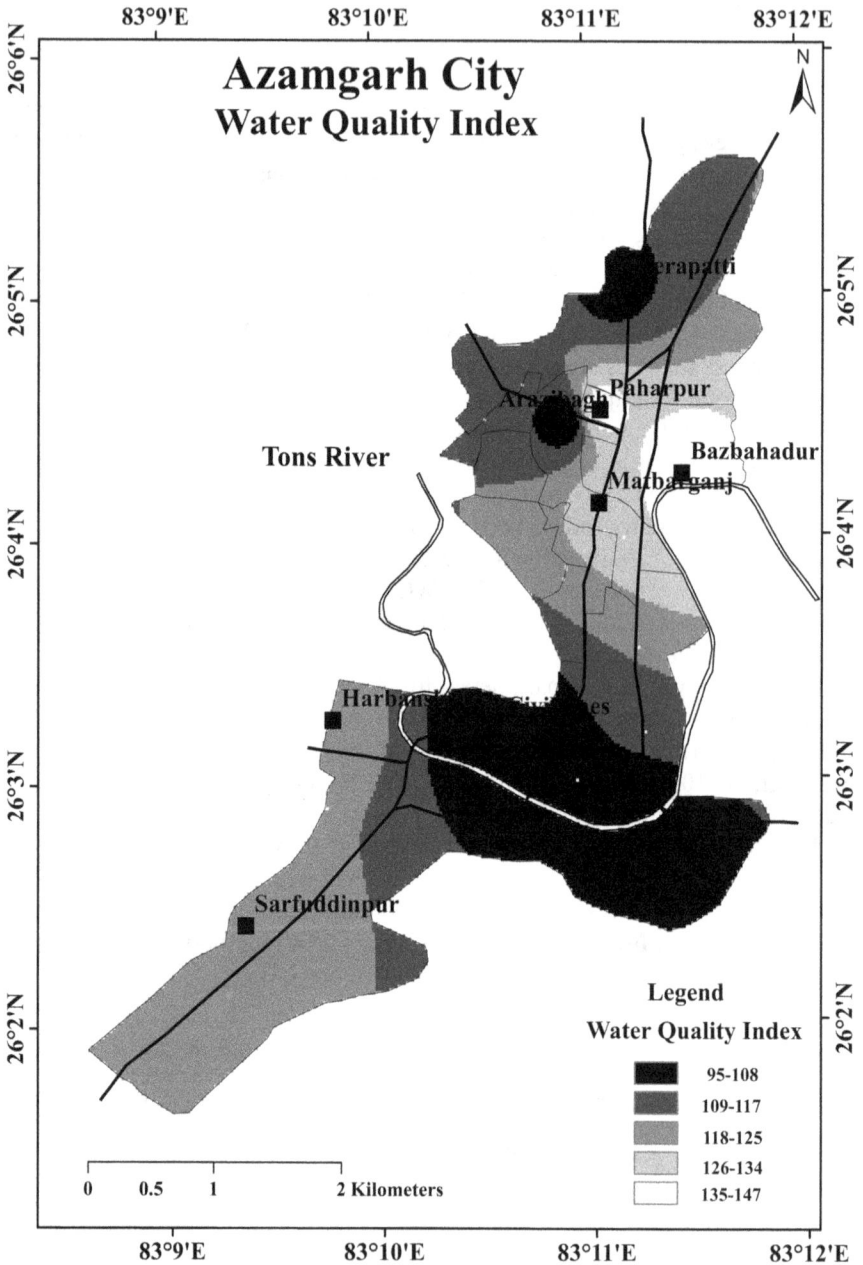

Figure 4.4 Azamgarh City: Water Quality Index.

Source: Calculated by Researcher in Environmental Engineering Lab, Civil Engineering, AMU, Aligarh, 2019.

The collected water samples have a WQI ranging from 95 to 147 with 117 an average WQI of the city's water. Total nine samples were collected, out of which five samples have emerged having "poor" quality of water while four samples represent water quality in the "good" category (Table 4.14). None of the water samples could reach up to the "excellent" category of water. An analysis of the table reveals that good quality water samples were collected from submersible pumps installed in the city while samples that fell into "poor" category of water were collected from municipal water supply sources and from hand pumps. The rationale behind this phenomenon could be the depth of the water table from which water is pumped. Water in submersible pumps comes from 180 feet below ground level while hand pumps draw water from 70–80 feet only. It is assumed that water from the upper acquifers is polluted as it faces a high risk of contamination due to leaching of pollutants from the surface. Similar finding was also recorded by Abdullah and Sarfuddin (2012) and they concluded that water from upper acquifers from Azamgarh city is not suitable for drinking (Abdullah and Sarfuddin, 2012). Although, municipality also fetches water with the help of submersible from much deeper acquifer; however, since the water supply pipes run about 4–5 feet below ground level, these are susceptible to breaking and mixing of dirt, sewage and sand in it.

The problem of water quality was also tried to examine during the field survey. Regarding the maintenance of the quality of water, it was reported by the municipality that 50-litre chlorination is done per tube well per week. Household survey revealed that about 47% of residents from the city have reported problem in the quality of water in the form of dirt, sand and smell in the water, etc. (Table 4.15). These problems occur because of improper cleaning of water tanks and pipes. Old, rusted and breached pipes also add problem in this regard. Water pipes sometimes break due to heavy vehicles stepping onto them, resulting in the mixing of dirt and sand in water. Problem with smell especially intensify in summer and rainy seasons due to increase in

Table 4.15 Neighbourhood-Wise Water Quality Problem (Resident's Perception) (in Percentages) in Azamgarh City

Neighbourhoods	Water Quality*	
	Good	Bad
HI/HD	58.33	41.67
HI/MD	56.78	43.22
HI/LD	58.86	41.14
MI/HD	48.45	51.56
MI/LD	53.87	46.13
LI/HD	48.63	51.37
LI/MD	45.61	54.39
Total	52.93	47.07

Source: Based on Field Survey, 2016–2017.
* Based on Resident's Perception.

bacterial activity in the water. Chlorination however helps to get rid of the bacteria and pathogens; a small amount of it still finds its way to houses.

Households from high-income neighbourhoods have water purifiers in their houses; however, residents from low-income neighbourhoods have to suffer and compromise with water quality. Households from all the neighbourhoods reported problem in the quality of water. Although residents of high-income neighbourhoods do not consume water without running it through filter whether obtained from in-house borings or municipal pipes, a considerable proportion of them still reported that breach in quality was found in the first place; therefore they use RO to treat the water before consumption.

4.2.2 Neighbourhood Service Environmental Problems

Neighbourhoods have a propensity to be environmentally degraded for many reasons. Many of these problems are area-specific. For example, low-income neighbourhoods tend to be situated in surrounding of polluted areas, prone to inadequate water supply, drainage, waterlogging, infestation with pests, lack of public services etc. This section of the chapter is mainly concerned with indigenous problems in the neighbourhood service environment, where services may vary significantly in different neighbourhoods. These problems are interrelated.

Municipal bodies in India are accountable to provide public health services to the residents in the form of water supply, sewerage and sanitation as well as eradication of communicable diseases. Major environmental problems identified in the city resulting from the absence of municipal services are insufficient supply of water, drainage problems and waterlogging as well as heaps of garbage in the neighbourhoods leading to spread of communicable diseases in the city. It has been reported that poor neighbourhoods suffer from territorial injustice in terms of the level of services provided by the municipality and the actual need for the services (Hastings, 2009). These problems are discussed as follows:

4.2.2.1 Inadequate Water Supply

WHO estimated that 29% of the world population or 2.1 billion people still lack safely managed drinking water, meaning the availability of safe water at home. As per the data of 2015, 88% of the total Indian population had access to improved water sources, which is 96% in urban areas and 85% in rural areas (WHO and UNICEF, 2017). In the most under developed countries, unclean water exposes billions of men, women and children to several diseases, weakens them and significantly reduces their productivity. These diseases even cause the death of those with weak immune systems like small children, the malnourished and HIV patients. A significant cause of lack in the water supply is rapid urbanisation with expanding population as it has been even more difficult to provide water to every household of the city.

Safe potable water supply is vital to human development and well-being. Access to safe drinking water is one of the most successful ways to promote health and reduce poverty. Adequate water source also means smaller expenditure on health, as people are less expected to fall ill and suffer medical expenses and can stay economically productive. For children, access to improved supply of water can result in improved health with positive long term impact on their lives.

In the previous chapter, it was discussed that groundwater is the primary source of water in Azamgarh city. Public water supply includes piped water supply, roadside hand pumps and roadside pipes while private supply includes motor pumps, submersible borings and hand pumps, etc., inside houses. Out of the total sampled households, 92.80% have water connection inside their premises, while 7.20% have to fetch water from outside their premises. Of the households having water supply inside houses, about half of them have their submersible borings and other half have piped connections. The main source of water supply outside the premises is roadside public hand pump providing water to 6.26% of the total households, and 0.67% households take water from roadside water pipes installed by the municipality (Table 3.8). It was also found that water supply pipelines do not cover all parts of the city.

Residents that have their own private water supply systems enjoy a regular supply of water while municipal water is supplied for fixed hours. Municipal water supply timing is, morning 5 am to 10 am and in the evening from 4 pm to 10 pm. During festivals, the evening time gets extended from 4 pm to 12 pm. A perusal of Table 4.16 reveals that about 59 (59.13)% of the total sampled households have reported regular supply of water inside their houses while remaining 41% households do not get this advantage. Neighbourhood-wise analysis reveals that about 70–80% households from high-income neighbourhoods enjoy a regular supply of water while the remaining population avail

Table 4.16 Neighbourhood-Wise Inadequate Water Supply (in Percentages) in Azamgarh City

Neighbourhoods	State of Water Supply		Duration of water supply			
	Regular	*Irregular*	*1–6 hrs.*	*7–12hrs.*	*13–18hrs.*	*24 hrs.*
HI/HD	78.3	21.7	2.7	11	8	78.3
HI/MD	73.93	26.07	5.55	13.68	6.81	73.96
HI/LD	81.72	18.28	3.49	5.29	9.5	81.72
MI/HD	48.47	51.53	10.35	20.59	20.59	48.47
MI/LD	54.83	45.17	27.59	15.08	2.5	54.83
LI/HD	41.56	58.44	16.14	31.74	10.56	41.56
LI/MD	35.09	64.91	23.96	34.37	6.58	35.09
Total	59.13	40.87	12.83	18.82	9.22	59.13

Source: Based on Field Survey, 2016–2017.

water supply for limited hours. About half of the population of high-income neighbourhoods have their own boring while remaining households have public water supply connection inside their houses. It was noted that in high-income neighbourhoods, most households use motor pumps to draw water from municipal pipes; therefore, they could get water even after the official supply hours. Despite that, they store their water in overhead tanks with higher storing capacity, which lasts for longer duration; therefore deficit of water is not generally experienced by these households. Data from low- and medium-income neighbourhoods do not show a good picture as only about 35–41% households from low-income, and 48–54% from medium-income neighbourhoods have reported regular supply of water. Residents that have reported regular supply of water are those that have their own water supply sources inside their houses. Apart from them, about 12% residents reported that they get water for 1–6 hours only, 19% reported 7–12 hours and 9% reported 13–18 hours. Residents of the elevated central part of the city, like Ailval, have reported that water supply pipelines do not reach to them.

Similarly, since water from pipes is drawn with the help of motor pumps by some wealthy households, it runs out earlier and other households are left deprived of it. Another problem is related to water storage. Households that do not have overhead tanks to store water, use containers of various sizes for the same but water in containers do not last for long, and if it ran out earlier, residents are left in a pathetic condition without water. Some parts of the city practically do not get water supplied by municipal pipes like Narauli, *Harijan basti* in Raidopur ward, Purajodhi in Heerapatti ward and Kaleenganj in Farashtola ward. Residents in these areas either fetch water from municipal hand pumps, installed outside their houses like in *Harijan basti* of Raidopur ward, *Mallah basti* of Madya, Kaleenganj of Farashtola ward or forced to have their water supply connection either hand pumps or motor pumps inside houses like in Purajodhi area of Heerapatti ward and in Narauli ward. Since Raidopur, Madya and Heerapatti are high-income areas, majority of the households have their own boring systems but these are the poor that suffer and are dependent on public hand pumps or forced to have their own boring systems.

Since the ground water level is decreasing, water table decreases up to the depth of 70 feet in summers (Field survey, 2017–2018) for which high capacity submersible pumps are required which are quite expensive for poor population. It has been found that irregularity in the water supply is most prevalent in low- and medium-income neighbourhoods.

4.2.2.2 *Improper Drainage and Waterlogging*

In the previous chapter, an analysis of wastewater management in Azamgarh city showed that about 10.53% households do not have drainage system around their houses (Table 3.10). Problem of inadequate drainage was the highest in LI/MD, LI/HD, HI/MD, and MI/LD neighbourhoods, i.e. in Farashtola, *Prajapati colony* in Arazibagh, *Harijan basti* in Sidhari east, *Mallah basti* in

Madya, *Harijan basti* in Raidopur and *Qasaibada* in Paharpur. Households that do not have drainage system around their houses dispose of wastewater either in surrounding water bodies, surrounding fields or in *kachchanalis* that fall either in main drains or in open spaces around houses.

In this chapter, the drainage system of the city has been examined based on the type of drains, state of drains and the periodic cleaning of drains. The situation of the existing drainage has been found far from satisfactory as out of the total sampled households 5.44% reported *kachcha* or informal drains around their houses, 58.05% reported closed drains while 41.95% households reported the presence of open drains in their neighbourhoods (Table 4.17). Neighbourhoods with the highest percentage of open drains were LI/HD, LI/MD and MI/HD, i.e. Katra, Paharpur, Bazbahadur, Gurutola, Pandeybazaar and Seetaram wards. However, in some areas like in Ailval, households deliberately do not let the main drains close, due to fear of choking and difficulty in proper cleaning.

Open drains get choked with waste from the homes, fallen leaves, dust and debris. An inefficient solid waste management system also adds to this problem. Proliferated solid waste from the roads and plastic gets accumulated in open drains, blocking the drains and thus resulting in waterlogging sites due to spilling of wastewater.

The drainage system in the city is meant to remove the waste and storm water from the city but for drains to work proficiently, they need to be well maintained and cleaned regularly. Periodical cleaning of water is an important means to keep the water flowing smoothly in the drains. Data from the Table 4.17 reveals that only 26.21% households have reported proper cleaning of drains around their houses while remaining 73.79% households (84.34% from LI/MD, 82.70% from LI/HD, 73.33% from MI/LD, 69% from HI/HD and 68.17% from HI/LD neighbourhoods) have reported of spilt over as well as choked drains around their houses due to irregular cleaning. Drains were

Table 4.17 Neighbourhood-Wise Inadequate Drainage (in Percentages) in Azamgarh City

Neighbourhoods	Type of Drains		State of Drains		Cleaning of Drains	
	Kachcha	*Pucca*	*Open*	*Closed*	*Periodical Cleaning*	*No Cleaning*
HI/HD	0.00	100	10.00	90.00	31.00	69.00
HI/MD	1.00	99	34.44	65.56	26.67	73.33
HI/LD	2.83	97.17	42.22	57.78	31.83	68.17
MI/HD	7.53	92.47	45.00	55.00	34.00	66.00
MI/LD	4.60	95.4	30.00	70.00	27.00	73.00
LI/HD	9.53	90.47	63.00	37.00	17.30	82.70
LI/MD	12.6	87.4	69.00	31.00	15.66	84.34
Total	5.44	94.56	41.95	58.05	26.21	73.79

Source: Based on Field Survey, 2016–2017.

either cleaned in a month or in two or three months or mostly at the time of festivals. Improper cleaning of drains results in choking of the drains, hindering the flow of water and spilling it in the surrounding areas.

Improper drainage system fails to remove household waste as well as storm water which leads to the problem of waterlogging in the cities. Waterlogging is the most common phenomenon in most parts of India, due to the seasonal nature of rainfall. With the onset of monsoon, rain makes various parts of the city to suffer from waterlogging. Waterlogging leads to low-lying areas get inundated, roads blocked, resulting in traffic jams and left people to walk through flooded streets. The main reason behind waterlogging is choking of drains due to plastic garbage.

A perusal of Table 4.18 reveals that about 50% of the total sampled households have reported the presence of waterlogging in their neighbourhoods. Of the total waterlogging sites, 30.38% were developed due to rainwater while 19.88% due to spilling of sullage. As far as the place of waterlogging is concerned, 24.39% households reported waterlogging in open spaces, 16.55% on the roads and 9.32% reported it around the houses.

Waterlogging due to sullage was found in *Prajapati* colony of Arazibagh, *Qasaibada* in Paharpur, in Bazbahadur and Matbarganj. Waterlogging in open spaces and around the houses was found in Bazbahadur, Prajapati colony of Arazibagh, *Qasaibada* in Paharpur. In these areas, due to unavailability of proper drainage network, wastewater gets collected around houses and in low-lying open areas. Waterlogging along roads was found in Matbarganj where open nala is the main source of the problem which remains choked most of the time, resulting in spilling of water to the surrounding areas. Problem of waterlogging due to sullage intensified in the rainy season and in Matbarganj, water even enters into low-lying houses and shops.

Waterlogging due to rainwater was seen in almost all the neighbourhoods however it was most prevalent in Narauli, where low-lying streets get submerged in water during rainy season, in Asifganj, where roads get

Table 4.18 Neighbourhood-Wise Waterlogging (in Percentages) in Azamgarh City

Neighbourhoods	Presence of Waterlogging		Type of Waterlogging (If Present)		Place of Waterlogging (if Present)		
	Yes	No	Rainwater	Sullage	Around the Houses	On the Roads	Open Spaces
HI/HD	39.78	60.22	22.78	17	5.08	34.7	0
HI/MD	41.67	58.33	18.43	23.24	11.06	13.61	17
HI/LD	33.33	66.67	29.21	4.12	0	13.36	19.97
MI/HD	51.98	48.02	36.68	15.3	0	14.75	37.23
MI/LD	56.46	43.54	39.65	16.81	7.85	21.58	27.03
LI/HD	61.25	38.75	25.75	35.5	19.09	11.85	30.31
LI/MD	67.33	32.67	40.13	27.2	22.14	6	39.19
Total	50.26	49.74	30.38	19.88	9.32	16.55	24.39

Source: Based on Field Survey, 2016–2017.

submerged in water due to overflowing of drains, and in Raidopur, Ailval, Matbarganj, Bazbahadur, Ghulami ka pura and Civil Lines due to accumulation of rainwater on the roads and in open spaces. Water stays for about 2–3 hours or sometimes takes the whole day to drain off from the roads. Rainwater after mixing with wastewater and solid waste becomes extremely unhygienic and exacerbate the likelihood of many waterborne and vector-borne diseases.

Due to increase in urbanisation and mushrooming population of the city, pressure on the existing drainage system has increased. The population of the city has doubled in the last 50 years but the capacity of the drains is still the same. Therefore even moderate rainfall results in overflowing of drains leading to waterlogging related issues. Other important reasons behind waterlogging were found as lack of drains, siltation and choking of drains due to irregular cleaning.

There is no provision of separate sewer line in Azamgarh city. Therefore, excreta too is disposed in open drains as toilets are directly connected to the drains of the city. The inadequate excreta disposal may result in groundwater contamination and faeces could find their way to the solid waste, to the open lands, into the drains and may come in contact with people. The resulting disease could be typhoid, cholera, diarrhoea, dysentery and several other intestinal and parasitic infections.

Another problem regarding the drainage system in the city is the disposal of the wastewater. Water is directly disposed in the water bodies (Tons river and Dharmu nala) without any treatment. Every day, 17.3 million litres of water is disposed in the Tons river (CPCB, 2009). Wastewater from the drains/*nalas* is pumped into the river with the help of pumping sets. However, at some places, the capacity of pumping stations is not enough to discharge all the water into the river and in rainy seasons it results in flooding situation on the roads and surrounding areas. The river surrounds the city from three sides and Dharmu nala from the North East side. Open disposal of wastewater, contaminated with faeces not only pollutes river water and soil but also produces breeding grounds for various insects and leading to the occurrence of various types of water as well as vector-borne diseases.

It has been found that the existing drainage system in Azamgarh city lacks proper maintenance, adequate carrying capacity and proper disposal of the wastewater, resulting in flooding of roads, streets and low-lying areas, producing stagnant water sites which becomes breeding water grounds for various disease vectors and may contaminate shallow water aquifers. Several diseases like malaria, dengue, chikungunya, typhoid, jaundice and amoebiasis are related to improper drainage and waterlogging.

4.2.2.3 Accumulation of Solid Waste

In the previous chapter, it was discussed that the municipal waste collection services do not cover the entire city and almost 20% of the total sampled households either burn their waste or dispose it into adjacent open fields, water bodies or backyards. Around 80% household waste is collected by municipal workers of which 14.35% waste is collected directly from the resident's houses, for which they pay some extra money to the municipal workers and around 65% waste is collected from the roads. In the present chapter, an attempt has been made to discuss the overall problems related to solid waste management in the city (Table 4.19). Field survey has revealed that provision of community dustbins by the municipality was almost absent in the city and only 1.72% households reported availability of dustbins in their neighbourhoods. In the absence of dustbins, residents drop their waste on the roads for sanitation workers to collect. Neighbourhood survey revealed that no system of segregation of waste into biodegradable and no-biodegradable was present in the city. Kitchen waste, plastic materials and all other waste is mixed at the household level and thrown on the roads. Besides providing separate dustbins for biodegradable and non-biodegradable waste, even common dustbins were lacking, to dispose of waste in the city. Accumulation of waste in the neighbourhoods was the most prominent problem of the city. Table 2.9 reveals that 74.20% households (88% from MI/LD, 84% from LI/MD, 79% from LI/HD, 70% from HI/MD, 70% from MI/HD, 66.66% from HI/HD and 60% from HI/LD neighbourhoods) have reported accumulation of garbage in their neighbourhoods. Regarding the site of waste, 28.28% reported of waste spilled over the roads, 24.79% in open spaces and 21.13% reported of waste collected in the drains.

Solid waste that remains uncollected in the neighbourhoods not only degrade the aesthetic value of neighbourhoods but also leaves the residents vulnerable to pungent smell, germs and bacteria, harmful gasses and pests. One of the major problems associated with waste accumulation in the neighbourhood is the presence of stray animals and pests at the waste accumulation sites. Stray animals like dogs, pigs, cattle, etc., feed on this waste and consume polythene and other harmful materials resulting in health issues for them. These animals and pests are generally poorly cared and are often carriers of various diseases (Trotman, 2018). Diseases transmitted by animals are called zoonotic diseases. Some modern zoonotic diseases are Ebola virus disease and salmonellosis. Most common pests associated with waste sites were rats, mice, cockroach and mosquitos. Many of these pests are harmful to human. Dust mites can cause allergies and asthma; mosquito bites can cause infections, itching and allergies. Flies may also breed in the solid waste and contaminate the food. Regarding the presence of pests and stray animals about 51.26% households (71.65% from LI/HD, 64% from LI/MD and 58.62% from MI/HD neighbourhoods) reported problem of stray animals and pests in their neighbourhoods.

Inspection of the waste collection services in the city has revealed that the frequency of waste collection is highly disappointing in the city. Only 46.93% residents (80% from HI/HD, 57% from MI/HD, 55% from HI/LD, 54% from HI/MD, 34% from LI/HD, 25% from LI/MD and 21% from MI/LD neighbourhood) reported that waste is collected from the roads daily. Total 53.07% residents have reported inadequate waste collection, of which 21.07% reported weekly, 21.76% bi-weekly and 9.58% have reported even monthly collection of

Table 4.19 Neighbourhood-Wise Waste Accumulation Conditions (in Percentages) in Azamgarh City

Neighbourhoods	Waste Segregation				Community Dustbin		Waste Accumulation in Neighbourhood		Problem of Stray Animals/pests due to Waste	
	At Household Level		At Neighbourhood Level							
	Yes	No	Yes	No	Available	Unavailable	Yes	No	Yes	No
HI/HD	0.00	100.00	0.00	100.00	9.65	90.35	66.67	33.33	37.48	62.52
HI/MD	0.00	100.00	0.00	100.00	0.00	100.00	70.00	30.00	49.65	50.35
HI/LD	0.00	100.00	0.00	100.00	2.36	97.64	60.00	40.00	39.63	60.37
MI/HD	0.00	100.00	0.00	100.00	0.00	100.00	70.00	30.00	58.62	41.38
MI/LD	0.00	100.00	0.00	100.00	0.00	100.00	88.33	11.67	37.35	62.65
LI/HD	0.00	100.00	0.00	100.00	0.00	100.00	79.71	20.29	71.65	28.35
LI/MD	0.00	100.00	0.00	100.00	0.00	100.00	84.66	15.34	64.44	35.56
Total	0.00	100.00	0.00	100.00	1.72	98.28	74.20	25.80	51.26	48.74

Neighbourhoods	Site of Waste Accumulation			Frequency of Waste Collection					Satisfaction with Waste Collection Service	
	Spilled on the Road	In open Space	Collects in the Drain	Daily/Adequate	Biweekly	Weekly	Monthly	Inadequate/not daily	Satisfied	Dissatisfied
HI/HD	17.00	23.78	25.89	80.00	10.00	10.00	0.00	20.00	65.00	35.00
HI/MD	23.76	19.98	26.26	54.44	24.61	6.78	14.17	45.56	46.67	53.33
HI/LD	24.00	21.00	15.00	55.83	24.56	16.28	3.33	44.17	47.78	52.22
MI/HD	25.00	20.00	25.00	57.50	20.00	22.50	0.00	42.50	45.00	55.00
MI/LD	25.00	38.33	25.00	21.67	13.33	30.00	35.00	78.33	15.00	85.00
LI/HD	37.04	23.10	19.57	34.06	25.00	34.69	6.25	65.94	28.25	71.75
LI/MD	46.13	27.33	11.20	25.00	34.83	31.84	8.33	75.00	25.00	75.00
Total	28.28	24.79	21.13	46.93	21.76	21.73	9.58	53.07	38.96	61.04

Source: Based on Field Survey, 2016–2017.

the solid waste (Table 4.19). Most of the residents reported that sanitation workers daily collect waste from the roads and on weekly/biweekly or monthly basis from the streets. Some households from the MI/LD neighbourhoods, of Sarfuddinpur and Harbanshpur, have also reported of the complete absence of waste collection services. The previous analysis has shown that waste collection service in the city is pathetic. Although the problem of accumulation of waste was found in all the neighbourhoods, their severity varies greatly.

One reason behind inadequate waste management in the city could be the lack of manpower for accumulation services as only 173 sanitation workers are appointed for the job, which means one sweeper has to cover on an average 94 houses other than the waste generated by commercial and industrial sites, hospitals, hotels and restaurants and construction and demolition sites. For effective solid waste management in a city, the anticipated strength of workers is 2 to 3 workers per thousand persons (NEERI, 1996). With this standard in mind, if we expect 2.5 workers per thousand population, the required strength of sanitation workers in the city will be 278 and with the present strength of 173 workers, 105 workers are still needed in the city.

Residents have reported non-satisfactory cleaning by municipal workers. On the other hand, municipal workers have reported irresponsible behaviour of residents i.e. throwing of the garbage on the roads after the cleaning which gets accumulated and spilled over till the next cleaning time showing their lack of cooperation to achieve cleaner neighbourhood environment. It has been found that out of the total sampled households, only 38% were satisfied with the waste collection services in their neighbourhood.

All the open spaces and empty plots inside the city have been turned into waste dumping sites due to continuous waste disposal in them. Municipal workers collect garbage from the roads but do not care about the pseudo dumping sites that have been developed in all around the city in various neighbourhoods. With the blowing of wind and rain showers, heaps of solid waste get carried away and spread in larger parts. In the rainy season, the solid waste accumulated on the streets produces foul smell, floats on roads, streets and even on the doorsteps of various houses. In case of open drains, solid waste gets stuck in the drains leading to choking of the drains and resulting in stagnant water or waterlogging sites. The capacity of the drains also gets reduced due to continuous accumulation of waste in it. Because of the waste thrown on the roadsides, streets, low-lying areas, vacant places and in and outside drains, not only the environment becomes annoying and unhygienic but it also leads to serious environmental and human health hazards.

Vehicles that transport the waste are also not designed appropriately. They are not equipped with tools to collect the entire waste nor adequately covered, so the solid waste scatters here and there during the process of collection and transportation.

Another problem is related to the disposal of solid waste. Like in most of the Indian cities, in Azamgarh too, open dumping method is used as a means for disposal of waste material. After sometime, when vast heaps of garbage get created, it is burnt down by the municipality. Earlier, solid waste was disposed in the low-lying area near the river Tons but that site was criticised on the ground that it was located inside the city. Although new waste dumping site, outside the city, has been identified the practice of dumping inside the city has still not stopped.

Most of the material that ends up into the dumping sites is usually organic material, including food waste which pollutes the area and environment. Almost two-third of the waste in landfill sites is generally biodegradable which rots, decomposes and produces poisonous gasses like CO_2 and Methane resulting in bad odour as well as contributing to global warming. Open dumping sites also pollute the local environment leading to water and soil pollution. Burning of the waste produces a huge cloud of smoke as well as several poisonous and harmful gasses. Residents thus suffer from many environmental problems due to the dumping of waste within the city.

Overall solid waste management system in the city exhibits a range of problems including little collection coverage, inefficient collection services, open dumping and burning of waste without air and water pollution control.

People that live near the accumulated solid waste are at high risk of infectious diseases as the waste produces bad odour and the rotting waste material is highly infectious. Mosquitos and flies which breed in the accumulated waste are transporters of diseases like malaria and dengue etc.

4.2.2.4 Unequal distribution of Facilities and Amenities

Another important problem identified in the city is unequal distribution of amenities and facilities as resident's access to quality of community services, health care services, recreational services, educational and employment opportunities, transportation and other public services, greatly depends upon how near or far these are located. A concentration of various health, educational and recreational facilities have been seen in the northern part of the city which is not equally accessible to all the residents living in different areas of the city. Unequal distribution of public goods and services across neighbourhoods lowers the overall well-being of the residents in a country (Peluso and Michelangeli, 2016). Differences across neighbourhoods in various educational and employment opportunities may result in further increase in neighbourhood disadvantages, creating disparities in health along socio-economic lines (Williams & Collins, 2001). Neighbourhoods that typically lack educational and employment opportunities also lack chances of upward social and economic mobility. There could be lesser role models and lesser community members with ample resources too to provide support to those in need. Studies have concluded that local facilities and public services available at the neighbourhood level may have an impact on resident's well-being (Aaberge et al., 2017).

Density maps of all the facilities and amenities have been prepared to evaluate the access of these facilities to the residents of various neighbourhoods. Kernel density estimation technique has been used to generate density maps.

Four maps including health facilities density, educational facilities density, recreational facilities density and religious facilities density have been prepared. Recreational facilities density map has included all the recreational facilities including gyms, restaurants, libraries, cinema halls as well as shopping malls.

Further a composite density map of all the facilities has been prepared by combining the maps of educational, health, recreational and religious densities (Figure 4.5). Raster calculator tool in Arc Map 10.2.1 has been used to generate the final composite map. The unequal nature of the distribution of facilities is very clear in the map. It has been found that major hotspot of all these facilities can be spotted near the city centre, covering wards namely Asifganj, Paharpur, Pandeybazar, Mukeriganj, Arazibagh and Matbarganj. Density of amenities and facilities is also high in the Civil Lines area of the city while the lowest density of educational, health as well as recreational facilities has been observed in MI/LD neighbourhood, mainly in the wards Sarfuddinpur and Harbanshpur. Therefore, these are basically the residents of Sarfuddinpur and Harbanshpur that face the problem of unavailability of facilities and amenities in their neighbourhoods. Density of the facilities is also low in the Sidhari east and west ward of HI/MD and HI/LD neighbourhoods; however, these are the high-income counterparts and their distance from the city centre is somewhat suppressed by presence of modern vehicles in majority of the houses.

4.2.3 Neighbourhood Social Environmental Problems

While measuring neighbourhood problems, social cohesion in the neighbourhood has emerged as an essential feature of the neighbourhood context (Fisher et al., 2004). Major environmental problems that came across while analysing the social environment of the neighbourhoods are residential segregation and neighbourhood disorder. These problems are discussed in the following sections:

4.2.3.1 Residential Segregation

"Social relations are so frequently and so inevitably correlated with spatial relations" (Park, 1926). The spatial separation of two or more social groups within a specific terrestrial area, such as a census tract, a municipality or a metropolitan area is generally referred to as residential segregation (Timberlake and Ignatov, 2014). Residential segregation is a kind of segregation that categorise population groups into different localities and outlines their living environment at the community level (Kawachi and Berkman, 2003). While residential segregation has conventionally been linked with racial segregation, it can be any type of categorisation based on characteristics of the population, i.e. race, ethnicity, income, religion, family structure as well as socio-economic status (Uslaner, 2000; Timberlake and Ignatov, 2014). Residential segregation is believed to benefit population groups with the high level of various forms of capital like the racial majority and prosperous, while it poses adverse outcomes

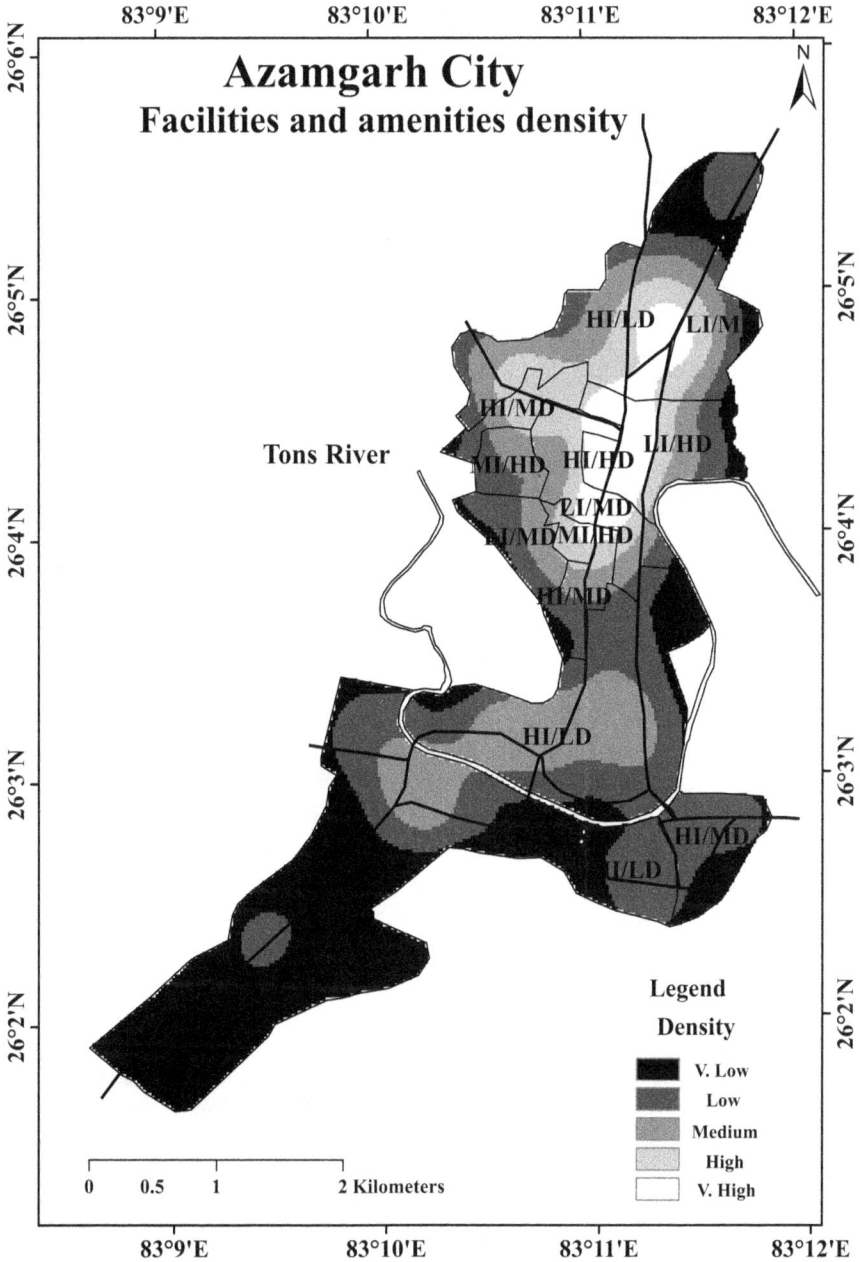

Figure 4.5 Azamgarh City: Composite Facilities and Amenities Density.

Source: Municipal Office, Azamgarh, 2016–2017; Field Survey, 2016–2017; Google Maps, 2019.

to the groups with low level of capital like minority groups and impoverished, mainly by the effects of exposure of neighbourhood wealth or poverty. Residential segregation tends to occur due to suburbanisation, discrimination and personal choice. In the Indian scenario, residential segregation is shaped by the caste structure of the region. Indian societies are traditionally been divided into hierarchical structure along the lines of caste.

Spatial segregation and discrimination have been one of the fundamental aspects of the caste system (Desai, 1994). In this way, the arrangement of society along the caste line has made inequality and exclusion an in-built character of the Indian society (Chandra and Mukherjee, 2015). The constitution of India recognised the term Scheduled Caste and Scheduled Tribe for disadvantaged groups in modern India, which are the main sufferers of spatial segregation in the country. Although residential segregation along the caste lines is a rural phenomenon, high inequality still prevails in smaller cities (Desai and Dubey, 2012).

In Azamgarh city, about 12.91% population belong to Scheduled Caste and 0.33% to Scheduled Tribe (Census of India, 2011). Residential segregation in the city has been studied in terms of SC (Scheduled Caste) population in the city, as they represent a considerable share of the total population. From Table 4.20, it is clear that the proportion of SC population is the highest in the ward Narauli, i.e. 41% followed by Pandeybazar and Harbanshpur, i.e. 22% and 19%, respectively. The proportion of SC was the lowest in Jalandhari, i.e. 0.55% followed by Bazbahadur and Sadavarti, i.e. 0.61% and 1.36%, respectively. Hotspot analysis has been used to identify clustering of SC population in the city.

The hot spot analysis revealed significant areas of clustering for high proportions of SC population in Azamgarh City (Figure 4.6). It shows the level of significant clustering of high proportions of the SC population in the city. The map indicates that high proportions of *the* scheduled caste tend to cluster at the outer limits of the city, along the northern and southern banks of the river Tons. It is visible that with 99% confidence wards Narauli and Harbanshpur belong to a statistically significant cluster of high proportion of SC population. Table 4.20 reveals that 41% population of Narauli and 19.52% population of Harbanshpur, respectively, belong to scheduled caste. Wards with 95% significant clustering are Civil Lines, Madya and Sidhari West with 18%, 15% and 9% SC population, respectively. It is easily perceived that the majority of scheduled caste population remains clustered in the outer part of the city along the river. Significant cold spots of SC population have been found near the city centre. Wards with 99% significant cold spots are Asifganj, Paharpur, Jalandhari, Seetaram, Farashtola, Sadavarti and Pandeybazaar. It has been found that only 0.55% population of Jalandhari, 0.61% of Bazbahadur, 1.36% of Sadavarti and 1.96% of Farashtola belongs to Scheduled Caste. Wards with cold spots of 95% confidence are Badarka, Bazbahadur, Ailval and Katra. It has been found that the largest proportion of scheduled caste population is still found to be clustered in the outskirts of the city following the traditional

Table 4.20 Distribution of Scheduled Caste Population in Different Wards of Azamgarh City

Ward No	Ward Name	Total Population	SC population	Percentage SC Population
1	Farashtola	1991	39	1.96
2	Sidhari West	3544	536	15.12
3	Seetaram	4968	319	6.42
4	Badarka	6405	617	9.63
5	Jalandhari	3289	18	0.55
6	Gurutola	3361	651	19.37
7	Sidhari East	5907	622	10.53
8	Arazibagh	4465	386	8.65
9	Bazbahadur	7411	45	0.61
10	Katra	3395	292	8.6
11	Asifganj	3727	103	2.76
12	Harbanshpur	6383	1246	19.52
13	Ghulami ka pura	5914	1083	18.31
14	Mukeriganj	3764	543	14.43
15	Heerapatti	4254	306	7.19
16	Sarfuddinpur	3872	317	8.19
17	Raidopur	2676	133	4.97
18	Narauli	4067	1683	41.38
19	Matbarganj	5020	887	17.67
20	ChaklaPaharpur	2967	318	10.72
21	Civil Line	9039	1639	18.13
22	Pandey Bazaar	2947	669	22.7
23	Ailval	3670	545	14.85
24	Sadavarti	2873	39	1.36
25	Madya	5047	502	9.95

Source: Census of India, 2011.

spatial structure of rural India. In traditional rural India, such segregated arrangements delimit caste group's access to public goods such as village well, grazing fields, etc.

However, the field survey revealed a very different phenomenon in Azamgarh city. In the city, segregation was found between wards and between neighbourhoods but the problem of segregation was most prominent within wards and within the neighbourhoods. The major caste groups in Azamgarh city are *harijan*s, *dom*, *mallah*, *Prajapati*, *Mauurya* and *Yadav*. *Yadav* is one of the largest caste groups in the city and comes under OBC category and no segregation was observed regarding this caste, therefore it was excluded from the analysis. Out of remaining castes, *Mallah* and *Parajapati* castes though come under OBC category, however Social Welfare department of Uttar Pradesh has demanded to issue Scheduled caste certificate to them based on their current social backwardness. Segregated colonies of these castes termed as *Harijan bastis, Mallah bastis, Prajapati* were found nested within wards. Various colonies termed as *Harijan bastis, Mallah bastis, Prajapati* colony based on their caste were found

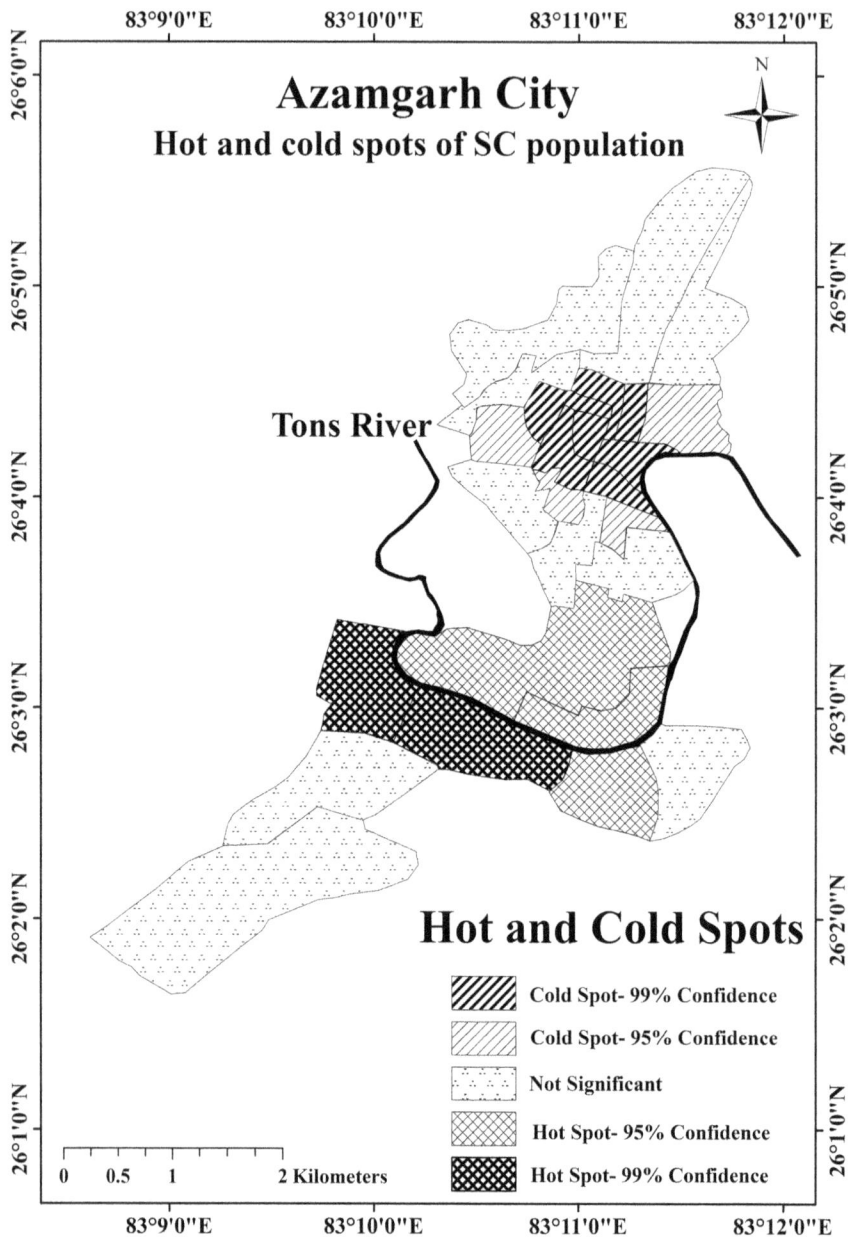

Figure 4.6 Azamgarh City: Hot and Cold Spots of SC Population.
Source: Census of India, 2011.

Table 4.21 Neighbourhood-Wise Distribution of Segregated *Bastis* in Azamgarh City

Neighbourhoods	Percentage SC Population	Harijan Bastis (Number)
HI/HD	2.76	No
HI/MD	12.28	Yes (3)
HI/LD	11.63	Yes (4)
MI/HD	9.12	Yes (1)
MI/LD	23.03	Yes (2)
LI/HD	4.57	No
LI/MD	13.09	Yes (3)

Source: Based on Field survey, 2016–2017.

segregated within the neighbourhoods (Table 4.21). For example in HIMD neighbourhood covering wards namely Sidhari East, Arazibagh and Matbarganj (with 12.28% SC population), two *Harijan basti*s and one *Prajapati* colony were spotted. These *basti*s were totally segregated from rest of the neighbourhood. The environmental condition was worst, and services like water supply, drainage and sewerage, waste collection were pathetic. Dilapidated housing and poor environmental condition were prominent features of these *bastis*. A perusal of the Table 4.21 shows that these types of bastis were present in almost all the neighbourhoods, i.e. four bastis were found in HI/LD neighbourhood (11.63% SC population; three *Harijan bastis* and one *Mallah basti*), three *harijan bastis* in LI/MD neighbourhood (13.09% SC population), two *harijan bastis* in MI/LD (23.03% SC population) and one in MI/HD neighbourhood (9.12% SC population) were found. *Harijan bastis* were absent in HI/HD neighbourhood (2.76% SC population) covering ward Asifganj and in LI/HD neighbourhoods (4.57% SC population), wards Paharpur, Jalandhari, Seetaram and Bazbahadur.

It has been found that these *basti*s are not only found in the hotspots of the city but are prevalent in the cold spots as well, as small *harijan basti*s have been found abutted in central wards like Farashtola, Seetaram and Katra, remained segregated having no social ties with the majority population of the ward. Scheduled caste population remain segregated even in hotspots as well, where they have a major share; they remain segregated from the rest of the ward population, having their separate locations and unique names, i.e. *harijan bastis*, etc.

4.2.3.2 Neighbourhood Disorder

Neighbourhood disorder can be understand as awful activities in public such like drunk people, drug dealing, fighting, people loitering, rowdy groups and gang activity on the street as well as street prostitution. Neighbourhood disorder or social disorganisation in the neighbourhood that is an indication of the collapse of order and social control could threaten the quality of life as well (Gracia, 2014). Social disorganisation may be harmful to both the physical and mental health of the residents (Latkin and Curry, 2003). Mental well-being is affected by the consistent experience of criminality, vandalism, drug dealing on the streets, noise and other forms of the disorder. In a neighbourhood where social order has damaged, people are confronted with an unsafe and harmful setting, which could be distressing (Ross, 2000). The most common impact of the disorder on resident's health is stress which results from the fear of crime or fear of being attacked and can damage the health in many ways. The regular stress related to living in a neighbourhood where threat, trouble, misconduct, crime and incivility are common may arouse recurrent fear, frequently overflowing the body with hormones that directly weaken health. Neighbourhood disorder can be studied in two forms, i.e. physical disorder and social disorder. Physical disorders are abandoned buildings, noise, graffiti, vandalism, filth and shabbiness whereas social disorders include crime, i.e. theft, robbery, pickpocketing, people loitering, public drinking or drug use, rowdy groups as well as conflict and indifferences. The present study is concerned with social disorders predominant in Azamgarh city. Table 4.22 shows the prevalence of crime in Azamgarh city for the year 2017. The Table revealed that major crimes that took place in 2017 in the city are burglary, chain snatching, severe injuries by fighting, kidnapping, eve-teasing and stalking etc. of which a significant share of theft, gangster act, gambling, burglary etc. was found.

The typical approach in measuring disorder has been to ask residents how much of a problem they perceive disorder to be; the standard finding is that perception of disorder predicts fear of crime (Skogan, 1990; Perkins et al.,1996). Residents were asked, what are the problems, they believe that exist in their

Table 4.22 Prevalence of Crime in Azamgarh City

Serial Number	Crimes	Percentage
1	Burglary	6.89
2	Chain snatching	6.68
3	Dowry deaths	2.71
4	Eve teasing	7.65
5	Gambling	9.86
6	Gangster act	13.63
7	Illegal weapon	4.15
8	Kidnapping	3.21
9	Loot road	6.58
10	Murder	4.23
11	Rape	0.98
12	Serious injury	7.63
13	Sexual harassment	3.28
14	Stalking	6.52
15	Theft	11.35
16	Vehicle theft	4.65
Total	Total	100

Source: SP office, Azamgarh.

neighbourhoods and their response is shown in Table 4.23. The table shows the prevalence of theft, robbery, pickpocketing, people drinking, drug dealing, people loitering, rowdy groups, street fighting and prostitution in different neighbourhoods.

It is observed that people living in LI/HD, LI/MD and MI/HD have reported almost all of the problems in their neighbourhoods i.e. in LI/HD (theft 55%, robbery 57.5%, pick pocketing 51.5%, People drinking 71.86%, liquor stores 66.23%, drug dealing 64.98%, people loitering 77.97% and rowdy groups and fighting 80.97%), LI/MD (theft 43.76%, robbery 33.81%, pick pocketing 34.76%,

Table 4.23 Azamgarh City: Neighbourhood Disorder

Neighbourhoods	Specific Location	Urgent Problems
HI/HD	Core of the city	Overcrowding, Narrow Streets, Noise pollution, Water Quality problem, Unsatisfactory cleaning of drains, Accumulation of waste
HI/MD	Core of the city	Overcrowding, Narrow Streets, Water Quality problem, Unsatisfactory cleaning of drains, Waterlogging, Accumulation of waste, Residential segregation
HI/LD	Outer part of the city	Water Quality problem, Open drains, Unsatisfactory cleaning of drains, Accumulation of waste, Residential segregation
MI/HD	Core of the city	Overcrowding, Narrow Streets, Water Quality problem, Irregular water supply, Open drains, Unsatisfactory cleaning of drains, Waterlogging, Accumulation of waste, Residential segregation, Neighbourhood disorder
MI/LD	Outer part of the city, newly included parts	Noise pollution, Water Quality problem, Irregular water supply, Unsatisfactory cleaning of drains, Waterlogging, Accumulation of waste, Residential segregation
LI/HD	Core of the city	Overcrowding, Narrow Streets, Water Quality problem, Irregular water supply, Open drains, Unsatisfactory cleaning of drains, Waterlogging, Accumulation of waste, Neighbourhood disorder
LI/MD	Core of the city	Overcrowding, Quality problem, Irregular water supply, Open drains, Unsatisfactory cleaning of drains, Waterlogging, Accumulation of waste, Residential segregation, Neighbourhood disorder

Source: Based on Field survey, 2016–2019.

People drinking 42.27%, liquor stores 45.6%, drug dealing 96.66%, people loitering 90.93% and rowdy groups and fighting 96.11%) and in MI/HD (theft 60%, robbery 55%, pick pocketing 52.30%, people drinking 75.40%, liquor stores 68.20%, drug dealing 30.59%, people loitering 39.88% and rowdy groups and fighting 39.98%).

These are mainly low-income neighbourhoods, occupied by the poor. Mostly these neighbourhoods are situated in the highly congested central old part of the city, along the river Tons. They cover the wards namely Bazbahadur, Seetaram, Jalandhari and Paharpur predominated by low-income households with slums and substandard housing conditions. As this is a socio-economically backward area, unemployed and underemployed people in these wards are mainly engaged in loitering, fighting as well as theft. Drinking and drug dealing is also common. MI/HD constitutes two wards, i.e. Katra and Badarka. This neighbourhood is the hub of rowdy group activity as well as fighting where loitering and drug dealing is also prevalent. Prostitution has been found in only LI/MD neighbourhood which is a historical phenomenon in Farashtola ward leading to drinking, loitering as well as fighting. Liquor consumption and fighting was also reported from Pandey Bazar ward. However, other wards of these neighbourhoods, i.e. Ailval and Sadavarti are somewhat peaceful. It was observed that in a neighbourhood where one problem is found, other problems are also prevalent indicating that all forms of the disorder are interrelated.

Neighbourhoods such as MI/LD, HI/LD and HI/MD have reported less disorder than LI/HD, LI/MD and MI/HD neighbourhoods, i.e. MI/LD (38.89%), HI/LD (25.63%) and HI/MD (22.21%). HI/HD neighbourhood has reported the least disorder, i.e. 10.16%. These neighbourhoods cover wards, namely, Civil Lines, Raidopur, Madya, Asifganj, Sidhari East, Arazibagh and Matbarganj. The major part of these neighbourhoods is occupied by high-income counterparts of the City inhabited by business and service class residents. These neighbourhoods are mainly peaceful with very less disorder. Mostly these neighbourhoods are located in outer parts of the city; however, some are located in the inner city as well.

4.3 Urgent Problems in Different Neighbourhoods

In the previous section, an attempt was made to address different neighbourhood environmental problems in Azamgarh city. It has been found that major environmental issues in the city are narrow or congested streets, insufficient water supply, water quality problem, improper drainage, heaps of uncollected garbage, neighbourhood disorder as well as air and noise pollution. Furthermore, an attempt is made to identify urgent problems in different neighbourhoods as all the neighbourhoods have different locations, characteristics and different environmental issues. In this regard, if an environmental problem is reported by more than 40% of its residents, it has been considered as an urgent problem of the neighbourhood as it affects more than two third of the population of a neighbourhood (Table 4.24).

Table 4.24 Urgent Problems in Different Neighbourhoods

Neighbourhoods	Theft	Robbery	Pick Pockeing	People Drunk	Liquor Stores	Drug Dealing	People Loitering	Rowdy Group And Fighting	Prostitution	Total
HI/HD	11.1	13.3	11.2	13.3	11.1	13.2	11.1	7.2	0	10.16
HI/MD	6.66	17.76	17.76	35.53	35.53	24.43	31.1	31.1	0	22.21
HI/LD	35.55	24.71	21.54	35.55	36.93	24.44	30.27	21.66	0	25.63
MI/HD	60	55	52.3	75.4	68.2	30.59	39.88	39.98	0	57.93
MI/LD	38.91	36.96	37.66	54.17	50.71	36.97	48.26	46.41	0	38.89
LI/HD	55	57.5	51.5	71.86	66.23	64.98	77.97	80.97	0	58.45
LI/MD	43.76	33.81	34.76	42.27	45.6	96.66	90.93	96.11	100	53.76
Total	35.85	34.15	32.39	46.87	44.9	41.61	47.07	46.2	14.29	38.14

Source: Based on Field Survey, 2016–2019.

A perusal of the Table 4.24 reveals that almost all the neighbourhoods are loaded with numerous environmental issues. The neighbourhoods that have reported almost all the problems identified in the city are LI/MD, LI/HD and MI/HD neighbourhoods while number of urgent environmental problems are relatively lower in HI/LD and HI/HD neighbourhoods. Environmental problems that are common in all the neighbourhoods are accumulation of solid waste, water quality problem and unsatisfactory cleaning of drains while environmental problem reported by least number of neighbourhoods was neighbourhood disorder which was an urgent problem in MI/HD, LI/HD and MI/LD neighbourhoods.

4.4 Summary

In the present chapter, an analysis of major neighbourhood environmental problems of Azamgarh city has been presented. This chapter has been divided into two sections. In the first section, an attempt has been made to understand what actually neighbourhood problems are. In the second section, an identification of major neighbourhood problems in Azamgarh City is made and further the identified neighbourhood environmental problems of the city are discussed comprehensively under three major categories, i.e. neighbourhood physical environmental problems, neighbourhood service environmental problems as well as neighbourhood social-environmental problems.

An analysis of major neighbourhood environmental problems in Azamgarh city revealed that narrow or congested streets, insufficient water supply and water quality problem, improper drainage, heaps of uncollected garbage and neighbourhood disorder are the most urgent problems of the city.

Problems identified in the physical environment include overcrowding, narrow or congested streets, substandard housing and slums, air pollution, noise pollution and water quality problem. Sense of overcrowding was found the highest in HI/HD, MI/HD, LI/HD and LI/MD in the old central parts of the city covering the wards namely Badarka, Katra, Bazbahadur, Paharpur, Gurutola, Jalandhari, Asifganj and Sadavarti. Another major problem prevalent in these neighbourhoods was narrow and congested streets. In these wards, houses are made without proper guidelines on how much open space should be left and what should be the adequate width of streets for proper flow of traffic as well as wind.

Neighbourhood survey has revealed that about 26% of the total sampled households have reported living in substandard houses and this percentage was the highest in LI/MD, i.e. 36.80% followed by MI/LD, i.e. 36.44, MI/HD, i.e. 29.50, LI/HD, i.e. 24.95 and HI/LD, i.e. 21.98%. Substandard housing was found as a common phenomenon in *Harijan bastis* of Farashtola, Sidhari East, Katra, Harbanshpur, Ghulami ka pura, Mukeriganj, Raidopur, Narauli, Pandeybazaar, in Prajapati colony in Arazibagh and in *Mallah basti* in Madya. These bastis were basically developed in the central part of the city as well as along the banks of the river Tons. Slum like condition has also been found in

Kaleenganj in Farashtola, Kundigarh in Badarka and in parts of Katra and Ghulami ka pura ward.

Regarding air pollution in Azamgarh city, values of PM_{10} and $PM_{2.5}$ at all the monitored stations were higher than national standards for ambient air quality. The highest values were recorded in Paharpur in LI/HD neighbourhood and Narauli in MI/LD neighbourhoods. Air quality was considerably fair in Civil Lines but the value exceeded the national average standard.

Noise pollution analysis found that noise level is within the standard limits for the residential areas; however, it exceeds the prescribed standards at commercial and silence zones as well as traffic intersections. Traffic has been found to be the major source of noise pollution in the city. Households located along the major roads as well as markets complained the problem of higher noise in their neighbourhoods. Neighbourhoods that have complained the major problem of noise pollution are HI/HD and MI/LD with 47.67% and 43.85%, respectively. The HI/HD neighbourhood is located in the downtown of the city and presence of a central market, i.e. *Takiya* and constant traffic on the major Gorakhpur Allahabad road, makes it the most busy and noisy places of the city. The neighbourhood MI/LD is located in the southern part of the city and includes Railway Station, Taxi Stand as well as major roads of the city; therefore exposure to noise problem is higher in this neighbourhood.

The problem in water quality was also reported during the survey; therefore, an attempt was made to check physico-chemical characteristics of water. It was found that all parameters like pH, EC, TDS, alkalinity, hardness, TSS, chloride and chlorine in all the samples were within the permissible limits except the samples collected from Bazbahadur, Paharpur, Sarfuddinpur and Matbarganj. Water Quality Index of the samples revealed that the water quality of 5 samples was poor out of 9 samples. Analysis has revealed that water samples collected from submersible pumps exhibited better water quality than those from hand pumps and municipal taps.

Problems in service environment included inadequate water supply, inadequate drainage system as well as accumulation of solid waste in the neighbourhoods. An analysis of water supply services reveals that about 60% of the total sampled households have reported regular supply of water inside their houses. From the remaining 40% households, about 12% reported that they get water for 1–6 hours only, about 19% reported 7–12 hours, and 9% reported 13–18 hours. It has been found that about 47% residents from the city have reported problem in the quality of water in the form of dirt, sand, smell in the water, etc.

Drainage condition analysis showed that out of the total sampled households 5.44% households reported the presence of kachcha drains in their neighbourhoods, 58.05% reported closed drains while 41.95% households reported presence of open drains in their neighbourhoods. Neighbourhoods with the highest percentage of open drains were LI/HD, LI/MD and MI/HD where problem of open drains was mainly prominent in Katra, Paharpur, Bazbahadur, Gurutola, Pandeybazaar and Seetaram wards. Another problem related to drainage was waterlogging. About 51% of the total sampled households have reported the presence of waterlogging in their neighbourhoods. Of the total waterlogging sites, 30.46% was developed due to rainwater while 20.65% due to spilling of sullage. Waterlogging was mainly prevalent in Paharpur, Bazbahadur, Arazibagh, Narauli and Matbarganj areas of the city.

Inadequate waste collection was another problem in the city. The practice of waste segregation both at household and neighbourhood level was absent in the city. Only 1.72% household reported the presence of community dustbin in the neighbourhood. It has been found that 74.20% households (88% from MI/LD, 84% from LI/MD, 79% from LI/HD, 70% from HI/MD, 70% from MI/HD, 66.66% from HI/HD and 60% from HI/LD neighbourhoods) have reported accumulation of garbage in their neighbourhoods. And with the accumulation of garbage in the neighbourhood, about 51% households reported problem of stray animals and pests around their houses. Frequency of waste collection was also found unsatisfactory in the city and out of the total sampled households, only 46.93% residents (80% from HI/HD, 57% from MI/HD, 55% from HI/LD, 54% from HI/MD, 34% from LI/HD, 25% from LI/MD and 21% from MI/LD neighbourhood) reported that waste is collected from the roads daily. Out of the total 55% residents that have reported inadequate waste collection, 25% reported weekly, 21% bi-weekly and 9% had reported even monthly collection of solid waste. Another important problem identified in the city is unequal distribution of amenities and facilities as major hotspot of all these facilities can be spotted near the city centre, covering wards namely Asifganj, Paharpur, Pandeybazar, Mukeriganj, Arazibagh and Matbarganj. Therefore these are basically the residents of Sarfuddinpur and Harbanshpur that face the problem of unavailability of facilities and amenities in their neighbourhoods.

Problems in the neighbourhood social environment include the problem of residential segregation and neighbourhood disorder. Residential segregation with respect to Scheduled Caste population was measured by hotspot analysis. Hotspot analysis revealed that significant hot and cold spots of SC population are prevalent in the city and majority of the SC population is living inwards, near the outer boundary of the SC, repeating the historical phenomena of segregation of SC population in the outer area of the settlements. However, field survey revealed that the problem of segregation in the city was more prominent within the wards and neighbourhoods than between the wards and neighbourhoods. Separate *harijan bastis*, *Mallah bastis*, based on caste have been developed in different parts of the city in which environmental conditions are very pathetic.

Another problem identified in the city was neighbourhood disorder. It was mainly prevalent in the central, congested, old parts of the city in LI/HD, LI/MD and MI/HD neighbourhoods, i.e. in LI/HD (theft 55%, robbery 57.5%, pick pocketing 51.5%, people drunk 71.86%, liquor stores 66.23%, drug dealing 64.98%, people loitering 77.97% and rowdy groups and fighting 80.97%), LI/MD (theft 43.76%, robbery 33.81%, pick pocketing 34.76%, people drunk 42.27%, liquor stores 45.6%, drug dealing 96.66%, people loitering 90.93% and rowdy groups and fighting 96.11%) and in MI/HD (theft 60%, robbery 55%, pick pocketing 52.30%, people drunk 75.40%, liquor stores 68.20%, drug dealing 30.59%, people loitering 39.88% and rowdy groups and fighting 39.98%. It covered wards namely Badarka, Katra, Bazbahadur, Seetaram, Jalandhari and Narauli.

In the third section, an attempt is made to identify urgent problems in different neighbourhoods and the problem which was reported by more than 40% of the residents of a neighbourhood has been considered as an urgent problem of the neighbourhood. The neighbourhoods that have reported almost all the problems identified in the city are LI/MD, LI/HD and MI/HD neighbourhoods while number of urgent environmental problems are relatively lower in HI/LD and HI/HD neighbourhoods.

References

Aaberge, R., Langørgen, A., & Lindgren, P. (2017). The distributional impact of public services in European countries. *Monitoring Social Inclusion in Europe*, 159.

Abdullah, Alauddin S, & Sarfuddin (2012). Seasonal variability and physico- chemical characteristics of ground water at Azamgarh. *s*, *1*(1), 1–4.

Anwar, K. M., & Aggarwal, V. (2014). Analysis of groundwater quality of Aligarh City (India): using water quality index. *Current World Environment: An International Research Journal of Environmental Sciences*, *9*(3), 851.

Bhat, S. A., & Pandit, A. K. (2014). Surface water quality assessment of Wular Lake, a Ramsar site in Kashmir Himalaya, using discriminant analysis and WQI. *Journal of Ecosystems*, *2014*, 1–18.

BIS. (2012). *Specification for Drinking Water.IS: 10500*. New Delhi, India.

Blake, K. S., Kellerson, R. L., & Simic, A. (2007). *Measuring Overcrowding in Housing*. Washington, DC: Department of Housing and Urban Development, Office of Policy Development and Research.

BS 3452. (1966). Method for measurement of noise emitted by motor vehicles.

Casey, J. A., James, P., & Morello-Forsch, R. (2017). Urban noise pollution is worst in poor and minority neighborhoods and segregated cities. *PBS*. Published October 7, 2017.

Chandra, R., & Mukherjee, S. (2015). Urban transformations and new dynamics of exclusions: a mixed method study of health and well-being in an expanding city of India. *Current Urban Studies*, *3*(02), 135.

CPCB. (2009). Status of water supply, wastewater generation and treatment in class-I cities & class-Ii Towns of India, *Control of Urban pollution*, SERIES: CUPS/ 70 / 2009 – 10.

CPCB, Guide Manual: Water and Waste Water, Central Pollution Control Board, New Delhi. http://www.cpcb.nic.in/upload/Latest/Latest_67_guidemanualw&wwanalysis.pdf (Accessed 12 July 2013).

Crothers, C. Kearns, R., & Lindsey, D. (1993) Housing in Manukau City: overcrowding, poor housing and their consequences working papers in *Sociology* No. 27 University of Auckland.

Desai, A. R. (1994). *Rural Sociology in India*. PopularPrakashan, Mumbai.

Desai, S., & Dubey, A. (2012). Caste in 21st century India: competing narratives. *Economic and Political Weekly*, *46*(11), 40.

Diez-Roux, A. V. (1998). Bringing context back into epidemiology: variables and fallacies in multilevel analysis. *American Journal of Public Health*, 88(2), 216–222.

Environmental Protection Agency (EPA) of the U.S. Website. (2005). http://www.epa.gov

Fawell, J. K., Lund, U., & Mintz, B. (2003). Total dissolved solids in drinking-water. In *Background document for development of WHO guidelines for drinking-water quality*. World Health Organization, Geneva.

Fisher, K.J., Li, F., Michael, Y., & Cleveland, M. (2004).Neighborhood-level influences on physical activity among older adults: a multilevel analysis. *Journal of Aging and Physical Activity 12* (1), 45–63.

Gove, W. R., Hughes, M., & Galle, O. R. (1979). Overcrowding in the home: an empirical investigation of its possible pathological consequences. *American Sociological Review, 44*, 59–80.

Gracia, E. (2014). "Neighbourhood Disorder". In *Encyclopaedia of Quality of life and Well-Being Research*, pp. 4325–4328. https://rd.springer.com/referenceworkentry/10.1007percent2F978-94-007-0753-5_2751. (Accessed 14 January 2017).

Gray, A. (2001). Definitions of crowding and the effect of crowding on health. *A Literature Review Prepared for the Ministry of Social Policy.*

Hastings, A. (2009). Neighbourhood environmental services and neighbourhood 'effects': exploring the role of urban services in intensifying neighbourhood problems. *Housing Studies, 24*(4), 503–524.

Hogan, C. M., & Latshaw, G. L. (1973). The relationship between highway planning and urban noise. In *Proceedings of the ASCE Urban Transportation Division Environment Impact Specialty Conference*, May 21–23, 1973, Chicago, Illinois. (No. Proceeding).

International Occupational Safety and Health Information Centre (CIS), Chlorine, in International Chemical Safety Cards. (2009). 31 March. International Programme on Chemical Safety (IPCS) and European Commission (EC). (Accessed 5 September 2019).

Jazwinski, C. (1998). Crowding. http://condor.stcloud.msus.edu/~jaz/psy373/7.crowding.html

Kawachi, I., & Berkman, L. F. (Eds.). (2003). *Neighborhoods and health*. Oxford University Press.

Kumar, M., & Puri, A. (2012). A review of permissible limits of drinking water. *Indian Journal of Occupational and Environmental Medicine, 16*(1), 40.

Latkin, C. A., & Curry, A. D. (2003). Stressful neighborhoods and depression: a prospective study of the impact of neighborhood disorder. *Journal of Health and Social Behavior, 44*(1), 34–44.

McGowan, W. (2000). *Water Processing: Residential, Commercial, Light-industrial*, 3rd ed. Water Quality Association, Lisle, IL.

Mishra, B., Singh, R. B., & Anupama, M. (2001). *Delhi Metropolis: Housing and Quality of Life*, Ed. R. P. Mishra, Million Cities of India, Vikas Publishing, New Delhi, Vol. 1, pp. 196–228.

Mohsin, M., Safdar, S., Asghar, F., & Jamal, F. (2013). Assessment of drinking water quality and its impact on residents health in Bahawalpur city. *International Journal of Humanities and Social Science, 3*(15), 114–128.

NEERI Report "Strategy Paper on Solid Waste Management in India", pp. 1–7. (1996).

Noise Pollution (regulation and Control) Rules. (2000).

Park, R. E. (1926). The urban community as a spatial pattern and a moral order. *Urban Social Segregation*, 21–31.

Peluso, E., & Michelangeli, A. (2016). Cities and inequality. *Region: The Journal of ERSA*, *3*(2), 47–60.

Perkins, Douglas, & Ralph B. Taylor. (1996). Ecological assessments of community disorder: their relationship to fear of crime and theoretical implications. *American Journal of Community Psychology*, 24, 63–107.

Perkins, H. C. (1974). *Air Pollution*. McGraw Hill Book Company, New York, p. 15.

Perlin, S. A., Wong, D., & Sexton, K. (2001). Residential proximity to industrial sources of air pollution: interrelationships among race, poverty, and age. *Journal of the Air & Waste Management Association*, *51*(3), 406–421.

Pickett, K. E., & Pearl, M. (2001) Multilevel analyses of neighbourhood socioeconomic context and health outcomes: a critical review. *Journal of Epidemiology and Community Health*, *55*, 111–122.

Radberg, J. (1988). *Doktrinochtäthetisvensktstadsbyggande 1875–1975*. Byggforsknings-rådet, Stockholm.

Rahman, A. (1998). *Household Environment and Health*. B R Publishing Corporation, Delhi.

Ross, C. E. (2000). Neighborhood disadvantage and adult depression. *Journal of Health and Social Behavior*, *41*(2), 177–187.

Seasonal Weather Averages. (2010). Weather underground. December. Temperature data from Weather Underground. (Accessed 22 December 2010).

Semiromi, F. B., Hassani, A. H., Torabian, A., Karbassi, A. R., & Lotfi, F. H. (2011). Water quality index development using fuzzy logic: a case study of the Karoon River of Iran. *African Journal of Biotechnology*, *10*(50), 10125–10133.

Seng, J. J. B., Kwan, Y. H., Goh, H., Thumboo, J., & Low, L. L. (2018). Public rental housing and its association with mortality–a retrospective, cohort study. *BMC Public Health*, *18*(1), 665.

Skogan, Wesley. (1990). *Disorder and Decline: Crime and the Spiral of Decay in American Cities*. University of California Press, Berkeley.

Srinivas, J., Purushotham, A. V., & Murali Krishna, K. V. S. G. (2013). Determination of water quality index in industrial areas of Kakinada, Andhra Pradesh, India. *International Research Journal of Environment Sciences*, *2*(5), 37–45.

Stansfeld, S., Haines, M., & Brown, B. (2000). Noise and health in the urban environment. *Reviews on Environmental Health*, *15*(1–2), 43–82.

Thangval, C, Jayapal, P, & Kulkami, K.M. (1987). "Spatial Patterns of Some Infectious Diseases-A Case Study of Ahmedabad City". Ed. Yadav, C.S., *Contemporary Urban Issues*, Concept Pub. Company, New Delhi, p. 235.

Timberlake, J.M., & Ignatov, M.D. (2014). Residential segregation. *Oxford Bibliographies*. https://doi.org/10.1093/OBO/9780199756384-0116. https://www.oxford bibliographies.com/view/document/obo-9780199756384/obo-9780199756384-0116.xml

Trotman, M. (2018). *Regional realities: Impact of stray dogs and cats on the community impact on economy, including tourism impact on livestock, wildlife and the environment*. 2006.

Tyagi, S., Sharma, B., Singh, P., & Dobhal, R. (2013). Water quality assessment in terms of water quality index. *American Journal of Water Resources*, *1*(3), 34–38.

United State EPA 816-F-09-004, May 2009, http://water.epa.gov/drink/contaminants/upload/mcl-2.pdf (Accessed 12 July 2013).

Uslaner, E. M. (2000). Producing and consuming trust. *Political Science Quarterly*, *115*(4), 569–590.

Weather Online. (2019), August 17. https://www.weatheronline.in/UttarPradesh/ Azamgarh/Wind.htm

WHO. (2004). Health & Environment Tools for Effective Decision-Making.

WHO (2009). Unsafe Drinking Water, Sanitation and Waste Management.

WHO (2010). Why urban health matters. World Health Organisation.

WHO. (2012). *Guidelines for Drinking-Water Quality*, Fourth Edition, World Health Organization ISBN 978 92 4 154815 1.

WHO and UNICEF. (2017). *Progress on Drinking Water, Sanitation and Hygiene: 2017 Update and SDG Baselines*. World Health Organization (WHO) and the United Nations Children's Fund, Geneva.

Williams, D. R., & Collins, C. (2001). Racial residential segregation: a fundamental cause of racial disparities in health. *Public Health Reports, 116*(5), 404.

5   Addressing Health Problems Associated with Neighbourhood Environment in Azamgarh City

It is estimated that by 2030, six out of every ten people will be living in cities and at present one out of three urban people, live in slums. Speedy, unplanned and unsustainable patterns of urbanisation is making cities and towns of the developing countries a centrepiece for many environmental and health threats. In case of the Indian cities, rapid urbanisation and increase in the population has led to serious shortage in housing, public and community services. The urban environment has degraded, giving birth to haphazard land use, heavy population concentrations and slums. Rapid urbanisation has surpassed the capacity of most of the cities to make available adequate essential facilities such as housing, water and sanitation, drainage, sewerage, lighting, transport and recreational as well as welfare facilities to its residents (Aftab, 2015). Population and industrial growth, in-migration of people and poor environmental services etc. are the reasons that deteriorate the quality of the urban environment. Environmental quality is a crucial factor in the well-being of people, as people's health is strongly influenced by the health of their neighbourhood environment (Coan and Holman, 2008). Environmental factors, particularly in developing countries, are the basic cause of a considerable burden of death and disease, as estimated 25% of all avoidable illnesses are caused by environmental factors. This includes environmental threats in the work, home and wider community/living environment. Environmental hazards and related diseases kill millions worldwide every year (WHO, 2004). Urban environment generally leads to decreasing physical activities due to factors like overcrowding, heavy traffic, poor air quality and lack of safe public places. Incidence of tuberculosis is also high in urban areas due to overcrowding. A substantial proportion of the overall disease burden in developing countries can be accredited to relatively smaller key areas of the risk. These are unavailability of good quality water, sanitation, poor outdoor and indoor air quality and global environmental changes. Developing countries are particularly burdened by communicable diseases like typhoid, malaria, diarrhoea, amoebiasis, helminthic infections, influenza, filariasis, cholera, hepatitis and jaundice. The health impact of environmental problems is heaviest upon the poor and disadvantaged groups in the underdeveloped countries. Poor people are more vulnerable to environmental threats and health problems such as water and

DOI: 10.4324/9781003442486-6

vector borne diseases. Other neighbourhood issues include overcrowding, inadequate solid waste and waste water management etc. Health risks related to socio-economic condition involve inadequate housing, water supply and quality problems, problems related to cooking fuels and place of cooking, poor sanitation as well as inadequate disposal of waste.

This chapter is in continuity with the previous chapters. In chapter 4 an attempt was made to identify environmental problems at the neighbourhood level. It was found that major neighbourhood environmental problems in Azamgarh city are irregular water supply and water quality problem, over-crowding, inadequate collection and accumulation of waste in the neighbour-hoods, open drains, improper cleaning of drains, air and noise pollution as well as neighbourhood disorder. Environmental problems were prevalent in almost all the neighbourhoods but a domination of environmental issues was seen in the low-income neighbourhoods of city.

In this chapter an attempt has been made to understand the health condi-tion of the city residents with a special focus on the prevalent diseases and their association with environmental problems. The chapter is divided into three sections. In the first section, most frequent diseases in the city that have occurred during the last two years have been identified and analysed thor-oughly. In the second section, risk factors in the neighbourhood environment are identified and their association with the prevalent diseases is examined. Karl Pearson's coefficient of correlation has been used for analysis. In the third section, hypotheses of the study are tested using Karl Pearson's coefficient of correlation.

5.1 Health Status of the Residents

The World Health Organization (1948) defines health as a "State of complete physical, mental, and social wellbeing, and not merely the absence of disease or infirmity" (Grad, 2002). Health can be influenced by several factors ranging from individual to social, cultural as well as environmental factors. People's health is largely affected by their environment. A number of diseases can be attributed to unsafe environmental conditions such as waste accumulation and water logging around houses, air, water and soil pollution, presence of animals as well as poor housing etc.

Among the various health issues around the world, disease is the most com-mon issue faced by each and every human. Communicable diseases like malaria, tuberculosis, AIDS/HIV, both viral and bacterial, cause millions of death every single year (Shah, 2014).

The information regarding the health status of the residents was collected during field survey. To obtain the overall view of prevalent diseases in the city, Out Patient Departments of various government hospitals i.e. District Hospital/Sadar Hospital, Mahapandit Rahul Sankrityayan Mahila Hospital, Chief Medical Office-Azamgarh as well as various private clinics in the city were visited and interviews of the health officials were conducted.

5.1.1 Most Frequent Diseases (Diagnosed) Occurred in the Last Two Years

During the field survey, households were asked to mention the diseases that they have experienced and were diagnosed by health practitioners, during the last two years. From the household's responses, 12 most frequent diseases as mentioned by them are identified for the analysis. These diseases in the descending order are cold and flu (46.83%), malaria (44.49%), diarrhoea (41.30%), cholera (39.74%), skin infections (scabies, ringworm) (39.20%), jaundice (39.03%), dengue (38.32%), typhoid (37.76%), measles (33.51%), chicken pox (25.71%), tuberculosis (4.34%) and asthma (1.65%) (Table 5.1).

Figure 5.1 shows that three most frequent diseases are cold and flu, diarrhoea and malaria reported by 40–50% households while least common diseases, tuberculosis and asthma were found within less than 10% households. Table 5.1 shows that diseases show an increasing trend of diseases moving from high- to low-income neighbourhoods depicting that people living in low-income neighbourhoods are the major sufferers from these diseases. A comprehensive analysis of all the disease has been made to understand their nature and distribution in different neighbourhoods of the city.

5.1.1.1 Common Cold and Flu

Rhino virus is the most common virus, causing common cold. These viruses spread through the air, while in close contact with infected people or with things contaminated with virus. Common cold comes with symptoms like runny or blocked nose, cough and congestion, sneezing, headache, low-grade fever, and a general feeling of malaise. It is the most common acute problem in the US and is accountable for around 37 million (3%) doctor visit every year. The cases of common cold per child per year are parallel in both developed and developing nations. Major victims of common cold are children below six; however adults can also experience two to three colds annually. Common cold is mostly common in winter and spring seasons as it leads people to spend more time inside the houses, where they are in closer contact with persons who are infected. Crowding in the house thus plays an important role in the spread of diseases. Cold are generally harmless and leave without any serious impact. However sometimes after a viral infection, bacteria can spread through the airways and could result in further complications such as pneumonia and sinus infection.

Influenza, which is also known as flu, is a communicable disease and it is caused by an Influenza virus. It is a respiratory illness affecting nose and throat. Flu is highly infectious and it normally spreads by the coughs and sneezes of an ill person. Flu can also be transmitted by touching like shaking hands with the infected person. It comes with symptoms like fever, chills, cough, body ache, headache and fatigue.

Flu differs with common cold at the first place by its causing virus. Although symptoms of both common cold and flu are similar, the main difference

Table 5.1 Neighbourhood-Wise Distribution of Most Frequent Diseases (Diagnosed) as Reported by Residents of Different Neighbourhoods in Azamgarh City (in Percentages)

Neighbour-hoods	Cold and Flu	Typhoid	Malaria	Dengue	Diarrhoea	Skin Infections	Cholera	Jaundice	Chicken pox	Measles	Tuberculosis	Asthma
HI/HD	37	34.67	31	31	33.37	28.76	35	34	26.8	28.95	2.1	2.03
HI/MD	41.46	33.5	37.7	35.89	36.56	37.32	39.41	39	27.9	24.3	1.33	0.98
HI/LD	39.98	29.21	41.52	34.87	34.52	33.8	31.98	31.89	18.71	19.95	3	0
MI/HD	51.98	38.76	41.98	37.67	40.32	44.89	43.45	43.97	28.86	51.65	6.9	1.38
MI/LD	48.98	41.56	47.76	39.86	43.9	41.96	42.57	37.8	20.89	27.42	5.6	2.65
LI/HD	52.66	44.06	52.54	41.31	51.86	42.05	41.8	44.97	31.43	43.65	5.2	3.21
LI/MD	55.75	42.54	58.91	47.67	48.56	45.62	43.98	41.56	25.36	38.62	6.23	1.29
Total	46.83	37.76	44.49	38.32	41.3	39.2	39.74	39.03	25.71	33.51	4.34	1.65

Source: Based on field Survey, 2016–2017.

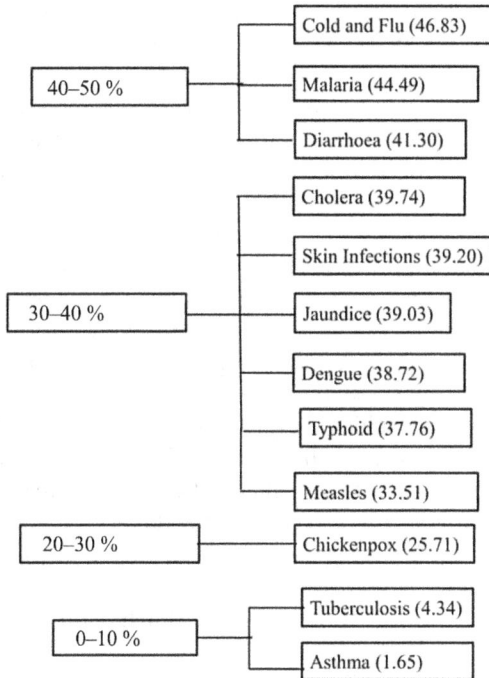

Figure 5.1 Most Frequent (Diagnosed) Diseases as Reported by the Residents of the Azamgarh City.

Source: Based on Field Survey, 2016–2017.

between them is intensity. Flu is more intense and kind of worse than common cold. Flu can also result in very serious other associated complications like viral pneumonia, bacterial pneumonia or sinus infection. The influenza virus that infects the nose and throat sometimes reaches to the lungs too and at times can result in death as well. High-risk groups like infants, pregnant women, elderlies and people with previous respiratory history are more likely to hospitalise or die from the illness

Though common cold and flu were prevalent in all the neighbourhoods of the city, their significant concentration was seen in the low-income neighbourhoods of the city. From LI/MD neighbourhood, 55.75% and from LI/HD neighbourhood, 52.66% households reported constant prevalence of common cold and flu in their houses. Cases from other neighbourhoods include 48.98% from MI/LD, 51.98% from MI/HD, 41.46% from HI/MD, 39.98 per cent from HI/LD and 37% from HI/HD neighbourhoods (Table 5.1).

5.1.1.2 Typhoid

Typhoid also known as typhoid fever is a bacterial infection, caused by *Salmonella typhi*. Symptoms of the typhoid fever are daily fever reaching up to 104°F, headache, weakness and fatigue, muscle pain, sweating, loss of appetite, rashes, swollen abdomen, diarrhoea or constipation and weight loss. Fever, if not treated on time can last up to weeks and months and can give rise to further complications. Typhoid fever can be life threatening in case of one-third of infected persons. A typhoid infection spreads through faecal-oral route. Infected food and water, poor sanitation or direct contact with infected person is the main reasons causing typhoid. People diagnosed with typhoid can contaminate the water supply through their faeces, containing a great concentration of the microbe. Contamination of the water supply can also pollute the food supply. The bacteria can last for weeks in water or sewage. According to the WHO, world-wide, every year, between 11 and 21 million people are diagnosed with typhoid and around 128,000 to 161000 people die due to it (WHO, 2018a). Typhoid cases are the most common ones in underdeveloped countries. In fact, in some Asian countries, incidence of typhoid is as high as 1600 per 1 lakh population. In India alone, in year 2015, 18, 45,997 people were infected and 393 died due to typhoid (Chrisy, 2017). Incident of typhoid reaches to its peak in the rainy season. In fact, it is also called an endemic disease in India. Typhoid is one of the most common diseases in the country and so, in the Azamgarh city. It was reported by 44.06% households of LI/HD neighbourhood followed by 42.54% in LI/MD and 41.56% from MI/LD neighbourhood (Table 5.1).

5.1.1.3 Malaria

Malaria is a vector borne disease caused by a parasite belonging to plasmodium group. It is an infectious disease and affects both humans and animals. Malaria is transmitted by the bite of infested Anopheles mosquito. Plasmodium parasite is transmitted by these infected mosquitoes. With the mosquito bite, the parasite is released into human bloodstream. Symptoms of malaria include fever, fatigue, vomiting, shaking chills, muscle pain, profuse sweating and headache.

Malaria is generally found in tropical and subtropical countries where the parasites can survive. Approximately 219 million people were infected from malaria worldwide in the year 2017 and approximately 435000 people died from the disease (WHO, 2018b).

It has been found that 44.49% households reported of being infected with malaria in the previous two years. Highly affected neighbourhoods were LI/MD (58.91%), LI/HD (52.54%), MI/LD (47.76%), MI/HD (41.98 %) and HI/LD with 41.52 %.

5.1.1.4 Dengue

Dengue is an arboviral or mosquito borne disease caused by dengue virus. Numerous species of the *Aedes type* of female mosquitos, particularly *A.aegypti*, are responsible for the spread of dengue. Symptoms of dengue include sudden, high fever, severe headache, severe joint and muscle pain, fatigue, nausea, pain behind eyes and vomiting. Dengue generally develops in poor urban areas, slums, suburbs and the rural areas however even wealthy neighbourhoods are not immune of it. Social and environmental factors, development of poor areas without basic health services mainly due to increasing urbanisation are associated with revival of dengue disease. Inadequate drainage and waste disposal services facilitate dengue transmission. Dengue causing virus is generally associated with poor water services and sanitation (WHO, environmental management). Climate change may also enhance dengue transmission, as in high temperatures, mosquitos reproduce more rapidly and bite more often. World-wide, every year between 50 and 528 million people become the victims of dengue virus and around 10,000–20,000 people die (Carabali et al., 2015). Dengue was reported by 38.32% of the total sampled households but its highest prevalence was found in LI/MD and LI/HD neighbourhoods, i.e. 47.67% and 41.31%, respectively. In the high-income neighbourhoods, it was reported as 35.89% from HI/MD, 34.87% from HI/LD and 31% from HI/HD neighbourhood (Table 5.1).

5.1.1.5 Diarrhoea

Diarrhoea is the passing of loose and watery stool three or more times a day. Acute diarrhoea is generally caused by *salmonella bacteria*, r*otavirus* or *norovirus*. Symptoms of diarrhoea include passing of watering tools, abdominal pain and cramping, change in the colour of stool, vomiting and general body weakness. In case of diarrhoea, lining of the intestine becomes unable to absorb fluids and keeps on secreting it. This is also known as gastrointestinal infection. It is commonly caused by consumption of infected food or water or from person to person due to poor hygiene. Serious diarrhoea results in fluid loss and may be fatal, particularly in infants and malnourished or non-immune people.

Diarrhoeal disease is the second important cause of under-five children's death. Each year around 525,000 children die due to diarrhoea. Worldwide around 1.7 billion children become the victims of diarrhoea and it is the main cause of child malnutrition. Furthermore, malnourished or non-immune children as well as people suffering with HIV are more prone to lethal diarrhoea. Diarrhoea can be prevented by consumption of clean drinking water, better sanitation conditions and hand washing with soap. Regular and thorough hand washing, after using toilet and before meals, is one of the most efficient ways to stop the spread of diarrhoea.

A perusal of Table 5.1 reveals that diarrhoea was one of the most prevalent diseases in Azamgarh city. About 41.30% of the sampled households reported incidence of diarrhoea in their houses. Neighbourhood-wise analysis revealed that it was most common in LI/HD neighbourhood i.e. 51.86% followed by LI/MD, MI/LD and MI/HD, i.e. 48.56%, 43.90% and 40.32%, respectively.

5.1.1.6 Skin Infections

The term skin infection in the present analysis has been used to describe the skin problems like scabies and ringworm. These are highly contagious skin infections characterised by inflamed skin with severe itching. Scabies is caused by *sarcoptes scabiei*, an eight-legged microscopic mite. It spreads easily in crowded condition from person to person through close physical contact. These are water-washed disease which is caused by poor availability of water through poor personal hygiene. Scabies is estimated to be infecting over 300 million humans worldwide each year. Ringworm is a skin infection that is caused by different types of fungi like Trichophyton, *Microsporum* and *Epidermophyton*. These fungi live on the dead tissues of skin, hair and nail. Ring worm involves red, itchy and scaly patches or raised areas of skin called plaques. The most important preventive measure for these infections is personal hygiene which is greatly affected by availability of water.

Table 5.1 reveals that about 39.20% households reported occurrence of skin infections. Prevalence of skin problems was the highest in LI/MD neighbourhood, i.e. 45.62% followed by MI/HD, LI/HD and MI/LD neighbourhoods, i.e. 44.89%, 42.05% and 41.96%, respectively.

5.1.1.7 Cholera

Cholera is a critical diarrheal disease commonly spreading through infected water. It causes extreme condition of diarrhoea and dehydration. If not cure within time, cholera can be deadly and can kill even the previously healthy people. Cholera is caused by bacteria called *Vibreo Cholerae*. Common sources of the bacteria include public water supplies, foods and drinks purchased from the street sellers, vegetables grown in faeces contaminated water, raw or under-cooked sea food developed in swage contaminated waters. Bacteria after entering in human body along with contaminated food or water, releases a toxin in the intestines and produces severe diarrhoea.

Cholera is a universal peril to public health and remains an indicator of inequality and dearth of social development. It has been assessed that each year around 1.3 to 4 million people become the victims to cholera and around 21000 to 143000 people worldwide die due to it. Availability of safe water and sanitation is crucial to control the diffusion of cholera and other water related diseases (Ali et al., 2015)

Occurrence of Cholera was reported by 39.74% of the total sampled households with the highest prevalence in LI/MD and MI/HD neighbourhoods, i.e. 43.98% and 43.45% followed by MI/LD neighbourhood (42.57%) and LI/HD neighbourhood (41.80%) (Table 5.1). Risk of cholera is higher among poor people who live in crowded settings and without proper sanitation facilities. Common at-risk areas for the cholera are urban slums, where clean drinking water and sanitation are not available to the people.

5.1.1.8 Jaundice

Jaundice is a disease in which skin colour and eye whites turn yellow. It happens due to high bilirubin levels, which occurs because of liver diseases, excessive breakdown of red blood cells. It can also be associated with *hepatitis* or inflammation of liver. The viruses that cause hepatitis A and E can be spread through water and food as well as from person to person. Symptoms of Jaundice include yellow trace on the skin and eye whites, vomiting, high fever, loss of appetite, pale coloured stool and urine, abdominal pain and weakness. Jaundice is commonly linked with itchiness. The major route for jaundice transmission is faecal-oral route. Poor sanitation, crowding and faecal contamination of water and food are the common causes of the infection. Jaundice can spread from person to person in the houses with poor hygiene, insufficient washing after defecation, shared drinking and eating utensils. In the developing nation, poor sanitary and hygienic conditions are the main reason behind jaundice. Prevalence of Jaundice reaches to its peak in rainy season due to deteriorating sanitation conditions. Jaundice ranked 7th out of the 13 most common diseases and was reported by 39.03% of the total sampled households. Jaundice was found the highest in LI/HD neighbourhood, i.e. 44.97% closely followed by MI/HD neighbourhood, i.e. 43.45% (Table 5.1).

5.1.1.9 Measles

Measles is an extremely transmittable infectious disease caused by the *measles virus*. Symptoms of measles include high fever, cough, runny nose, sore throat, red, watery eyes (conjunctivitis). Symptoms appear after 7 to 14 days of infection. After 2–3 days of infection, a tiny white spot also known as koplik spot appears in the mouth and afterwards red rash spreads to the whole body. It is more common among children. Measles is an airborne disease and it spreads through the wheezes, sneezes and coughs of the infected persons. Saliva and nasal secretions too act as carriers for the *measles virus*. Measles if not cured on time can lead to other complications like diarrhoea, middle air infection and pneumonia or some less common issues like seizures, blindness or inflammation of the brain. Measles have been an important cause of death among infants worldwide in spite of the availability of measles vaccine. Around 7 million people were infected by measles in the year 2016 (WHO, 2018). It is more common in the developing countries particularly in Africa and Asia where par-capita incomes are low and health infrastructures are weak. Urban slums and poor neighbourhoods with dilapidated and crowded housing are the victim areas for measles. Measles was reported by 33.51% of the total sampled households out of which the highest proportion was recorded from MI/HD, i.e. 51.65% followed by LI/HD and LI/MD, i.e. 43.65% and 38.62%, respectively (Table 5.1).

5.1.1.10 Chickenpox

Chicken pox, which is also known as varicella, is caused by *varicella zoster virus*is, an extremely infectious disease. It is characterised by small, inflamed, red blisters all over the body. However, the symptoms that appear before the rashes are, a general feeling of being sick, fever, muscle pain, loss of appetite and in some cases, feeling of nausea. After several days of appearance of blisters, crust appears over them and they finally start healing. This usually takes five to seven days. Chickenpox, in case of complications can lead to pneumonia, inflammation of the brain and bacterial skin infections. Chickenpox generally affects children but can affect elders too. In case of elders, it is more severe than children. Once chickenpox infection is over, the virus remains inactive in the human body and in most of the cases infection never happens again. Reactivation of the *varicella zoster virus*, which is generally rare, can result in *herpes zoster. Herpes zoster* happens mostly to the adults.

Chickenpox is an airborne disease and it spreads from an infected person to the healthy ones through the coughs and sneezes. It can also spread from touching of the blisters or saliva of the infected persons. Chickenpox is generally common in low-income neighbourhoods with overcrowded houses. Chickenpox takes place all around the world. In the year 2013, more than 140 million cases of chickenpox and *herpes zoster* were recorded worldwide (Vos et al., 2016). Table 5.1 reveals that 25.71% sampled respondents reported occurrence of chickenpox out of which the highest percentage belonged to the high-density neighbourhoods. Chickenpox was reported by 31.34% households from LI/HD, 28.86% from MI/HD and 26.80% from HI/HD neighbourhoods. Its prevalence was the lowest in the HI/LD neighbourhood, i.e. 18.71%.

5.1.1.11 Tuberculosis

Tuberculosis is a contagious disease caused by *Mycobacterium Tuberculosis Bacteria*. Tuberculosis generally affects lungs, but other parts of the body can also get affected by it. Tuberculosis could be active or latent and about 10% latent infections, if not treated, can develop into active TB. Common symptoms for the active TB are bad cough, loss of appetite, weight loss, fever, weakness, night sweats and coughing off blood or mucus.

Tuberculosis is an airborne disease and its bacteria spread through the air from one person to another. The bacteria spread in the air, through the minute drops released in the air, when the infected person coughs, sneezes or talks. Tuberculosis, if not treated properly, can be fatal (Park, 2007). Approximately 10.4 million new tuberculosis cases were recorded in the year 2016 and around 1.7 million people died of it in the same year. More than 90 % of tuberculosis cases are found in the developing countries with poor health care infrastructure and deficit resources available. Tuberculosis is the number one among the infectious disease causing death. Over 95 % of the deaths take place in under-developed countries and over 50% in India, Indonesia, Philippines, China and

Pakistan (WHO, 2018c). Only 4.34% households reported incidence of TB in their houses out of which 6.23% belonged to LI/MD and 5.6% to MI/LD neighbourhoods. Tuberculosis in the high-income areas was almost negligible (Table 5.1).

5.1.1.12 Asthma

Asthma is a chronic disease of lung characterised by inflammation of airways. The disease causes swelling and narrowness inside the lung, restricting air supply. Symptoms of asthma involve coughing, wheezing and breathlessness. Symptoms can get worse or even bring an asthma attack, if come in contact with asthma triggers. Asthma can be caused by a person's genetic makeup as well as the environment. In the previous studies asthma has been significantly linked with traffic related air pollution (Perez et al., 2013). Each year about 250,000 people die globally due to Asthma (Felman, 2018). Air pollution both in and out the homes can impact the development and triggers of Asthma. Indoor air pollution from burning of cow dung and other solid fuels has also been related with an elevated risk of Asthma (Singh and Jamal, 2013). Only 1.65% households reported incidence of asthma in their houses out of which 3.21% belonged to LI/HD and 2.65% to MI/LD and 2.03% to HI/HD neighbourhood (Table 5.1).

5.1.2 Other Health Problems (Symptomatic)

Other health problems reported by residents (Symptomatic, not diagnosed by doctor, residents were just asked if they are facing these problems) of Azamgarh city were stress (38.66%), sleep disturbances (31.80%), annoyance (29.75%), headache (26.83%), shortness of breath (17.39%), coughing and wheezing (16.15%) and deafness (0.93%) (Table 5.2). These problems though do not get counted into chronic or acute disease but they do lead to serious

Table 5.2 Neighbourhood-Wise Incidence of Most Frequent (Symptomatic) Diseases as Reported by the Residents of Azamgarh City (in Percentages)

Neighbour- hoods	Stress	Deafness	Annoyance	Headache	Sleep Disturbances	Shortness of Breath	Coughing and Wheezing
HI/HD	11	1.67	34.62	29.52	36.52	21.02	18.56
HI/MD	35.05	0.65	30.22	20.13	31.2	14.32	13.23
HI/LD	24.88	1.2	29.65	25.06	34.52	15.23	14.23
MI/HD	50.4	0.96	28.56	29.53	32.56	17.86	16.23
MI/LD	42.83	0.84	34.21	35.56	37.56	18.96	18.58
LI/HD	53.66	1.19	25.89	26.52	29.52	13.23	14.95
LI/MD	52.83	0	25.09	21.52	20.69	14.86	13.25
Total	38.66	0.93	29.75	26.83	31.8	16.49	15.57

Source: Based on Field Survey, 2016–2017.

illness if experienced for longer duration. **Stress** is the most common impact of disorder on resident's health which results from the fear of crime or fear of being attacked and it can damage the health in many ways. It is a mental and biological reaction experienced on coming across a threat that a person can feel but doesn't have means to deal with. Stress can lead to anxiety and further depression. Stress hormones cause blood pressure, heart rate, and blood sugar levels to go up. Prevalence of stress was reported by 38.66% respondents which was the highest in the neighbourhood LI/HD (53.66%) and the lowest in the HI/HD neighbourhood (11%). **Sleep disturbances, annoyance, headache and deafness** are the most common impacts of noise pollution. These can damage physiological and psychological health of the people along with hypertension, high stress levels, increasing blood pressures and incidence of coronary artery disease (Stansfeld and Matheson, 2003). Among all these problems, sleep disturbance was reported the highest (31.80) while deafness was reported the lowest (0.93%). Among the health problems associated with short-term exposure of air pollutants, most remarkable are irritation of eyes, nose and throat, coughing, chest tightness and shortness of breath. Causes of shortness of breath or breathing difficulty include asthma, bronchitis, pneumonia, COPD or allergic reaction. However, it is not necessarily caused by a medical condition and could be the result of exercise, altitude or sedentary lifestyle. Some people may experience shortness of breath for a short time while others may experience it for weeks or more. About 16.49% respondents reported shortness of breath while 15.57% reported problem of coughing and wheezing. Causes of coughing and breathing involve cold, allergies as well as asthma or COPD.

5.2   Risk Factors in the Neighbourhood Environment and Associated Health Issues

In the previous two chapters a thorough analysis of the neighbourhood environment in Azamgarh city has been provided. It has been found that overall city in general and some low- and medium-income counterparts of the city in particular are facing a number of environmental problems. Major neighbourhood environmental problems in the city as identified and discussed in chapter two are neighbourhood overcrowding, narrow or congested streets, traffic congestion, air and noise pollution, substandard housing and slums, insufficient supply of water, heaps of garbage in the neighbourhoods, inadequate drainage and water logging as well as prevalence of neighbourhood disorder.

Risk assessment is the process of spotting and investigating potential issues that could negatively affect a system. Its basic role is identification and evaluation of risks and in turn it also helps in managing those risks. To carry our risk assessment, one needs to find out the possible threats that can harm the system and also an estimation of the likelihood that those threats would reveal themselves. The overall process of risk assessment involves

- Identification of hazards and risk factors that have the prospective to produce harm
- Analysis and association of the risk associated with the harm
- Determination of appropriate ways to eradicate the hazards

Risk factors in the neighbourhood environment are the factors that cause deterioration of the environment and in turn harm the health of the residents. Risk factors are identified with a comprehensive field survey. Following are the risk factors that play catalysing role in harming the environmental quality and resident's health.

- Irregular Water Supply
- Water Quality Problem
- Open drains
- Inadequate cleaning of drains
- Water logging
- Inadequate waste collection
- Neighbourhood Disorder
- Overcrowding
- Air Pollution
- Noise Pollution (Table 5.3)

To test the relationship between risk factors and diseases, Karl Pearson correlation co-efficient technique was applied. "t" test was applied to examine the level of significance.

For the sake of analysis risk factors in the neighbourhood have been divided into two categories.

- Risk factors associated with water, drainage and sanitation
- Risk factors associated with overcrowding, neighbourhood disorder, air and noise pollution

5.2.1 Risk Factors Related to Water, Sanitation and Associated Diseases

Inadequate water supply, water quality problem, open drains, inadequate cleaning of drains, water logging and inadequate waste collection are included in this category. Safety and quality of water are vital to human development and well-being. Many environmental problems are associated with water availability, quality and proper provision for disposal. Most of the water borne diseases like diarrhoea, jaundice, hepatitis A, typhoid, worm-infestation are caused by poor sanitation. In case of inadequate supply, people are compelled to store water by insufficient means which could result in development of microorganisms in the water. Some of the disease vectors like dengue breed in

Table 5.3 Risk Factors in the Neighbourhood Environment of Azamgarh City

Neighbourhoods	Over crowding	Irregular Water Supply	Water Quality Problem	Open Drains	No Cleaning	Water logging	Inadequate Waste Collection	Neighbour hood Disorder	Noise Pollution	Air Pollution
HI/HD	66.66	21.7	41.67	10	69	39.78	20	10.16	47.67	24.48
HI/MD	60	26.07	43.22	34.44	73.33	41.67	45.56	22.21	32.22	18.68
HI/LD	34.17	18.28	41.14	42.22	68.17	33.33	44.17	25.63	35.06	17.24
MI/HD	95	51.53	51.56	45	66	51.98	60	57.93	36.65	19.68
MI/LD	18.33	45.17	46.13	30	73	56.46	78.33	38.89	43.85	26.33
LI/HD	77.6	58.44	51.37	63	82.7	61.25	65.94	58.45	32.5	15.5
LI/MD	64.33	64.91	54.39	69	84.34	67.33	75	53.76	26.23	13.25
Total	59.44	40.87	47.07	41.95	73.79	50.25	55.57	38.14	36.31	19.31

Source: Based on Field Survey, 2016–2019.

Table 5.4 Correlation Coefficient (r) Between Water and Sanitation Related Problems and Associated Diseases

	Irregular Water Supply	Water Quality Problem	Open Drains	Inadequate Cleaning of Drains	Water logging	Inadequate Waste Collection
	(X)	(X_2)	(X_3)	(X_4)	(X_5)	(X_6)
Typhoid(Y_1)	.924**	.836*	0.531	0.686	.959**	0.744
Malaria(Y_2)	.854*	.805*	.883**	.809*	.861*	.876**
Dengue(Y_3)	.884**	.853*	.854*	.808*	.899**	.868*
Diarrhoea(Y_4)	.919**	.844*	.787*	.835*	.931**	.815*
Skin Infections(Y_5)	.897**	.841*	.757*	0.48	.831*	.910*
Cholera(Y_6)	.890**	.858*	0.521	0.499	.885*	.787*
Jaundice(Y_7)	.853*	.870*	0.65	0.506	.777*	0.607

Source: Based on Field Survey, 2016–2019.
** Correlation is significant at the 0.01 level (2-tailed).
* Correlation is significant at the 0.05 level (2-tailed).

clean water, rather than dirty water. In this way, household water storage containers aid as breeding grounds for them. Irregular water supply also forces people to fetch water from unsafe sources, whose quality is not reliable.

Results given in Table 5.4 show a strong positive correlation between the risk factors (6) and occurrence of associated diseases (7). A highly complex relationship was observed with various interacting pathways and non-linear relationships between risk factors and health. The exposure to risk factors is very much significant and sometimes holds long impacts on the residents' health. A perusal of Table 5.4 showing the dimension of relationship between risk factors in the neighbourhood environment and occurrence of associated diseases reveals that the risk factors were found positively and strongly co-related with specific diseases.

- A positive relationship between **irregular water supply** and 7 associated diseases was found. A very strong positive association with typhoid (Y_1) (r= .924**), diarrhoea (Y_2) (r= .919**), skin infections (Y_5)(r=0.897**), cholera, (Y_3) (r=0.890**), dengue (Y_4) (r=0.84**) and jaundice (Y_6) (r= 0.853*) is found. Since irregular water supply compels households to store water, it is strongly associated with the water borne diseases. Irregular water supply is also associated with sanitation related disease like skin infections, typhoid and vector borne diseases like dengue.
- **Problem in water quality** is another risk factor that can threaten the health of the residents. About 47% have reported water quality in the form of dirt, colour and smell. Physico-chemical analysis of the water also revealed that concentration of total dissolved solids, total suspended solids, electrical conductivity and total hardness exceeds the desirable limit in most of the

samples. Problem of smell in the water was also reported which can indicate presence of biological contaminants in the water. A positive relationship between water quality problem and 7 associated diseases was found. A very strong positive association has been found with jaundice (Y_7) (r= 0.870*), cholera (Y_6) (r=0.858*), diarrhoea (Y_4) (r= 0.844*), skin infections (Y_5) (r= 0.841*), typhoid (Y_1) (r= 0.836*).

- A number of diseases like malaria, dengue, chikungunya, typhoid, jaundice and amoebiasis are related with improper drainage system like **open drains**. The most common diseases that are associated with insufficient drainage and water logging are dengue and malaria. Other diseases could be helminthic infections, typhoid, viral, diarrhoea, amoebiasis and ascariasis, etc. A positive relationship between open drains and associated diseases has been shown in Table 5.4. A very strong positive association with malaria (Y_2) (r= 0.883**) and dengue (Y_3) (r= 0.854**) has been found. Association is also strong with diarrhoea (Y_4) (r= 0.844*) and skin infections (Y_5) (r = 0.841*).
- Relationship between **Improper cleaning of drains** and associated diseases has also been shown in Table 5.4. A glance of the table shows that inadequate cleaning of drains is strongly associated with diarrhoea ($_{Y4}$) (r= 0.835*), malaria ($_{Y2}$) (r= 0.80^{9*}) and dengue ($_{Y3}$) (r= 0.80^{8*}).
- The problem of **water logging** is another striking problem found in the city. Relationship between water logging and associated diseases has also been shown in Table 5.4. A strong positive association of water logging has been found with typhoid (Y_1) (r= 0.959**), diarrhoea (Y_4) (r= 0.931**), dengue (Y_3) (r= 0.899**), cholera (Y_6) (r= 0.885*), malaria (Y_2) (r=0.861*).
- **Inadequate waste collection** is a major risk factor that is common in almost all the Indian cities. The problem of inadequate waste collection is a major threat in Azamgarh city where more than 55% people have reported that waste is not collected properly from the streets and heaps of garbage can be seen here and there. Because of the waste thrown on the roadsides, streets, low-lying areas, vacant places and in and outside drains, not only the environment becomes annoying and unhygienic but it also leads to serious environment and health hazards to people. The diseases that could be caused are typhoid, fever, dysentery, diarrhoea, worm-infestation and cholera. A positive relationship between inadequate waste collection and associated diseases has been shown in Table 5.4. A very strong positive association with malaria (Y_2) (r= 0.876**) and dengue (Y_3) (r= 0.868*) has been found. Association is also strong with diarrhoea (Y_4) (r= 0.815*), skin infections (Y_5) (r = 0.910*) and cholera (Y_6) (r= 0.787*).

5.2.2 Risk Factors Related to Overcrowding, Neighbourhood Disorder, Air Pollution and Noise Pollution and Associated Diseases

- Environmental problems associated with **overcrowding** are traffic congestion, worsening air quality, potential reduction of outdoor spaces and noise problem. Diseases that are most related with overcrowding are airborne diseases that spread by the coughs and sneezes of the infected. Since over-crowding is generally prevalent in poor neighbourhood, in those areas there are more chances for diseases to spread from one person to another. Rela-tionship between overcrowding and associated diseases has been presented in Table 5.5. A strong positive association has been found between over-crowding and chickenpox (Y_1) (r= 0.860*) and measles (Y_2) (r= 0.796*). Association of overcrowding is not strong with tuberculosis (Y_{11}) (r= 0.238) and asthma (Y_{10}) (r= 0.119) as incidence of these diseases was not much strong in the city.

- In a neighbourhood where theft, robbery, pick pocketing are common, drunk people roam on the streets and fight, rowdy activities take place very frequently, street prostitution is a common phenomenon, one cannot feel safe either in or outside the house and cannot enjoy complete sense of well-being. Stress is the most common impact of **neighbourhood disorder** on resident's health which results from the fear of crime or fear of being attacked and can lead to health damages in many ways. Stress is a mental and biological reaction experienced on coming across a threat that a person can feel but doesn't have means to deal with. Stress can lead to anxiety and further depression. Since neighbourhood disorder was reported by around 40% respondents of the city, stress was a common response that was recorded. Regarding the association between neighbourhood disorder and stress a very strong positive association has been found between (Y_3) (r= 0.947**) (Table 5.5).
- **Air pollution** has emerged as a major environmental issue in the city as shown by the Climate Agenda report. It has been found that values of both

Table 5.5 Correlation Coefficient (r) between Neighbourhood Overcrowding, Neigh-bourhood Disorder, Air Pollution, Noise Pollution and associated diseases

	Neighbourhood Disorder (X_1)	Overcrowding (X_2)	Noise Pollution (X_3)	Air Pollution (X_4)
Chicken pox (Y_1)	0.368	.860*	−0.21	−0.266
Measles (Y_2)	0.817	.796*	−0.253	−0.296
Stress (Y_3)	.947**	0.295	−0.634	−0.49
Deafness (Y_4)	−0.467	0.041	0.738	0.507
Annoyance (Y_5)	−0.733	−0.49	.916**	.951**
Headache (Y_6)	0.04	−0.286	.785*	.791*
Sleep Disturbances (Y_7)	−0.544	−0.388	.874*	.852*
Shortness of breath (Y_8)	−0.634	−0.115	0.652	0.75
coughing and wheezing (Y_9)	0.048	0.164	0.749	0.723
Asthma (Y_{10})	0.338	0.119	0.302	0.296
Tb (Y_{11})	0.897	0.238	−0.246	−0.194

Source: Based on Field Survey, 2016–2017.

$P_{M2.5}$ and P_{M10} exceeded the national ambient standard at all the monitoring stations of the city. Resident's judgement regarding air pollution however was not found much strong as per the air quality data of Climate agenda report. However, their responses were in conformity with the major pollution hotspots of the city as households located near the traffic intersections and markets as well as along the major roads have reported that air is not good enough in their neighbourhoods. Relationship between air pollution and associated diseases has been presented in Table 5.5. Association of air pollution is not strong with asthma ($_{Y10}$) (r= 0.296) and tuberculosis ($_{Y11}$) (r= 0.-194). Therefore, the weak association suggests that air pollution and air-borne disease are not a major problem in the city. However, data was also obtained regarding the incidence of short term problems associated with exposure of air pollution like shortness of breath, coughing and wheezing, etc. A strong positive association has been found with shortness of breath ($_{Y8}$) (r= 0.750) and coughing and wheezing ($_{Y9}$) (r= 0.723). Since shortness of breath, coughing and wheezing are significant symptoms of major respiratory diseases like asthma, bronchitis, pneumonia and COPD, incidence of these symptoms cannot be neglected and proper attention is necessary.

- An analysis of problem of **noise pollution** in the city revealed that although noise level is within the standard limits for the residential areas however, it exceeds the prescribed standards at commercial and silence zones as well as traffic intersections, therefore households located along the major roads as well as markets complained problem of higher noise in their neighbourhoods. The highest noise pollution was reported from the neighbourhood HI/HD due to the presence of central market, i.e. *Takiya* and constant traffic on the major Gorakhpur Allahabad road and from MI/LD which includes railway station, Taxi Stand as well as major roads of the city. Impact of noise pollution on health has been studied in the form of sleep disturbances, annoyance, headache and deafness. A positive relationship between noise pollution and associated diseases has been shown in Table 5.5. A very strong positive association with annoyance (Y_5) (r= 0.916**), sleep disturbances (Y_7) (r= 0.874*) and headache (Y_6) (r= 0.785*) has been found. Association is also strong with deafness (Y_4) (r= 0.738*). Linear relationship of noise pollution with associated diseases has also been presented with the help of scatter plot (fig 5.12).

5.3 Hypothesis Testing

Hypothesis (H_1): *Neighbourhood environment is significantly associated with resident's health.*

Null Hypothesis (H_0): *There is insignificant effect of neighbourhood environment on resident's health.*

Table 5.6 Correlation between Neighbourhood Environmental Problems and Health
Problems

Variables	N	Mean	Std. Deviation	Correlation (r)	P Value
Neighbourhood Environmental Problems	7	0.00	0.518	0.897**	.006
Health Problems	7	0.00	0.562		

Table 5.6 shows the Karl Pearson's correlation coefficient of neighbourhood environmental problems and health problems. Here, the r value is close to 1, so there exists a strong positive correlation between two variables. A positive relationship between neighbourhood environmental problems and health problems suggests that with increasing neighbourhood environmental problems health problems increase. It shows that prevalence of health problems is higher in those areas with higher environmental problems. Therefore, the null hypothesis of the study mentioned as *"There is insignificant effect of neighbourhood environment on resident's health"* is failed to accept.

Summary

This chapter has attempted to get an overall view of the health condition of the sampled households, identify risk factors in the neighbourhood environment and assess the relationship between neighbourhood environment and prevalent diseases. The chapter has been divided into three sections. In the first section, most frequent diseases in the city that have occurred during last two years have been identified and analysed thoroughly. In the second section, risk factors in the neighbourhood environment are identified. Furthermore, an attempt was made to understand the association between risk factors in neighbourhood environment and prevalent diseases. In the third section, hypothesis of the study are tested using Karl Pearson's coefficient of correlation.

Most common (diagnosed) diseases that were reported by residents are cold and flu (46.83%), malaria (44.49%), diarrhoea (41.30%), cholera (39.74%), skin infections (39.20%), jaundice (39.03%), dengue (38.32%), typhoid (37.76%), chicken pox (25.71%), measles (33.51%), tuberculosis (4.34%) and asthma (1.65%). Other health problems (symptomatic) reported by residents of Azamgarh city were stress (38.66%), sleep disturbances (31.80%), annoyance (29.75%), headache (26.83%), shortness of breath (17.39%), coughing and wheezing (16.15%) and deafness (0.93%). It was found that diseases show an increasing trend moving from high-income to low-income neighbourhoods depicting that people living in low-income neighbourhoods were the major sufferers of these diseases.

Major risk factors identified in the neighbourhood environment were over-crowding, irregular water supply, water quality problem, open drains, improper cleaning of drains, water logging, improper collection of solid waste, over-crowding, neighbourhood disorder, air pollution and noise pollution. Karl Pearson's coefficient of correlation and scatter plots have been used to study the association between these risk factors and prevalent diseases. It has been found that risk factors related to water and sanitation are associated with dis-eases like typhoid, cholera, jaundice, diarrhoea and skin infections. Over-crowding is associated with measles and chickenpox; neighbourhood disorder is associated with prevalence of stress; air pollution is associated with short-ness of breath, coughing and wheezing; and noise pollution is associated with annoyance, sleep disturbances and headache, as explained with significant val-ues of r. Furthermore, hypothesis testing has been performed by using Karl Pearson's coefficient of correlation. It has been found that null hypothesis of the study, i.e. "There is insignificant effect of neighbourhood environment on resident's health", failed to be accepted as suggested by "r" and "p" values of correlation.

References

Aftab, S. (2015). Status of quality of urban environment with special reference to urban planning policy in Aligarh city. Published thesis, Dept. of Geography, Aligarh Mus-lim University, Aligarh. http://hdl.handle.net/10603/70229

Ali, M., Nelson, A. R., Lopez, A. L., & Sack, D. A. (2015). Updated global burden of cholera in endemic countries. *PLoS Neglected Tropical Diseases*, 9(6), e0003832.

Carabali, M., Hernandez, L. M., Arauz, M. J., Villar, L. A., & Ridde, V. (2015). Why are people with dengue dying? A scoping review of determinants for dengue mortal-ity. *BMC Infectious Diseases*, 15(1), 301.

Chrisy, N. (2017). Enteric fever (typhoid) - prevalence & deaths in India. https://www.medindia.net/health_statistics/diseases/typhoid-enteric-fever-india-healthstatistics.asp. (Accessed 07 March 1993.

Coan, T. G., & Holman, M. R. (2008). Voting green. *Social Science Quarterly*, 89(5), 1121–1135.

Felman, A. (2018). What is asthma? https://www.medicalnewstoday.com/articles/323523.php

Grad, F. P. (2002). The preamble of the constitution of the World Health Organization. *Bulletin of the World Health Organization*, 80, 981–981.

Park, K., 2007, *Prevention and Social Medicine*, Banarsidas Bhanot Publisher, Jabalpur, India.

Perez, L., Declercq, C., Iñiguez, C., Aguilera, I., Badaloni, C., Ballester, F., ... & Fors-berg, B. (2013). Chronic burden of near-roadway traffic pollution in 10 European cities (APHEKOM network). *European Respiratory Journal*, 42(3), 594–605.

Shah, Anup (2014). Health issues. *Global Issues*, 5 January.

Singh, A. L. & Jamal, S. (2013). Prevalence of asthma and risk factors inside the poor homes in India: A study. *International Journal of Scientific Research*, 2(10), 1–4.

Stansfeld, S. A., & Matheson, M. P. (2003). Noise pollution: non-auditory effects on health. *British Medical Bulletin*, 68(1), 243–257.

Vos, T., Allen, C., Arora, M., Barber, R. M., Bhutta, Z. A., Brown, A., ... & Coggeshall, M. (2016). Global, regional, and national incidence, prevalence, and years lived with disability for 310 diseases and injuries, 1990–2015: a systematic analysis for the Global Burden of Disease Study 2015. *The Lancet, 388*(10053), 1545–1602.

WHO. (2004). Health & Environment Tools for Effective Decision-Making.

WHO. (2018). https://www.who.int/news-room/fact-sheets/detail/measles

WHO. (2018a). https://www.who.int/immunization/diseases/typhoid/en/

WHO. (2018b). Environmental management. https://www.who.int/denguecontrol/control_strategies/environmental_management/en/

WHO. (2018c). Global tuberculosis report. World Health Organization. Retrieved 2017-11-09.

6 Vulnerable Neighbourhoods

Looking for the Way Forward

Vulnerability assessment has emerged as a complicated area of research in studies related to environment and it has a great scope in the developing countries. Vulnerability can be understood as exposure to certain threat and the incapability to avoid or fight with the expected harm (Lavell, 2003). Most vulnerable are those people, classes and places that have the most likelihood of getting harmed from exposure and have the weakest capability to absorb the harm and recover from it De Sherbinin et al., 2007). In developing countries, a place could be vulnerable due to problems it face owing to unplanned settlements, lack of basic facilities like water and sanitation, insufficient housing provision, air and noise pollution and poverty. Vulnerable places are continuing to increase despite the measure taken to reduce vulnerability (Singh and Jamal, 2012). Cities are exposed to a multitude of environmental problems which disproportionately affect poor communities from vulnerable neighbourhoods. Studies have revealed that with increasing urbanisation, the population of the cities has grown tremendously; however, provision of services has not increased with the same pace and a significant share of the population lives in life-threatening environmental conditions with inadequate essential services. These are mostly poor, living in the disadvantaged neighbourhoods, who are the most affected by the failure of the administration to cope with problems of urbanisation.

Gardon McGranahan in 1990s and his colleagues in 2001 developed a theory named as "Urban Environmental Transition Theory". The theory claims that urban environmental problems are associated with the wealth of the cities, such as in low income cities environmental problems are localised, instant and threat to the health of the people while as cities become wealthy their environmental problems shift from local to global and become a threat to the ecosystem. Thus it has been widely accepted that in the third world cities, main urban problems are local problems having immediate and health-threatening effect and mainly confined in poor urban neighbourhoods (McGranahan and Songsore, 1994). Several studies on neighbourhood effects on health support the notion that wealthy neighbourhoods have better health conditions while poorer neighbourhoods have poor health outcomes (Diez-Roux, 1998; Kawachi and Berkman, 2003).

DOI: 10.4324/9781003442486-7

Environmental problems affect poor and marginalised communities first and the hardest. Poor urban societies generally have less influence over local administration, and usually, their needs are overlooked in city development plans. Identifying neighbourhood vulnerability is an attempt to help government officials, understand a specific neighbourhood's vulnerability, recognise infrastructural gaps and involve urban poor in the planning and implementation process. Comprehensive and specific data at the city as well as neighbourhood level is crucial for a balanced development of the cities. Vulnerability identification is a bottom-up planning process, connecting local knowledge with city planning priorities. It can guide city officials and elected legislatives in designing policies and projects that better address the needs of the vulnerable areas.

This chapter is in continuation of the previous chapter, which has focused on health issues related to neighbourhood problems like typhoid, malaria, worm-infestation, cholera, flu, etc. Relationship between neighbourhood environmental problems and the incidence of diseases were examined, and it was observed that strong association existed between them. In this chapter, an attempt has been made to identify vulnerable neighbourhoods of the city to address their problems and provide plausible suggestions. The chapter has been divided into three sections. In the first section, socio-economic profile of the residents of different neighbourhoods has been examined. In the second section, attempt has been made to identify environmentally vulnerable neighbourhoods. In the third section, major neighbourhood problems and their possible solutions of the city are discussed to find a way forward.

6.1 Socio-Economic Profile of the Residents in Different Neighbourhoods

Socio-economic status refers to the position that an individual occupies in the structure of the society owing to his social and economic conditions (Galobardes et al., 2006). Socio-economic status affects complete human functioning, including both physical and mental health. Socio-economic status incorporates not only income but also educational achievement, financial security, as well as the general perception of social class and social status. Socio-economic status is a continuous and reliable predictor of a massive variety of outcomes through the life span, including physical and mental health. The effects of lower socio-economic status on health can be seen by the impact of poor nutrition, congested and unhealthy living conditions and inadequate health care. It is important to note that the association of socio-economic status and health can be seen at all levels of social hierarchy. Low-income families are significantly more disease prone and therefore need more medical attention. These families also have a lower ability to pay for desirable medical facilities. The poor social classes are more likely to have a variety of behavioural patterns that are not conducive to health i.e. a greater prevalence of smoking and drinking (Smith et al., 1990). A direct result of inadequate attention to health problems in the country is that the population is steadily exposed to high occurrence of infectious diseases. Prevalence of diseases, disabilities and premature deaths is higher in case of lower socio-economic groups (Kunst et al., 2004). There are undoubtedly numerous causal links between socio-economic status and health; income and education affects health, and health affects the capability to be educated and achieve skills for work. Other factors also affect both socio-economic status and health which contribute to the connection between them (Case and Deaton, 2005).

There are mainly two hypotheses that attempt to explain the relationship between socio-economic status and health. The poverty hypothesis states that poor health is a result of poor living condition. People with low income have less to eat, drink contaminated or polluted water and live in dilapidated houses. Consequently, due to their poverty, they may also not get medical services when needed, leading to poor health. Another hypothesis is behavioural hypothesis which states that poor people are involved in health-damaging behaviours such as alcoholism, smoking, use of narcotic drugs and domestic violence, etc. Partly, this may be because the poor also tend to be poorly educated. In urban slums and other areas where poor people live, generally, the behavioural hypothesis predominates. Even earlier definitions of urban slums involved physical, spatial, social and behavioural aspects of poverty (United Nations Human Settlements Programme, 2003).

An individual's health is deeply associated with its economic status and other social factors that are beyond one's control. These factors, also known as social determinants of health, include race, sex, migratory status, religion, and whether one lives in the rural or urban area. Social determinants are important factors affecting health (Wilkinson and Marmot, 2003). Azamgarh city has a heterogeneous structure due to different religions and migration. The favourable facilities of education as well as the availability of employment opportunity, attract people from the neighbouring areas of the city. It has been found that the level of education of a family defines the health status of its members. Discrimination based on caste, also plays a vital role in determining the health status of the family. Bad habits and addiction to harmful materials damages the health of the people.

In this section, general characteristic of socio-economic status (age, sex, religion, caste, income, educational and employment status, marital status, family type and size, migratory status) of the sampled households have been discussed. All these factors directly or indirectly not only affect the health of the people but their neighbourhood environment as well.

6.1.1 Religion and Caste

Religion defines the relation between human being and the sacred or divinity. It is a collection of beliefs that establishes moral values among humans. Religion is one of the most crucial determinants that determine the values, systems, philosophy, tradition and thoughts of people. Many studies have examined the effect of religion on health. The World Health Organization has determined four dimensions of health, viz. physical, social, mental and spiritual health. Certain religious beliefs could have both positive and negative effects on health and morbidity, and it also leads people to certain preferred lifestyle.

Multi-religiosity is an important characteristic found in Azamgarh city. Table 6.1 reveals that most of the sampled households belong to Hindu religion (59.66%) followed by Muslims (38.23%) and Christians (2.10%).

Caste System is one of the important forms of social association in India. The Government of India has classified its citizens into different castes depending upon their social and economic status. Communities from any religious group which are socio-economically advanced, come under the General Caste. Socially and economically backward communities are described as Other Backward Classes (OBC) while people belonging to lower economic strata come under Scheduled Caste (SC). The table reveals that about more than half the sampled respondents/households belong to the general caste (53.92%) followed by other backward classes (26.76%) and scheduled caste (19.32%). The overall picture of the caste shows that share of general caste is the highest in high-income neighbourhoods, i.e. in HI/HD (81.65%), in HI/MD (73.57%), and in HI/LD (69.61%) and vice versa.

6.1.2 Age, Sex and Marital Status

Age can be understood as the length of time that a person has lived. Age affects the decision making of an individual. Age is a crucial factor determining the health of an individual. Ageing deteriorates the health of people with problems like hearing loss, cataract, back and neck pain, diabetes, heart problem and depression. A perusal of Table 6.2 reveals that most of the surveyed respondents were from the age group of 35–44 (46.68%) followed by 45+ (27.48%) and 25–34 (20.69%). Proportion of age group 35–44 was found the highest as generally responsible members of the family belong to this age group.

Table 6.1 Neighbourhood-Wise Distribution of Religion and Caste (in Percentages) of the Sampled Households in Azamgarh City

Neighbourhoods	Religion			Caste		
	Hindu	Muslim	Christian	General	OBC	SC
HI/HD	31.65	67.44	0.91	81.65	16.23	2.12
HI/MD	59.16	36.64	4.20	73.57	11.85	14.58
HI/LD	65.55	31.04	3.41	69.61	21.64	8.75
MI/HD	67.23	32.77	0.00	47.86	34.01	18.13
MI/LD	90.75	3.04	6.21	23.07	41.02	35.91
LI/HD	49.56	50.44	0.00	41.86	35.01	23.13
LI/MD	53.75	46.25	0.00	39.85	27.55	32.6
Total	59.66	38.23	2.10	53.92	26.76	19.32

Source: Based on Field Survey, 2016–2017.

Table 6.2 Neighbourhood-Wise Distribution of Age, Sex and Marital Status (in Percentages) of the Sampled Respondents in Azamgarh City

Neighbour-	Sex		Age in Years				Marital status		
hoods	Male	Female	15–24	25–34	35–44	45+	Married	Unmarried	Widow
HI/HD	53.67	46.33	2.31	17.92	56.85	22.92	91.65	8.02	0.33
HI/MD	49.53	50.47	4.89	25.61	43.31	26.22	87.68	8.75	3.57
HI/LD	55.62	44.38	1.82	16.32	49.33	32.53	90.25	5.56	4.19
MI/HD	40.48	59.52	6.58	27.61	39.21	26.6	83.51	11.58	4.91
MI/LD	47.59	52.41	3.45	14.87	52.94	28.74	90.85	3.08	6.07
LI/HD	42.48	57.52	7.58	26.61	38.21	27.6	81.51	12.58	5.91
LI/MD	50.59	49.41	9.45	15.87	46.94	27.74	88.85	4.08	7.07
Total	48.57	51.43	5.15	20.69	46.68	27.48	87.76	7.66	4.58

Source: Based on Field Survey, 2016–2017.

Sex affects the health of the people by differential exposure to risk factors, access to and understanding of various diseases, attitude towards maintenance of one's health, patterns of services used, as well as perceptions of quality of care. Sex-wise distribution in the Table 6.2 reveals that the proportion of male and female was almost same in the sampled population (51.43% were female, while 48.57% were male).

Studies point out that married people are generally healthier than unmarried people (Schoenborn, 2004). However, many other studies confirmed that marriage had a mixed effect on health behaviours, i.e. it can either lead to behaviours good for health in some people like reduced drinking (Umberson, 1987) or behaviours not good for health in others like gaining of weight (Kahn et al., 1991). An analysis of marital status revealed that more than three fourth respondents were married (87.76%) while rest were either unmarried (7.66%) or widowed or divorced (4.58%).

6.1.3 Income Status

Income is the driving force behind the perceptible health differentials that many societies experience. Income and wealth directly lead to better health as wealthier people have enough money to access the resources that protect and improve health. Greater is one's income, the lesser gets one's possibility of sickness and premature death (National Centre for Health Statistics, USA, 2013). Income can influence health in many ways viz. in a materialistic way like money buys health-promoting belongings, in a psychological way like the stress of not having money, in behavioural manner like people living in deprived condition could be more likely to have unhealthy behaviour, etc. Income status also governs the living standard including social status, literacy, housing condition, nutrition, health and hygiene, directly and indirectly affecting health. Being in poor health further affects education and employment opportunities that subsequently affect health. A wide variation in income was observed among the households of Azamgarh city.

Table 6.3 Neighbourhood-Wise Distribution of Total Monthly Income (in Percentages) of the Sampled Households in Azamgarh city

Neighbourhoods	Total Monthly Income of the Household			
	Very Low	Low	Medium	High
	>5,000	5,001–15,000	15,001–30,000	<30,000
HI/HD	5.56	22.22	28.33	43.89
HI/MD	12.51	14.79	35.3	37.4
HI/LD	3.05	17.19	34.64	45.13
MI/HD	10.36	25	43.75	20.89
MI/LD	14.75	33.49	34.9	16.86
LI/HD	19.56	32.76	32.94	14.75
LI/MD	18.16	27.58	36.98	17.29
Total	11.99	24.72	35.26	28.03

Source: Based on Field Survey, 2016–2017.

Households have been grouped into four categories on monthly family income. The first is high-income category (>30,000 per month) which includes 28.03% households; the second is the medium-income category (25,001–30,000 per month) which includes 35.26% of the total sampled households; third is the low-income category (5001–15,000 per month) which includes 24.72% of the total sampled households; and the fourth one is very low income category (<5,000 per month) which includes 11.99% of the total sampled households. From the Table 6.3, it is clear that proportion of high-income households were higher in high-income neighbourhoods, i.e. 45.13% in HI/HD, 43.89% in HI/HD and 37.40% in HI/MD neighbourhood and vice versa which was also one of the most crucial criteria behind the identification of neighbourhoods.

6.1.4 Educational Status

Income, Education and Occupation are the three significant dimensions of Socio-Economic status while all other social and economic factors are seem to be influenced by these. Education determines the lifetime choices, job opportunities as well as resource availability among humans. It can affect people throughout their lifetime and has been found to increase healthy behaviours and improve health outcomes. Researches have also shown that more educated people tend to live longer (Meara et al., 2008). According to census of India, 2011, about 75% population of Azamgarh city is literate. Table 6.4 reveals that of the total sampled households, 87.50% were educated. The proportion of educated people was the highest in HI/HD (96.55%), HI/MD (94.67%) and HI/LD (93.65%). Of the total sampled households, 24.35% were graduate, 18.29% were postgraduate, 13.97% were educated up to intermediate, 13.31% were educated up to high school level, 10.56% were educated up to primary or middle school level while 19.53% had professional degrees (i.e. Doctors, Engineers, Professors, Pharmaceuticals, Managers and Accountants). The percentage of professionals

Table 6.4 Neighbourhood-Wise Distribution of Educational Status (in Percentage) of the Sampled Respondents in Azamgarh City

Neighbour-hoods	Educational Status		If Educated, up to					
	Educated	Uneducated	Primary/ Middle	High school	Inter-mediate	Graduate	PG	Professional
HI/HD	96.55	3.45	0	2.54	9.85	29.84	36.5	21.27
HI/MD	93.65	6.35	3.88	6.94	13.84	32.93	16.56	25.85
HI/LD	94.67	5.33	5.81	7.31	5.56	24.72	21.54	35.06
MI/HD	84.29	15.71	9.96	15.64	15.54	22.34	17	19.52
MI/LD	78.51	21.49	15.66	17.54	10.56	25.64	21.64	8.96
LI/HD	81.29	18.71	17.96	25.64	20.73	16.34	5.81	13.52
LI/MD	83.51	16.49	20.66	17.54	21.69	18.62	8.98	12.51
Total	87.5	12.5	10.56	13.31	13.97	24.35	18.29	19.53

Source: Based on Field Survey, 2016–2017.

was the highest in HI/LD neighbourhood (35.06%) followed by HI/MD (25.85%) and HI/LD neighbourhoods (21.27%). The percentage of uneducated respondents was the highest in MI/HD neighbourhood (21.49%) closely followed by LI/HD and LI/MD neighbourhoods, i.e. 18.71% and 16.49%, respectively.

6.1.5 Employment and Occupational Status

A perusal of Table 6.5 reveals the distribution of employment and occupational status of the respondents. It shows that of the total sampled households, 80.77 were employed, 14.87 were unemployed while 4.37% were retired. Employed individuals generally have better health than unemployed ones (Ross and Mirowsky, 1995). Occupational status is another critical dimension of socio-economic status and is also an essential device by which livelihood is earned. Better occupations give higher earnings, and higher earnings determine high rank in the society as well as better health.

Of the total employed respondents 29.54% were in different types of government services (teachers, doctors, professors, advocates, bank employees as well as police), 27.93% were engaged in various businesses, 19.79% worked as labourers as well as fruit and vegetable sellers, 6.73% were drivers, 4.45% were tailors while 10.56% were engaged in other activities like *beedi*-making, cultivation, etc. Household survey revealed that proportion of people in various services was the highest in HI/LD, i.e. 53.56% followed by HI/MD and HI/HD neighbourhoods, i.e. 49.64% and 44.21%, respectively; while people belonging to LI/HD, LI/MD and MI/LD neighbourhoods mainly worked as labourers, fruit and vegetable sellers, drivers, tailors and ran small shops (Table 6.5).

6.1.6 Family Type and Size

A family is a social unit comprising of two parents and their offspring living together in a household united by convictions or with common affiliations. The main family characteristics that were taken into consideration are the type and

Table 6.5 Neighbourhood-Wise Distribution of Employment Status (in Percentage) of the Sampled Respondents in Azamgarh City

Neighbour-hoods	Employment Status			If Employed					
	Employed	Unemployed	Retired	Service	Business	Labourer	Driver	Tailor	Other
HI/HD	88.63	7.03	4.34	44.21	31.45	8.13	0	3.21	13
HI/MD	95.01	2.63	2.36	49.64	29	12.89	2.56	0	5.91
HI/LD	89.65	4.58	5.77	53.56	20.77	10.58	4.23	3.09	7.77
MI/HD	78.65	18.56	2.79	18.92	29.65	14.77	17.1	14.56	5
MI/LD	76.89	15.09	8.02	15.62	24.22	30.64	6.25	11.2	12.07
LI/HD	69.32	26.32	4.36	11.62	22.45	28.26	11.36	6.11	20.2
LI/MD	67.23	29.85	2.92	13.2	38	33.23	5.62	0	9.95
Total	80.77	14.87	4.37	29.54	27.93	19.79	6.73	5.45	10.56

Source: Based on Field Survey, 2016–2017.

size of the family. Family could be either nuclear or joint type. A nuclear family consists of husband, wife and their children. While, joint family comprises of spouses, their children, grandparents, families of brothers or sisters, all living and eating together under the same roof.

A perusal of Table 6.6 shows that of the total sampled households, 78.93% comprised nuclear family and remaining 21.07% is joint family. Neighbourhood-wise distribution shows that nuclear families were more in HI/MD neighbourhood, i.e. 90.64, followed by HI/HD, i.e. 89.91%. Analysis of number of families in a joint family shows that two families were living together in 11.88% joint families, three families in 7.55% households while four families were living together in 1.84% households.

As far as number of persons living in a house is concerned, 58.10% houses comprised of 5–10 persons living together, 25.11% houses comprised 1–5 persons while in 16.79% houses comprised more than 10 persons living inside a house. It was observed that households in medium- and low-income neighbourhoods have

Table 6.6 Neighbourhood-Wise Distribution of Family Type and Size (in Percentages) of the Sampled Households in Azamgarh City

Neighbourhoods	Family Type		No. of Families in Joint Family			No. of Persons Living in a House		
	Nuclear	Joint	2	3	4	1 to 5	5 to 10	>10
HI/HD	89.91	10.09	7.86	3.04	0	39.65	60.03	0.32
HI/MD	90.64	9.36	4.55	4.81	0	35.1	55.25	9.65
HI/LD	83.56	16.44	7.75	7.69	1	30.25	56.12	13.63
MI/HD	75.64	24.36	10.85	10.02	3.49	15.64	59.78	24.58
MI/LD	69.53	30.47	20.56	5.6	4.31	23.58	51.31	25.11
LI/HD	68.56	31.44	17.75	11.65	0.56	11.89	68.44	19.67
LI/MD	74.64	25.36	13.85	10.02	3.49	19.64	55.78	24.58
Total	78.93	21.07	11.88	7.55	1.84	25.11	58.1	16.79

Source: Based on Field Survey, 2016–2017.

good proportion of larger family size, i.e. having more than 10 persons in a house, indicating pressure on the sleeping space, food, water, sanitation, health and hygiene, etc.

6.1.7 Migratory Status

An analysis of migratory status in Azamgarh city revealed that nearly three fourth of the respondents have been residing in the city since their birth and only 25.52% households had migrated (Table 6.7). Proportion of migrants was the highest in HI/MD neighbourhood (52.54%) followed by HI/LD neighbourhood (39.21%). The most significant reason found for the migration was employment (63.53%) followed by education (24.31%) and better environment (12.15%). In HI/MD and HI/LD neighbourhoods, migrants were officers of different administrative sectors, professors as well as bank employees that have migrated from different parts of the state as well as country. Education was a major reason for migration of the residents that have come from different parts of the district, to provide better education to their children. Better environment was the reason for migration again for the household that have migrated from different parts of the district. Table 6.7 shows that of the total sampled households 55.12% have been residing in the city for about 10–25 years, 30.43% for 0–10 years while 14.53% for more than 25 years.

6.2 Identification of Environmentally Vulnerable Neighbourhoods of Azamgarh City

In the previous chapters, we have identified many environmental problems as well as problems related to socio-economic conditions in different neighbourhoods of the city. In this part of the chapter, an attempt has been made to identify vulnerable neighbourhoods of the city.

Table 6.7 Neighbourhood-Wise Distribution of Migratory Status (in Percentages) of the Sampled Households in Azamgarh City

Neighbour-hoods	Migratory Status		Reasons for Migration			Years lived in the Neighbourhood		
	Migrant	Native	Employment	Education	Better Environment	0–10	10–25	>25
HI/HD	23.56	76.44	61.88	29.36	8.76	23.64	63.78	12.58
HI/MD	52.54	47.46	55.25	31.19	13.56	14.52	61.92	23.56
HI/LD	39.21	60.79	68.83	21.10	10.07	31.76	54.01	14.23
MI/HD	22.05	77.95	52.56	29.34	18.10	40.21	50.54	9.25
MI/LD	9.59	90.41	65.00	25.00	10.00	57.32	39.65	3.03
LI/HD	13.06	86.94	60.25	20.19	19.56	14.52	61.92	23.56
LI/MD	18.62	81.38	80.95	14.02	5.03	31.76	54.01	14.23
Total	25.52	74.48	63.53	24.31	12.15	30.53	55.12	14.35

Source: Based on Field Survey, 2016–2017.

Neighbourhood environment represents a daily setting for its residents, which can both enhance or limit their physical, mental and social well-being. Therefore neighbourhood living environment of the community should be in such a manner that, it should support hospitality and offer an environment that generates a habitable place. The fact that so many people reside in inadequate environmental conditions, and with speedy urbanisation, this number continues to grow, highlights the importance of assessing the vulnerability of cities in developing countries. Neighbourhood occupants suffer if their air is polluted, water and sanitation are inadequate, waste is not disposed of, and the urban environment is unhealthy (Jacobi et al., 2010). Understanding neighbourhood environment or immediate housing environmental conditions can play a significant role in identifying vulnerable areas and making improvement at decentralised levels.

Since environmental quality is a function of various interrelated as well as multidisciplinary parameters like distribution of open green spaces, built-up density, air quality, noise level, solid waste management, wastewater management, overcrowding, etc.; therefore, measuring environmental vulnerability is a complex problem having many uncertainties and subjective decisions. Hence, decision making in these problems is hard and naturally encompasses various parameters and possibilities. To handle such problems, multi-criteria decision-making method can be adopted due to its ability to define and evaluate objective and subjective measures. Multi-criteria decision making involves a number of options or behaviour patterns when the numbers of alternatives tend to clash with one another. The most popular method of MCDA is Analytical Hierarchy Process (AHP), which determines the weights of the decision factors chosen. Therefore to identify environmentally vulnerable neighbourhoods of Azamgarh city 14 major neighbourhood environmental problems of the city, i.e. irregular supply of water, water quality problem, open drains, poor cleaning of drains, waterlogging, inadequate waste collection, waste accumulation in neighbourhood, overcrowding, narrow streets, air pollution, noise pollution, substandard housing, neighbourhood disorder as well as unequal distribution of amenities in different neighbourhoods were identified as decision criteria (Figure 6.1).

For analysis, the sub-criteria of all the decision criteria were given different weights in the form of ranks, ranging from 1 (most vulnerable vulnerable) to 7 (least vulnerable) (Table 6.8). Fourteen decision factors, i.e. irregular water supply, open drains, improper cleaning of drains, waterlogging, waste accumulation, inadequate waste collection, narrow streets, substandard housing, overcrowding and neighbourhood disorder, water quality index, air pollution ($PM_{2.5}$ and PM_{10}), noise pollution (Sound levels (in dB)) and kernel density map of amenities and facilities were considered for the analysis.

All the 14 decision factors were assigned weights by using analytical hierarchy process through pairwise comparison by creating a ratio matrix (Table 6.8). The pairwise comparison elements were selected based on existing literature,

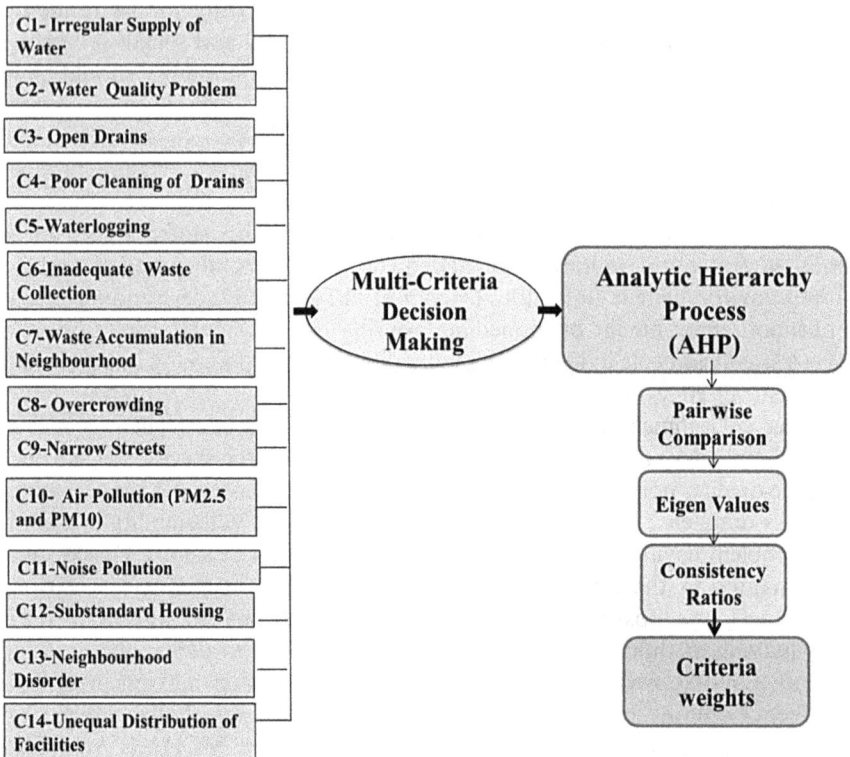

Figure 6.1 Criteria Selected to Measure Environmental Vulnerability in Azamgarh City.
Source: Based on Field Survey, 2016–2019.

Table 6.8 Weights of All the Sub-Criteria for Environmental Vulnerability in Azamgarh City

Serial Number	Decision Criteria	Neighbourhoods	Sub-Criteria	Weights (Ranks)
1	Irregular Supply of Water	HI/HD	21.7	6
		HI/MD	26.07	5
		HI/LD	18.28	7
		MI/HD	51.53	3
		MI/LD	45.17	4
		LI/HD	58.44	2
		LI/MD	64.91	1

(Continued)

Table 6.8 (Continued)

Serial Number	Decision Criteria	Neighbourhoods	Sub-Criteria	Weights (Ranks)
2	Open Drains	HI/HD	10	7
		HI/MD	34.44	5
		HI/LD	42.22	4
		MI/HD	45	3
		MI/LD	30	6
		LI/HD	63	2
		LI/MD	69	1
3	Improper Cleaning of Drains	HI/HD	75	4
		HI/MD	73.33	5
		HI/LD	54.17	7
		MI/HD	55	6
		MI/LD	95	1
		LI/HD	82.7	3
		LI/MD	84.34	2
4	Waterlogging	HI/HD	42.78	6
		HI/MD	46.67	5
		HI/LD	33.33	7
		MI/HD	51.98	4
		MI/LD	56.46	3
		LI/HD	67.33	1
		LI/MD	59.25	2
5	Inadequate Waste Collection	HI/HD	20	7
		HI/MD	45.56	5
		HI/LD	44.17	6
		MI/HD	60	4
		MI/LD	78.33	1
		LI/HD	65.94	3
		LI/MD	75	2
6	Waste Accumulation	HI/HD	20	7
		HI/MD	45.56	5
		HI/LD	44.17	6
		MI/HD	60	4
		MI/LD	78.33	1
		LI/HD	65.94	3
		LI/MD	75	2
7	Overcrowding	HI/HD	66.67	6
		HI/MD	70	4
		HI/LD	60	7
		MI/HD	70	4
		MI/LD	88.33	1
		LI/HD	79.71	3
		LI/MD	84.66	2
8	Narrow Streets	HI/HD	80	2
		HI/MD	54.99	3
		HI/LD	15.83	6
		MI/HD	100	1
		MI/LD	11.67	7
		LI/HD	45	4
		LI/MD	33.33	5

(*Continued*)

Table 6.8 (Continued)

Serial Number	Decision Criteria	Neighbourhoods	Sub-Criteria	Weights (Ranks)
9	Substandard Housing	HI/HD	7.77	7
		HI/MD	15.2	5
		HI/LD	13.8	6
		MI/HD	16.82	4
		MI/LD	26.4	3
		LI/HD	30.68	2
		LI/MD	35.53	1
10	Neighbourhood Disorder	HI/HD	10.16	7
		HI/MD	22.21	6
		HI/LD	25.63	5
		MI/HD	57.93	2
		MI/LD	38.89	4
		LI/HD	58.45	1
		LI/MD	53.76	3
11	Water Quality Index		93–103	5
			104–113	4
			114–122	3
			123–132	2
			133–142	1
12	Air Pollution	$PM_{2.5(\mu g/m^3)}$	114–162	5
			163–210	4
			211–258	3
			259–306	2
			307–354	1
		$PM_{10(\mu g/m^3)}$	250–370	5
			308–364	4
			365–421	3
			422–479	2
			480–536	1
13	Noise Pollution Sound Level (dB)		54.36–59.54	5
			59.55–64.52	4
			64.53–69.49	3
			69.5–74.47	2
			74.48–79.45	1
14	Facilities and Amenities Density		V. High	5
			High	4
			Medium	3
			Low	2
			V. Low	1

Source: Based on Field Survey, 2016–2019.

field knowledge as well as discussion with experts. Saaty's mathematical scale, ranging from 1 to 9, was used in the pairwise comparison matrix. The weights of all the decision factors are shown in Table 6.9, together with the consistency index (CI) and consistency ratio (CR) values. The value of consistency ratio is 0.08 which is below 0.1, i.e. acceptable (Saaty, 1980).

Table 6.9 Weights of All the Decision Criteria (Pairwise Comparison: Analytic Hierarchy Process) for Environmental Vulnerability in Azamgarh City

	Irregular Water Supply	WQI	Open Drains	Poor Cleaning of Drains	Water-logging	Inadequate Waste Collection	Waste Accumulation	Over-crowding	Narrow Streets	Air Pollution	Noise Pollution	Substandard Housing	Neighbour-hood Disorder	Unequal Amenit's Distribution	Normalised Weights
Irregular Water Supply	1	1	4	3	4	5	5	3	4	2	3	4	3	5	0.17
WQI	1	1	5	3	3	4	4	3	5	2	3	4	3	5	0.16
Open Drains	0.25	0.2	1	0.33	0.33	2	2	2	3	0.25	0.33	3	2	3	0.05
Poor Cleaning of Drains	0.33	0.33	3	1	2	2	2	2	3	2	2	3	2	2	0.08
Waterlogging	0.25	0.33	3	0.5	1	3	3	4	5	2	3	3	2	3	0.11
Inadequate Waste Collection	0.2	0.25	0.5	0.5	0.33	1	2	2	2	0.33	0.33	0.5	2	2	0.04
Waste Accumulation	0.2	0.25	0.5	0.5	0.33	0.5	1	3	3	2	3	2	2	2	0.07
Overcrowding	0.33	0.33	0.5	0.5	0.25	0.5	0.33	1	3	0.33	0.5	2	3	0.5	0.04
Narrow Streets	0.25	0.2	0.33	0.33	0.2	0.5	0.33	0.33	1	0.2	0.33	0.5	0.5	0.5	0.02
Air Pollution	0.5	0.5	4	0.5	0.5	3	0.5	3	5	1	4	4	3	3	0.09
Noise Pollution	0.33	0.33	3	2	0.33	3	0.33	2	3	0.25	1	4	3	2	0.06
Substandard Housing	0.25	0.25	0.33	3	0.33	2	0.5	0.5	2	0.25	0.25	1	0.33	0.2	0.03
Neighbourhood Disorder	0.33	0.33	0.5	2	0.5	0.5	0.5	0.33	2	0.33	0.33	3	1	1	0.04
Unequal Amenities Distribution	0.2	0.2	0.33	2	0.33	0.5	0.5	2	2	0.33	0.5	5	1	1	0.04

Source: Based on Field survey, 2016–2019.

CI 0.12 CR 0.08.

Calculated on the basis of Saaty.

Where CI – Consistency Index CR- Consistency Ratio.

CR and CI of 0.1 or below is considered acceptable. (Saaty, 1980).

Weighted linear combination technique was used to generate the final vulnerability map. It was performed after standardisation and calculation of weightage for each criterion using Analytical Hierarchy Process.

• Sub-Criteria weights (Ranks) were calculated by researcher, weight 1 equals to most vulnerable and 7 equals to least vulnerable

In the first step, weighted layers of decision criteria were produced using reclassify tool after assigning weights to different sub-criteria of the decision criteria. In the second step, weighted layers of all the decision criteria were combined while considering weights of each decision criteria calculated from AHP method (Figure 6.2).

The combination of weighted layers of different decision criteria, using weighted linear combination technique, produced the neighbourhood environmental vulnerability map of Azamgarh city. In the final vulnerability map, the weighted values have been divided into three classes with the use of classification analysis technique from "most" to "least" and following portrayals have been assigned from higher to lower values (Figure 6.3 and Table 6.10)

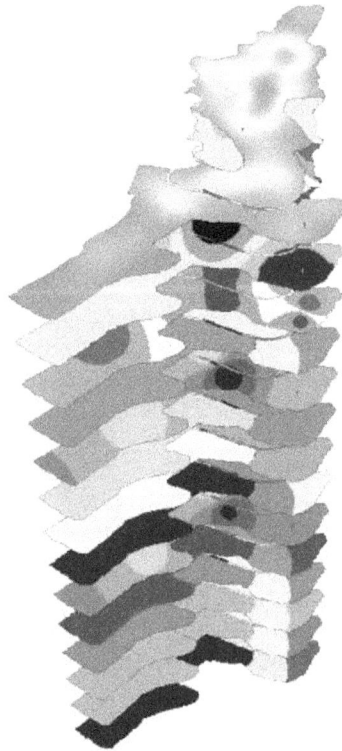

Figure 6.2 GIS Integration (Weighted Linear Combination) to Generate Environmental Vulnerability Map of Azamgarh City.

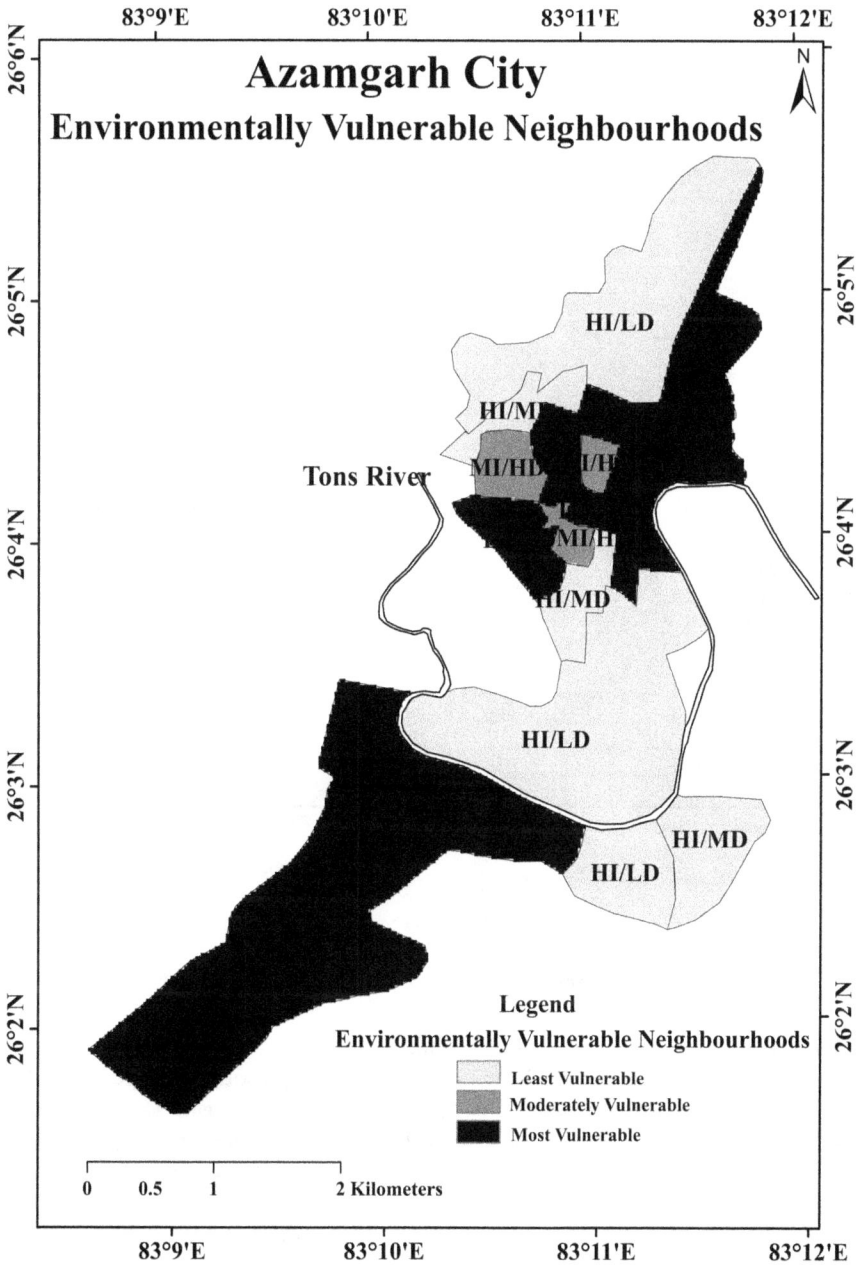

Figure 6.3 Azamgarh City: Identification of Environmentally Vulnerable Neighbourhoods.
Source: Based on Field Survey, 2016–2019.

Table 6.10 Identification of Environmentally Vulnerable Neighbourhoods by Weighted
Linear Combination Technique in Azamgarh City

Category	No of Neighbourhoods	Percentage of the Total Neighbourhoods	Name of the Neighbourhoods	Name of Wards
High (Most Vulnerable)	3	42.86	LI/HD, LI/MD, MI/LD	Bazbahadur, Seetaram, Jalandhari, Paharpur, Farashtola, Pandeybazaar, Ailval, Sadavarti, Ghulamikapura, Gurutola, Harbanshpur, Sarfuddinpur, Narauli,
Medium (Moderately Vulnerable)	2	28.57	MI/HD, HI/HD	Badarka, Katra, Asifganj
Low (Least Vulnerable)	2	28.57	HI/MD, HI/LD	Sidhari East, Arazibagh, Matbarganj Civil Lines, Raidopur, Mukeriganj, Heerapatti, Sidhari West, Madya

Source: Based on Field Survey, 2016–2019.

- Most vulnerable neighbourhoods
- Moderately vulnerable neighbourhoods
- Least vulnerable neighbourhoods

From the final environmental vulnerability map generated (Figure 6.3), it was found that the LI/HD and LI/MD and MI/LD neighbourhoods come under **the most vulnerable** category. LI/HD neighbourhood cover wards namely Bazbahadur, Seetaram, Jalandhari and Paharpur and LI/MD neighbourhood cover, Farashtola, Pandeybazaar, Ailval, Sadavarti, Ghulamikapura and Gurutola wards and MI/LD neighbourhood cover wards Harbanshpur, Sarfuddinpur and Narauli. These are basically low-income neighbourhoods, occupied mostly by poor and middle income population groups. These neighbourhoods are mostly situated in the highly congested central old part of the city, along the river Tons and in the southern extension of the city. In these neighbourhoods, there is a high density of low-income households living in dilapidated housing and slum-like conditions. These neighbourhoods face lots of environmental issues due to improper waste collection services by the municipality, inadequate water supply which is dependent upon municipal water system, improper drainage system (open drains and inadequate cleaning of drains) as well as water logging in the neighbourhood. Overcrowding and narrow streets are other problems of LI/HD and LI/MD neighbourhoods. These neighbourhoods have predominant environmental degradation and unhealthy conditions. It can be seen that the health impact of environmental risks is more upon the poor and vulnerable population. These are basically poor people that have least access to clean water, and more exposed to environmental problems like waterlogging, solid waste, overcrowding, etc. In MI/LD, although crowding condition was not found, but being away from the city centre, municipal services were poor in this neighbourhood. Waterlogging, air and noise pollution, open drains, overflowing wastewater, garbage dumps, etc., are the problems of this neighbourhood. Air and noise pollution was higher in MI/LD neighbourhood due to the presence of major taxi stand like Narauli in it. Provision of health, educational and recreational services is especially inadequate in this neighbourhood due to their distance from the city centre, as all the major amenities and facilities are located in the central part of the city. Majority of the households from these wards were found engaged in various unorganised activities like fruit and vegetable selling, working as labourers, auto drivers, beedi-making, running small shops at home as well as selling handmade crafts.

The **moderately vulnerable neighbourhood** include MI/HD and HI/HD neighbourhood covering two wards namely Badarka and Katra in MI/HD and Asifganj in HI/HD neighbourhood. MI/HD neighbourhood spreads over most crowded part of the city having water logging problem, open drains, overflowing wastewater, garbage dumps, etc. Overcrowding, narrow streets and neighbourhood disorder were other significant problems of this neighbourhood. In HI/HD neighbourhood, i.e. in Asifganj ward, although municipal services are satisfactory, but being located in the central part of the city, it is suffering from the issues like overcrowding and narrow streets. Air and noise pollution were also reported from this ward due to the presence of the central market, i.e. *Takia* in it. Other problems of this neighbourhood were accumulation of waste and unsatisfactory cleaning of drains. These neighbourhoods spread over most crowded part of the city having dilapidated housing condition in *Harijanbasti* and Kundigarh in Katra. However, housing condition was found better in Friends colony in Badarka ward.

The **least vulnerable category** includes HI/MD and HI/LD neighbourhoods. It incorporates wards namely, Sidhari East, Arazibagh and Matbarganj, Civil Lines, Raidopur, Mukeriganj, Heerapatti, Sidhari West and Madya. Major part of this kind of neighbourhoods is occupied by high-income counterparts of the city inhabited by business and service class residents. Municipal services like waste collection are comparatively better in these neighbourhoods, and these are the well-developed residential areas. Mostly these kinds of neighbourhoods are located in outer parts of the city, in northern and southern extension, in less crowded areas; however, Matbarganj and Arazibagh are located in the inner city. It is not the fact that neighbourhood environmental problems do not exist in these neighbourhoods, but their degree or intensity is low in comparison to other counterparts of the city.

Educational, health and other recreational facilities are very well distributed in these neighbourhoods. Some of the best residential colonies of the city, i.e. Millat Nagar, Hariaudh Nagar, Officers Colony, Judges Colony, Teachers Colony, Nagar Palika Colony, Ali Ausat Colony, Thandi Sadak Colony, Christians Colony, Police Line Colony, Nirala Nagar and Shivajinagar colony, etc., can be found in these neighbourhoods. Mostly officers, servicemen, professors, teachers, doctors and lawyers reside in these colonies. However, some *Harijanbastis* and *Mallahbastis* can also be seen in the wards Sidhari East, Arazibagh, Mukeriganj, Raidopur and Madya but a dominant character of high-income households is prominent.

However, some environmental problems prevail practically in all the neighbourhoods. These problems are accumulation of waste, presence of open drains around houses, poor cleaning of drains, waterlogging in the neighbourhoods and problem in quality of water. Their intensity varies among different neighbourhoods, but the situation was unsatisfactory in all of the neighbourhoods.

Since, lots of environmental problems were found in different neighbourhoods, often leading to threatening living conditions resulting in serious health issues, therefore to improve human health, enhancement in neighbourhood living environment can help to its maximum.

6.3 Major Neighbourhood Problems and the Way Forward

6.3.1 Water Supply and Quality

Under the Indian constitution, water supply and sanitation is the state's responsibility and in urban areas, urban local bodies, i.e. Municipalities are in charge of it. Data has revealed that municipal water was supplied to about half of the households while others, either have submersible connections inside houses or fetch water from outside the premises.

- It has been found that municipal water supply services do not cover the entire city and some low-income wards of the city, like Narauli ward, *harijanbastis* in Raidopur ward, Purajodhi in Heerapatti and Kaleenganj in Farashtola and parts of Ailval ward, are practically devoid of municipal water supply. Water supply facility should be extended to these areas to remove any kind of disparity. For elevated areas like Ailval, high-pressure water supply is suggested.
- Increasing water supply hours and ensuring water availability to households, restricting the use of illegal motor pumps to draw water from municipal pipes may work positively in ensuring clean and regular water supply.
- Proper cleaning of water tanks should be assured. Old and rusted pipes should be replaced and care should be taken to spot out any leakage from the water pipes so that immediate actions should be taken.
- Regular cleaning and chlorination of water tanks must be assured to check bacterial growth in the water, mainly in summers.

- Illegal water connections should be checked and restricted immediately.
- Dry hand pumps should be taken care of, especially in low-income neighbourhoods.

6.3.2 *Drainage and Solid Waste Management*

With the previous analysis, it has been found that drainage and solid waste management suffer from several drawbacks in the city. Waste collection and disposal services are not efficient, and heaps of garbage can be seen here and there. Open and choked drains and waterlogging sites are a regular feature in the city.

With rapid urbanisation, the city has experienced tremendous growth of population, but the drainage system has not developed with the same pace. Therefore increasing capacity of the drains is the foremost need of the city.

- Proper cleaning and timely de siltation of drains is prerequisite for the entire drainage system to work efficiently.
- Municipality needs to strengthen drainage network to cover every part of the city as, during the survey, proper drains were not found in some low-income neighbourhoods of the city.
- Disposal of wastewater is the major issue in the city as total wastewater generated is disposed of in the Tons River, which is environmentally as well aesthetically a jeopardy. Currently, there is no wastewater treatment plant in the city; however installation of STP has been passed recently in the city.
- Awareness among people to dispose of their wastewater in closed drains.

Since all the neighbourhood environmental problems are interrelated, no problem can be solved in isolation. Proper solid waste management is necessary for proper wastewater management. With efficient waste collection services, chances of drains to get choked due to solid waste would be reduced; enhancing the free flow of water and reducing waterlogging sites. The following measures could be taken to tackle the problem of solid waste management in the city:

- First and foremost action to tackle the solid waste problem is to reduce and reuse the waste. Reusing is most essential to reduce the waste generated. This is especially useful to handle plastic pollution. Use of plastic should be minimised, and plastic items should be reused at their fullest before dumping them into the garbage.
- Residents are needed to be encouraged for waste segregation at home and keep biodegradable and non-biodegradable waste in separate closed dustbins at home, before disposal.
- One of the main reasons behind the insufficient waste collection was the lack of sanitation workers. Therefore, every part of the city is not covered in a day as sanitation workers cover one part of the city one day and other parts on another day. Therefore, increasing staff of sanitation workers as well as providing more infrastructures could be a solution to this problem.

- Door to door collection services should be provided to curtail the number of disposal sites creating heaps of garbage in the neighbourhoods.
- Proper waste collection points were not found in the city. Dustbins need to be placed in residential areas, separate for biodegradable and non-biodegradable waste.
- Community participation is necessary for any action to be completed. Households need to cooperate with municipal workers to keep their surroundings clean.
- Neighbourhood-level disparity in waste collection system needs to be stopped, and every part of the city should be covered. Low- and medium-income neighbourhoods should not be left out by these services.
- All the tractors and trolleys involved in the transportation of solid waste must be covered properly to avoid littering on the roads.
- Waste disposal site in the city creates several health hazards ranging from water, soil and air pollution, etc. Since a new waste disposal site has been developed outside the city, disposal within the city needs to be stopped immediately.
- Burning of waste inside the city should be discouraged.
- Biodegradable waste can be processed by composting and vermicomposting.

6.3.3 Neighbourhood Overcrowding

Overcrowding is one of the most striking problems of Indian cities. Overcrowding is a consistent result of over-population in urban areas. Overcrowding both at the neighbourhood level as well as within the homes in the form of persons per bedroom and floor space per person was found in the city. It has been found that residential density and neighbourhood overcrowding is the highest in the old central part of the city consisting of wards Bazbahadur, Paharpur, Seetaram, Jalandhari, Gurutola, Badarka, Katra, Sadavarti and Asifganj. Overcrowding within the house measured with the help of persons per bedroom was also found prevalent in LI/HD, LI/MD and MI/HD neighbourhoods, i.e. wards Bazbahadur, Paharpur, Seetaram, Jalandhari, Gurutola, Badarka, Katraand Sadavarti, revealing the prevalence of overcrowding in the old central part of the city.

- The most crucial reason behind overcrowding in the central region is that almost all of the services like hospitals, educational and recreational facilities are concentrated in the central part of the city. Therefore development of infrastructure like houses, schools, supermarkets, hospitals, etc., in outer parts may help the movement of people from central to peripheral areas.
- The most important reasons for overcrowding in the city are natural density and migration. A considerable share of migrants in the Azamgarh city belong to surrounding villages from the district that have moved for educational facility and better infrastructure. Therefore development of better infrastructure in the district can help check the rate of migration in the city.

- Data on overcrowding can also be used to calculate the need for additional housing in the city. Development of housing facilities and infrastructure in outer parts of the city can help to move the population from inner to outer areas.

6.3.4 Air Pollution

Air Pollution is one of the emerging and most prominent problems in Azamgarh city. It was found that, values of PM_{10} and $PM_{2.5\ at}$ all the monitored stations were higher than national standards for ambient air quality. At some stations it is three to four times higher than the national standard. The highest values were recorded in Paharpur in LI/HD neighbourhood and in Narauli in MI/LD neighbourhoods. Air quality was considerably fair in the Civil Lines but the value exceeded than national average standard. Responses of the residents regarding air pollution were in conformity with the locations of their houses. Households located near the traffic intersections and markets as well as along the major roads have reported that air is not good enough in their neighbourhoods. These were basically HI/HD neighbourhood with the presence of central market *Takia* in it and MI/LD neighbourhood with the presence of a major taxi stand Narauli and major roads in it.

- It has been found that major sources of air pollution in the city are dust on the bumpy roads, diesel generators, weaker public transport, waste burning and uncontrolled construction activities.
- The very first strategy to combat air pollution in Azamgarh city is setting up continuous air quality monitoring stations for appraisal of severity of problem in the city.
- Road construction as well as other construction activities along roads needs to be completed at faster pace to help make the roads dust free.
- Maintenance of roads is necessary to reduce the transportation time of a vehicle moving on the poor roads.
- Auto-rickshaws are one of the major means of transport within the city and mostly they were found using kerosene mixed fuels which are the major contributors to particulate pollution in the air. Strict monitoring for usage of adulterated fuels will ensure less pollution.
- Introduction of CNG autos in Azamgarh city could be of great help for which setting up gas of stations is also required.
- Maximum use of e-rickshaw in the city should be encouraged.
- Use of battery-operated scooty is another sustainable solution.
- Another major source of pollution in the city is diesel generators mixed with kerosene. Since power cut is the reason behind maximum use of generators, therefore continuous supply of electricity can reduce this problem.
- Practice of waste burning in the city needs to be stopped.
- Strict vigilance and transparency should be deployed by pollution control agencies while providing PUC (Pollution under Control) certificate to the vehicles.

- Old vehicles should be repaired and replaced if needed.
- Mass awareness programmes for reduction of air pollution in the city should be incorporated. People are needed to be encouraged towards more sustainable ways of transport like bicycles, CNG vehicles, electric vehicles, e-Rickshaws, Car-pooling, etc.
- Greening of Azamgarh city by creating more green patches such as parks, planting of saplings and trees, may also reduce air pollution through pollution absorption.

6.3.5 Noise Pollution

Noise pollution analysis revealed that noise level is within the standard limits for the residential areas however, it exceeds the prescribed standards at commercial and silence zones as well as traffic intersections (Table 2.9). Traffic has been found the major source of noise pollution in the city. Households located along the major roads as well as markets complained of loud noise in their neighbourhoods. Neighbourhoods that have complained noise pollution are HI/HD and MI/LD. The HI/HD neighbourhood is located in the downtown of the city and presence of central market, i.e. *Takiya* and constant traffic on the major Gorakhpur Allahabad road, makes it the most busy and noisy places of city. The neighbourhood MI/LD is located in the southern part of the city which includes railway station, taxi stand as well as major roads of the city; therefore, exposure to noise pollution was higher in this neighbourhood. Since traffic has been found as the major source of noise pollution in the city, therefore;

- Restrictions should be posed on hydraulic horns.
- Use of silencers should be encouraged.
- Old and noisy vehicles should be banned or renewed.
- Awareness programmes should be organised at local levels about harmful effects of noise pollution.
- Plantation of noise-absorbing trees/noise barriers along major roads may be enhanced.
- Maintenance of roads can also help with low noise surface.
- Diverting traffic from inner Allahabad Gorakhpur highway that runs through the city to Baitholi bypass may reduce the existing problem.
- Since major sufferers of noise pollution in Azamgarh city are silence zones, therefore declaration of a no horn zone around hospitals and schools could help to solve the problem.

6.3.6 Neighbourhood Disorder

Safety is the forefront of every resident's mind, and it can be worrisome to learn about theft, robbery, pick-pocketing and rowdy activities in one's neighbourhood. Higher crime rate whether theft, pick-pocketing, robbery, drug dealing, and people fighting can affect the feeling of security at home. Neighbourhoods most affected by neighbourhood disorder are MI/HD, LI/HD and LI/MD covering wards namely Badarka, Katra, Bazbahadur, Seetaram, Jalandhari and Narauli. Living in a neighbourhood where theft, robbery, rowdy activity and other incivilities are common may result in recurrent fear which produces hormones that directly or indirectly weaken the health. Neighbourhood disorder is a community problem and can be solved by proper community action only.

- Healthy social relations among neighbours are prerequisite for a healthy social environment in a neighbourhood.
- Hosting community meetings to discuss neighbourhood disorder issues can also be a great help.
- Counselling of local youths to solve the problem.
- One of the primary strategies to fight neighbourhood disorder is employment generation as local crimes are mostly due to unemployed or underemployed people. Unemployment issues can cause potential dangers, i.e. psychological problems of the individuals to the society.
- Improvement of street lighting is a considerable measure to enhance neighbourhood security.
- Taking good care of homes, i.e., making sure that windows and doors are in good order and are locked properly. If a neighbour's house is empty for a while, it should also be taken care of.
- Involvement of local police can also help in the eradication or at least reduction of neighbourhood disorder.
- Neighbourhood watch programmes should be conducted by community members in the time of extreme threats.

6.3.7 *Inadequate and Unequal Distribution of Amenities and Facilities*

Unequal distribution of amenities and facilities is a crucial problem identified in Azamgarh city. Health and well-being of residents greatly depend upon the availability of various opportunities, services, facilities and amenities in the neighbourhoods. Resident's access to quality of the community services, educational and employment opportunities, transportation and other public services, greatly depends upon how near or far they are located. Density maps of educational, health, recreational and religious facilities reveal that major hotspot of all these facilities can be spotted near the city centre, covering wards namely Asifganj, Paharpur, Pandeybazar, Mukeriganj, Arazibagh and Matbarganj (Figure 2.17). The density of amenities and facilities is also satisfactory in the Civil Lines area of the city. It has been found that the lowest density of educational, health, as well as recreational facilities, has been observed in MI/LD neighbourhood, mainly in the wards Sarfuddinpur and Harbanshpur. Therefore, development of these facilities in this part of the city can help the residents. The density of the facilities was also found low in Sidhari East and West wards due to their outer location.

Inadequate availability of various public utility services is another important problem in the city. A perusal of Table 6.11 reveals that 11 inter colleges is

Table 6.11 Existing Facilities and Amenities in Azamgarh City

Name	Requirement According to Population	Present Requirement	Present Availability	Lack	Standard Area (Ha)	Total Required Land (Ha)	Extra Land required
Inter College (With primary, nursery schools)	1 per 10000	38	27	11	0.57		6.05
Degree Colleges	1 per 80000	5	8	0	1	8	0
Technical Institutions	1 per 100000	4	3	1	4	16	0.5
Health Centres	1 per 15000	25	25	0	0.08	2	0
Child Care and Maternity Centres	1 per 45000	9	1	8	0.2	1.8	1.6
FgmxgGeneral Hospital	1 per 100000	4	3	1	2	8	2
Post Offices	1 per 250000	2	1	1	0.25	0.5	0.25
Telephone Exchange	1 per 100000	4	2	2	0.4	1.6	0.8
Police Station	1 per 50000	8	2	6	0.4	3.2	2.4
Police Chowki	1 per 15000	25	10	15	0.15	3.75	2.25
Fire Station	1 per 2000000	2	1	1	0.8	1.6	0.8
Electricity Sub station	1 per 15000	25	6	19	0.4	10	7.6
Electricity Station	1 per 50000	8	2	6	1.4	11.2	8.4
Water Works		10	9	1	0.2	2	0.2
Community Centre	1 per 25000	16	2	14	0.1	1.6	1.4
Clubs		16	0	16	0.25	4	4
Sewage Treatment Plant		2	0	2	18	36	36
Solid Waste Management Centre		1	0	1	30	30	30
Cemetery					2	16.7	2
Total required Land (Ha)			14.7				106.25

Source: Master Plan, 2011–2031.

required in the city. Other required services are 1 technical institution, 8 government childcare and maternity centre (available services in the city run on private basis), 1 general hospital, 1 post office, 6 police stations, 15 police chowkis, 1 fire station, 19 electricity sub-stations, 6 electricity stations, 1 water-works department, 14 community centres, 16 clubs, 2 sewage treatment plants and 1 solid waste management plant for the present population.

Existing location of services suggests that the southern part of the city which was lately added into the municipal boundary, lack these facilities and need to be taken care in planning. Therefore new facilities should be developed at Harbanshpur and Sarfuddinpur wards of the city.

6.4 Summary

This chapter is in continuation of the previous chapters. In the chapter four, an attempt was made to identify major neighbourhood problems of the city. In continuation, in the fifth chapter, an effort was made to assess the health impacts of these problems. In this chapter, an attempt is made to identify vulnerable neighbourhoods of the city as well to tackle major neighbourhood problems of the city. The chapter is divided into three sections. In the first section, socio-economic profile of the sampled households has been discussed. The second section attempts to identify most vulnerable neighbourhoods of Azamgarh city while the third section deals with major environmental problems of the city. Environmentally vulnerable neighbourhood in the city are identified using 14 environmental problems of the city like irregular supply of water, water quality problem, open drains, poor cleaning of drains, waterlogging, inadequate waste collection, waste accumulation in neighbourhood, overcrowding, narrow streets, air pollution, noise pollution, substandard housing, and neighbourhood disorder as well as unequal distribution of facilities. Weighted linear combination technique has been used to categorise neighbourhoods in three categories, i.e. most vulnerable, moderately vulnerable and least vulnerable. It has been found that mostly low-income neighbourhoods (LI/HD, LI/MD and MI/LD) lie in the most vulnerable category and environmental problems are at their worst level in them. Medium- and high-income neighbourhoods (MI/HD, HI/HD, HI/MD and HI/LD) are in somewhat better condition.

In the second section, an attempt is made to address all the major problems identified in the city, i.e. water supply and quality, drainage and water logging, solid waste management, neighbourhood overcrowding, water supply and quality problem, air pollution, noise pollution, neighbourhood disorder and unequal distribution of amenities and facilities. Policy suggestions have been provided while considering existing schemes and policies running in the city.

References

Case, A., & Deaton, A. S. (2005). "Broken Down by Work and Sex: How Our Health Declines. *Analyses in the Economics of Aging*. University of Chicago Press, Chicago, pp. 185–212.

De Sherbinin, A., Schiller, A., & Pulsipher, A. (2007). The vulnerability of global cities to climate hazards. *Environment and Urbanisation*, *19*(1), 39–64.

Diez-Roux, A. V. (1998). Bringing context back into epidemiology: variables and fallacies in multilevel analysis. *American Journal of Public Health*, *88*(2), 216–222.

Galobardes, B., Shaw, M., Lawlor, D. A., Lynch, J. W., & Smith, G. D. (2006). Indicators of socioeconomic position (part 1). *Journal of Epidemiology and Community Health*, *60*, 7–12.

Jacobi, P., Kjellen, M., McGranahan, G., Songsore, J., & Surjadi, C. (2010). *The Citizens At Risk: From Urban Sanitation to Sustainable Cities*. Earthscan, Londan and Sterling, VA.

Kahn, H. S., Williamson, D. F., & Stevens, J. A. (1991). Race and weight change in US women: the roles of socioeconomic and marital status. *American Journal of Public Health*, *81*(3), 319–323.

Kawachi, I., & Berkman, L. F. (Eds.). (2003). *Neighborhoods and Health*. Oxford University Press, New York.

Kunst, A.E., K. Giskes & J.P. Mackenbach. (2004). *Socioeconomic Inequalities in Smoking in the European Union: Applying An Equity Lens to Tobacco Control Policies*. EU Network on Interventions to Reduce Socio-economic Inequalities in Health and Department of Public Health. ErasmusMedical Centre, Rotterdam, Netherlands.

Lavell, A., Wisner, B., Cannon, T., & Pelling, M. (2003). *The Vulnerability of Cities: Natural Disasters and Social Resilience*. Earthscan, London.

McGranahan, G. & Songsore, J. (1994). Wealth, health and the urban household. *Environment*, *36*(6), 4–11.

Meara, E. R., Richards, S., & Cutler, D. M. (2008). The gap gets bigger: changes in mortality and life expectancy, by education, 1981–2000. *Health Affairs*, *27*(2), 350–360.

National Center for Health Statistics US. (2013). Health, United States, 2012: With special feature on emergency care.

Ross, C. E., & Mirowsky, J. (1995). Does employment affect health?. *Journal of Health and Social Behavior*, *36*, 230–243.

Saaty, T. L. (1980). *The Analytic Process: Planning, Priority Setting, Resources Allocation*. New York: McGraw.

Schoenborn, C. A. (2004). *Marital status and health, United States 1999–2002* (No. 351). US Department of Health and Human Services, Centers for Disease Control and Prevention, National Center for Health Statistics.

Singh, A. L., & Jamal, S. (2012). Assessing vulnerability of women to indoor air pollution. *Research Journal of Environmental and Earth Sciences*, *4*(11), 982–989.

Smith, G. D., Bartley M., & Blane, D. (1990). The Black Report on socio-economic in-equalities in health 10 years on. *British Medical Journal*, *301*, 373–377.

Umberson, D. (1987). Family status and health behaviors: Social control as a dimension of social integration. *Journal of Health and Social Behavior*, 306–319.

United Nations Human Settlements Programme. (2003). *The Challenge of Slums: Global Report on Human Settlements, 2003*. UN-HABITAT, Earthscan Publications, London and Sterling, VA.

Wilkinson, R. G., & Marmot, M. G. (2003). *Social Determinants of Health: The Solid Facts*. WHO Publication, Denmark.

Conclusion

The book entitled "Neighbourhoods and Health: The impact of place in urban area" focuses on the environmental problems that people face in their neighbourhoods. Various environmental problems that are found in the neighbourhood can lead to numerous health hazards. Residents suffer if their air is polluted, their water and sanitation is inadequate, their waste is not disposed of and overall if the neighbourhood environment is unhygienic and unhealthy.

Major objectives of the study are to understand the concept of neighbourhoods over time and space, to examine the pathways by which neighbourhoods affect human health, to get an overview of neighbourhood environmental characteristics and problems in Azamgarh city, to examine the relationship between neighbourhood environmental problems and human health, to deal with vulnerable neighbourhoods in Azamgarh city and finally to compare the results of the current study with other global studies.

The first chapter of the book is devoted to first two objectives of the study, i.e. to examine the impact of place in urban areas and to understand the pathways by which neighbourhoods affect human health. Rest five chapters are devoted to case study conducted in Azamgarh city, India, fulfilling rest of the objectives. The case study is mainly based on primary as well as secondary sources of data. Stratified random sampling was used to select 1629 households from 7 neighbourhoods of Azamgarh city. For identification of different neighbourhoods, all 25 administrative wards of Azamgarh city were grouped into 7 neighbourhoods on the basis of (i) dominant income group in the ward, (ii) population density and (iii) household density. These neighbourhoods were HI/HD, HI/MD, HI/LD, MI/HD, MI/LD, LI/HD and LI/MD. Systematic social observation (SSO), schedule method, interview method, water quality monitoring, noise-level monitoring and GPS operation were used to collect primary data while secondary data have been collected from municipal office, Azamgarh City, Azamgarh Development Authority (ADA), Azamgarh city master plans, CMO office, district census handbook, regional office UPPCB, Azamgarh, various government and private hospitals, air pollution report "Air Kills" by NGO Climate Agenda, satellite data from Sentinel 2A and Google Earth. Statistical techniques used in the study were simple percentage, Karl

DOI: 10.4324/9781003442486-8

Pearson's coefficient of correlation and analytic hierarchy process (AHP) while geospatial techniques used in the study were choropleth mapping-natural breaks, inverse distance weighting, hotspot analysis, kernel density estimation and weighted linear combination.

Chapter-wise conclusion of the book is as follows.

Chapter 1 is devoted to different concepts of neighbourhood over space and time as well as an understanding of how neighbourhoods can impact health of its residents. The term neighbourhood has several meanings and usages. For example, neighbourhood can be used for a small group of houses in the immediate surroundings of one's home or a more substantial area with a similar type of housing and market value. It can also be defined as a census ward. This chapter has been divided into two sections. The first section deals with the concept of neighbourhood over space and time while the second section deals with the ways by which neighbourhoods can affect health of its residents. The major key points of this chapter are the concept of neighbourhood and its evolution as a planning unit. Apart from this, identification of neighbourhood boundaries, characteristic features of individual neighbourhoods, concept of neighbourhood in some major cities of the world as well as concept of neighbourhood in Indian cities are also covered. The analysis reveals that neighbourhoods have been identified since early times; however, their official recognition as a planning unit has started only after the publication of the idea of "Neighbourhood Unit" by Clarence Perry and "Neighbourhood" by Stein and Wright in 1929. In the modern world, neighbourhoods have not been given official status except that in the United States and Canada; however, the term is being comprehensively used for an informal division of the city and people have a certain boundary of their neighbourhood in their minds. The second section of the chapter deals with different forms of neighbourhood environment, i.e. neighbourhood physical environment, neighbourhood social environment as well as neighbourhood services environment and ways by which they can influence residents' health. Further, various methods used to measure neighbourhood impact on health have been discussed, ranging from ecological studies to contextual or multi-level studies and a comparison of certain number of well-defined neighbourhoods.

The second chapter deals with details about study area Azamgarh city. This chapter has been divided into two sections. The first part deals with geographical and other characteristics of study area, i.e. Azamgarh city, while the second part deals with identification and mapping of different neighbourhoods in Azamgarh city. In the first section, origin and evolution in medieval, British and modern period; physical setting in terms of terms of site and situation, drainage, soil, climate; demographic setting in terms of population growth, literacy level and sex ratio, occupational structure as well land use pattern in the city are discussed in detail. In the second section, first of all criteria selected for identification of different neighbourhoods, such as income-wise dominance, population density as well as household density, are discussed. Further, each neighbourhood of the city, along with its picture is discussed in detail.

In the third chapter, a full general overview of neighbourhood environment in Azamgarh city has been provided. Neighbourhood environment of Azamgarh city was divided into three forms, i.e. neighbourhood physical, social and service environment. Physical environment of the neighbourhoods included residential density, built-up area, open spaces, street lighting, solid waste management, waste water management and water supply conditions. Service environment included supply of various amenities and facilities in different neighbourhoods while social environment included social relation among residents of the neighbourhood. An analysis of **neighbourhood physical environment** in the city revealed that residential density and proportion of built-up area was the highest in the old central part of the city. Most of the parks were located in the high-income parts of the city. A study of **service environment** in Azamgarh city revealed that high-income neighbourhoods were well lit at the night. It was found that all the houses of the city were not covered by water supply pipelines and out of the total household waste generated in the city only about 80% waste was collected by the municipality while rest 20% was either collected by households themselves or left dumped to open fields, backyards, water bodies or burnt. There were 6 government and 93 private hospitals, nursing homes and clinics. There were 31 government, 93 private schools and 3 degree colleges in the city, and schools outside the city were also quite popular among residents. Market was developed along the Gorakhpur Allahabad highway. Shopping malls were spotted on the same road in the main market; however, a major concentration of malls was found in high-income neighbourhoods of the city. **Neighbourhood social environment** in Azamgarh city was measured by degree of trust and connectedness among neighbours. It was found that overall social environment in the city was good, but a big social gap between majority population and other marginalised communities like schedule caste was observed.

In the fourth chapter, an analysis of major neighbourhood environmental problems of Azamgarh city has been presented. **Problems identified in the neighbourhood physical environment** included overcrowding, narrow or congested streets; substandard housing and slums, air pollution, noise pollution, water quality problem and unequal distribution of facilities. Problem of **overcrowding** was found the highest in the old central parts of the city. Other major problem prevalent in these neighbourhoods was **narrow and congested streets**. In these wards, houses were found constructed without proper guidelines that how much open space should be left and what should be the adequate width of streets for proper movement of traffic as well as wind. Neighbourhood survey revealed that about one fourth of the total sampled households were living in **substandard houses** mostly in low- and medium-income neighbourhoods. Regarding **air pollution** in Azamgarh city, values of PM_{10} and $PM_{2.5}$ at all the monitored stations were higher than national standards for ambient air quality. **Noise pollution** analysis revealed that the noise level was within the standard limits for the residential areas; however, it exceeded the prescribed standards at commercial and silence zones as well as traffic intersections. Traffic has been found the major source of noise pollution in the city. Households located along the major roads, as well as in markets, reported the problem of noise pollution in their neighbourhoods. **Problem in water quality** was also reported during the survey; therefore, an attempt was made to examine the physico-chemical characteristics of drinking water in the city. Water Quality Index of nine samples collected from different neighbourhoods revealed poor water quality of five samples. Results revealed that water samples collected from submersible pumps were better in water quality than those of hand pumps and municipal taps. **Problems in service environment** included inadequate water supply, inadequate drainage system as well as accumulation of solid waste in the neighbourhoods. An analysis of **water supply services** revealed that about 40% residents do not get regular water supply. Regarding **drainage condition**, about half of the residents, mostly residing in low-income neighbourhoods, reported presence of open drains in their neighbourhoods. About half of the total sampled households have reported presence of water logging in their neighbourhoods. **Inadequate waste collection** was another major problem in the city. Practice of waste segregation, both at household and neighbourhood level was totally absent in the city. During the survey, Most of the households reported accumulation of garbage and problem of stray animals and pests due to garbage dumped around their houses. Frequency of waste collection was also found inadequate in the city and out of the total sampled households only about half of the residents reported daily waste collection from the roads and streets. **Unequal distribution of amenities and facilities** was another significant problem found in Azamgarh city. **Problems in the neighbourhood social environment** included problem of residential segregation and neighbourhood disorder. **Residential segregation** with respect to scheduled caste population was observed and measured by hotspot analysis. Hotspot analysis revealed that significant hot and cold spots of SC population were prevalent in the city and majority of the SC population was found living in wards near the outer boundary of the city. Another problem identified in the city was **neighbourhood disorder**. It was mainly prevalent in central, congested, old parts of the city in low- and medium-income neighbourhoods.

In the fifth chapter, an attempt has been made to get an overall view of the health condition of the sampled households, identify risk factors in the neighbourhood environment and to assess the relationship of prevalent diseases with neighbourhood environment. The chapter has been divided into four sections. **In the first section**, most frequent diseases in the city occurred during the last two years have been identified and analysed thoroughly. **Most common diseases** that were reported by residents as well as diagnosed by health practitioners were cold and flu, malaria, diarrhoea, cholera, skin infections, jaundice, dengue, typhoid, chicken pox, measles, tuberculosis and asthma. Other health problems (symptomatic), as reported by residents of Azamgarh city, were stress, sleep disturbances, annoyance, headache, shortness of breath, coughing and wheezing and deafness. Prevalence of the diseases was found to be most common in low-income neighbourhoods than that of high-income neighbourhoods. **In the second section**, an attempt was made to **identify risk factors in the neighbourhood environment**. Major risk factors identified in the neighbourhood environment were overcrowding, irregular water supply and water quality problem, open drains, improper cleaning of drains, water logging, improper collection of solid waste, overcrowding, neighbourhood disorder, air pollution and noise pollution. In the third section, an attempt was made to understand **the association between risk factors in neighbourhood environment and prevalent diseases**. Karl Pearson's coefficient of correlation and scatter plots have been used to measure the association between these risk factors and prevalent diseases. It has been found that risk factors related to water and sanitation, i.e. irregular water supply, water quality problem, open drains, improper cleaning of drains, waste accumulation, inadequate waste collection and water logging were associated with diseases like typhoid, cholera, jaundice, diarrhoea and skin infections, overcrowding was associated with measles and chickenpox, neighbourhood disorder was associated with prevalence of stress, air pollution was associated with shortness of breath, coughing, wheezing and noise pollution was associated with annoyance, sleep disturbances and headache , as explained with significant values of r. Furthermore, **in the fourth section**, hypothesis testing has been performed by using Karl Pearson's coefficient of correlation. It was found that null hypothesis of the study, i.e. "There is insignificant effect of neighbourhood environment on resident's health" failed to be accepted as suggested by "r" and "p" values of correlation.

The sixth and last chapter is divided into three sections. In the first section, socio-economic profile of the sampled households has been discussed. In the second section, an attempt has been made to identify most vulnerable neighbourhoods of Azamgarh city while in the third section an attempt has been made to tackle major environmental problems of the city. Environmentally vulnerable neighbourhoods in the city were identified using 14 major environmental problems of the city like, irregular supply of water, water quality problem, open drains, poor cleaning of drains, water logging, inadequate waste collection, waste accumulation in neighbourhood, overcrowding, narrow streets, air pollution, noise pollution, substandard housing, and neighbourhood disorder and unequal distribution of facilities. Weighted linear combination technique has been used to categorize neighbourhoods in three categories, i.e. most vulnerable, moderately vulnerable and least vulnerable. It has been found that the low-income neighbourhoods lie in most vulnerable category and environmental problems were at their worst level in them. Medium- and high-income neighbourhoods were in somewhat better condition. In the second section, an attempt is made to address all the major problems identified in the city, i.e. drainage and water logging, solid waste management, neighbourhood overcrowding, water supply and quality problem, air pollution, noise pollution, neighbourhood disorder and unequal distribution of amenities and facilities, and policy suggestions have been provided while considering existing schemes and policies running in the city.

The Overall important findings which have emerged from the foregoing study are as follows:

- Neighbourhood environment or the most immediate environment that surrounds humans can be one of the major determinants of resident's health.
- Major neighbourhood problems that could affect the health of the residents in a developing country are irregular water supply and quality, inadequate drainage and water logging, overcrowding, air and noise pollution, residential segregation, neighbourhood disorder as well as unequal distribution of amenities and facilities.
- Environmental problems are predominantly concentrated in low-income neighbourhoods.
- Strong positive correlation exists between neighbourhood environmental problems and common diseases like typhoid, diarrhoea, dengue, malaria, skin-infections, jaundice, cholera, measles, chickenpox, shortness of breath, coughing and wheezing, asthma, tuberculosis, deafness as well as stress.
- These are the poor people who suffer most with the major burden of diseases.
- These are mainly poor neighbourhoods which are both environmentally as well as socio-economically vulnerable.

Comparison of the Results from Global Studies

Study-1 "Neighbourhood environments and mortality in an elderly cohort: results from the cardiovascular health study", 2004

Authors – Ana V Diez Roux, Luisa N Borrell, Mary Haan, Sharon A Jackson, Richard Schultz

Place of Study – United States

Objectives – To examine the impact of neighbourhood environmental conditions on cardio-vascular disease-related mortality

Method – Cardio-vascular health study

Findings – The findings of the study revealed that of the persons died due to cardio-vascular diseases, the ones living in most deprived neighbourhoods were prone to higher rate of cardio-vascular deaths even after controlling for individual's socio-economic conditions.

Similarity/Difference with our study – The current study also reaches to conclusion similar to our study that people living in deprived neighbourhoods are more prone to deaths related to diseases (Roux et al. 2004)

Study-2 "Neighbourhood influences on health in Montréal, Canada", 2004

Authors – Nancy A Ross, Stephane Tremblay, Katie Graham

Place of Study- Montreal, Canada

Objectives – To examine the impact of neighbourhoods on health

Methods – 1652 respondents from Montreal health region sample of the 2000/1 Canadian Community Health Survey, Used census tract boundary as proxy to neighbourhood

Findings – The results of the study suggest that there does exist neighbourhood level variation in health status of the residents even after controlling for individual socio-economic and demographic behaviours.

Similarity/Difference with our study – The present study also used census tracts as proxy for neighbourhoods and suggests that present model of neighbourhood has similar results to natural neighbourhoods. Therefore, it proves that administrative boundaries can be used as neighbourhood for contextual analysis (Ross et al. 2004).

Study-3 "Neighbourhood environment and its association with self-rated health: evidence from Scotland and England", 2005

Authors – Steven Cummins, Mai Stafford, Sally Macintyre, Michael Marmot, Anne Ellaway

Place of study – Scotland and England

Objective – To examine the association between neighbourhood's social and material attributes and self-rated health

Methods – Self-rated health data for 13,899 male and female has been used from Scottish Health Survey and Health Survey of England.

Findings – The findings of the study revealed that attributes of the neighbourhood like poor physical neighbourhood environment (waste collection services, vacant houses or vacant lands in the neighbourhood), high unemployment rate and poor access to private vehicles are associated with poor self-rated health.

Similarity/Difference with our study – The results of this study support our findings as it also concludes that physical environment of the neighbourhood as well people's socio-economic conditions are associated with health(Cummins et al. 2005).

Study-4 "Do perceptions of neighbourhood environment influence health? Baseline findings from a British survey of aging", 2006

Authors Ann Bowling, Julie Barber, Richard Morris, Shah Ebrahim

Place of Study – Britain

Objectives – To investigate the association between neighbourhood environmental perceptions, social cohesion and support health of the people

Method – British Population Survey

Findings – The findings of the study revealed that perception of the neighbourhood environment regarding good quality services in the neighbourhood like leisure facilities, facilities for elderly, waste collection, health facilities, facilities for walk and proximity to shops as well as strong level of social cohesion is strongly associated with good health of the people.

Similarity/Difference with our study – The results of the current study too support our study as it also concludes that physical and service environmental features of the neighbourhoods are associated with health (Bowling et al. 2006).

Study-5 "Neighbourhoods and health: a GIS approach to measuring community resource accessibility", 2006

Authors – Jamie Pearce, Karen Witten, Phil Bartie

Place of Study – New Zealand

Objectives – Develop a new methodology for measuring access to community facilities associated to health

Method – Use of GIS to determine locational access to community facilities

Findings – The study concluded that there exists a geographical variation in accessibility to various community facilities like health, education, recreation and shopping in the entire country, but the variation was more prominent between rural and urban areas. Study further added that with the advancement in GIS technology it is viable to directly measure neighbourhood-wise accessibility.

Similarity/Difference with our study – The current study also made use of GIS in measuring accessibility to various community services along with emphasising role of access to amenities and facilities on the residents' health (Pearce et al. 2006).

Study-6 "Sources of stress in impoverished neighbourhoods: insights into links between neighbourhood environments and health", 2009

Authors – Deborah Warr, Peter Feldman, Theonie Tacticos, Margaret Kelaher

Place of Study- Victoria, Australia

Objectives – To examine the association between people's perception about physical and social disorders and health

Method – Primary Survey

Findings – The findings of the study revealed that physical and social disorders in the neighbourhood like drug and alcohol consumption, ill behaviour of people, rash driving, noise pollution and racism were associated with feeling unsafe which is further associated with poor health.

Similarity/Difference with our study – The results of the current study too support results of our study as how neighbourhood disorder gives birth the feeling of not being safe and a continuous stress among neighbours which ultimately affects their health (Warr et al. 2009).

Study-7 Associations between perceived stress, socio-economic status, and health-risk behaviour in deprived neighbourhoods in Denmark: a cross-sectional study, 2018

Authors – Maria Holst Algren, Ola Ekholm, Line Nielsen, Annette Kjaer Ersboll, Carsten Kronborg Bak & Pernille Tanggaard Andersen

Place of Study – Denmark

Objectives – To compare the level of stress in the residents of deprived neighbourhoods with people of non-deprived neighbourhoods

Methods – 14,868 samples from Danish Health and Morbidity Survey 2010

Findings – The results of the study revealed that perceived stress was found prevalent among the residents of deprived neighbourhoods. Residents of deprived neighbourhoods were also found engaged in unhealthy behaviours like less consumption of healthy diet, smoking and lack of physical activity.

Similarity/Difference with our study – The results of the current study also supports our results as prevalence of stress and unhealthy behaviours among the residents of low-income neighbourhoods (Algren et al. 2018).

Study-8 Associations between Neighbourhood Environment, Health Behaviours, and Mortality, 2018

Authors- Shaneda Warren Andersen, William J. Blot, Xiao-Ou Shu, Jennifer S. Sonderman, Mark Steinwandel

Place of Study – United States

Objective – To examine the combined influence of neighbourhood environment and people's health related behaviours on mortality

Methods – 77,896 samples from Southern Community Cohort Study

Findings – The results of the study revealed that there is a strong association between mortality due to any cause and living in low socio-economic neighbourhoods. However, individual living in disadvantaged neighbourhoods following healthy behaviours like less smoking and alcohol consumption, more physical activity and healthy diet and lifestyle are less vulnerable to mortality.

Similarity/Difference with our study – The results of the current study support our notion that living in disadvantaged neighbourhood is associated with mortality. The study also emphasised the role of individual health behaviour which is first and foremost in any health study. Neighbourhood effects do come after individual level impacts (Andersen et al. 2018).

Study-9 "Unequal impact of the COVID-19 pandemic on mental health: role of the neighborhood environment", 2022

Authors – Liang Ma, Yan Huang, Tao Liu

Place of Study – Beijing, China

Objectives – To examine the role of neighbourhood environment on differential impact of COVID-19 on mental health

Method – Primary Survey

Findings – The findings of the study revealed that residents of lower-income neighbourhoods experienced greater mental health impact than that of high-income neighbourhoods. The main features of neighbourhood environment that created the difference were proximity to parks and social cohesion and connectedness among neighbours.

Similarity/Difference with our study – The results of the current study support our study results as residents of high-income neighbourhoods recorded better mental health than that of low-income neighbourhoods even in pandemic. It also supported role of parks and social cohesion among neighbours in improving health (Ma et al. 2022).

Study-10 "Neighborhood Environment and Metabolic Risk in Hispanics/Latinos from the Hispanic Community Health Study/Study of Latinos", 2022

Authors – Linda C Gallo, Kimberly L Savin, Marta M Jankowska, Scott C Roesch, James F Sallis, Daniela Sotres-Alvarez, Gregory A Talavera, Krista M Perreira, Carmen R Isasi, Frank J Penedo, Maria M Llabre, Mayra L Estrella, Earle C Chambers, Martha L Daviglus, Scott C Brown, Jordan A Carlson

Place of Study – San Diego, California, United States

Objectives – To examine the association between neighbourhood environmental attributes and BMI, AbA1c and diabetes in Hispanic population

Method – Hispanic Community Health Study

Findings – The findings of the study revealed that Hispanic community members residing in lower socio-economic neighbourhoods were mostly diagnosed with higher BMI, Hba1c and have higher chances to be diabetic. However, they did not any association of said health issues to neighbourhood greenery, walkability or residential stability.

Similarity/Difference with our study – Although the current study focused on non-communicable diseases only, the results were in conformity with present study that residents of lower socio-economic neighbourhoods are more prone to diseases than that of high-income neighbourhoods (Gallo et al. 2022).

The analysis of all the selected global studies revealed that neighbourhoods play an important role in determining the health status of the residents. Now it is also clear that these environmental problems are mostly concentrated in deprived neighbourhoods of the city and these are the residents of deprived neighbourhoods that are more prone to deaths and diseases. However, a major difference that has been recorded between the selected studies and our study is that major urban problems in developing countries have still not progressed from water- and sanitation-related problems. The developed part of the globe has moved from communicable to non-communicable diseases and the developing countries in fact are facing dual burden of diseases. Non-communicable diseases also were not analysed in the study but are prevalent world-wide whether it's developed world or developing world and at the same time developing countries area also facing communicable diseases too.

The study concludes that Azamgarh, being a medium-sized growing city in a developing country, is associated with local environmental problems, which have a significant impact on resident's health, particularly from the low-income neighbourhoods. Therefore, the urban environmental plan for smaller cities of developing countries should be to alleviate their environmental issues by tackling local environmental problems, improving the residential conditions of the urban poor and lessening urban poverty. This could be achieved by giving priority to solutions applicable at the level of local neighbourhoods.

- The present study highlights that in order to improve the health and well-being of people, there is need to focus on their socio-economic conditions as well as the neighbourhood environment in which they live.
- Identification of vulnerable neighbourhoods has shown that there are differences in vulnerability among different neighbourhoods and environmental problems are basically concentrated in low- and medium-income neighbourhoods. Therefore, there is need to focus on vulnerable neighbourhoods of the city, and there is a necessity of better urban management which can be achieved by local plans rather than state and national plans.
- Areas comprising socio-economically backward population having unhealthy neighbourhood environment suffer the most burden of disease; therefore, special focus on them while making policy is recommended.

References

Algren, M. H., Ekholm, O., Nielsen, L., Ersbøll, A. K., Bak, C. K., & Andersen, P. T. (2018). Associations between perceived stress, socioeconomic status, and health-risk behaviour in deprived neighbourhoods in Denmark: a cross-sectional study. *BMC Public Health*, *18*(1), 1–12.

Andersen, S. W., Blot, W. J., Shu, X. O., Sonderman, J. S., Steinwandel, M., Hargreaves, M. K., & Zheng, W. (2018). Associations between neighborhood environment, health behaviors, and mortality. *American Journal of Preventive Medicine*, *54*(1), 87–95.

Bowling, A., Barber, J., Morris, R., & Ebrahim, S. (2006). Do perceptions of neighbourhood environment influence health? Baseline findings from a British survey of aging. *Journal of Epidemiology & Community Health*, *60*(6), 476–483.

Cummins, S., Stafford, M., Macintyre, S., Marmot, M., & Ellaway, A. (2005). Neighbourhood environment and its association with self rated health: evidence from Scotland and England. *Journal of Epidemiology & Community Health*, *59*(3), 207–213.

Gallo, L. C., Savin, K. L., Jankowska, M. M., Roesch, S. C., Sallis, J. F., Sotres-Alvarez, D., ... & Carlson, J. A. (2022). Neighborhood environment and metabolic risk in hispanics/latinos from the hispanic community health study/study of latinos. *American Journal of Preventive Medicine*, *63*(2), 195–203.

Ma, L., Huang, Y., & Liu, T. (2022). Unequal impact of the COVID-19 pandemic on mental health: role of the neighborhood environment. *Sustainable Cities and Society*, *87*, 104162.

Pearce, J., Witten, K., & Bartie, P. (2006). Neighbourhoods and health: a GIS approach to measuring community resource accessibility. *Journal of Epidemiology & Community Health*, *60*(5), 389–395.

Ross, N. A., Tremblay, S., & Graham, K. (2004). Neighbourhood influences on health in Montreal, Canada. *Social Science & Medicine*, *59*(7), 1485–1494.

Roux, A. V. D., Borrell, L. N., Haan, M., Jackson, S. A., & Schultz, R. (2004). Neighbourhood environments and mortality in an elderly cohort: results from the cardiovascular health study. *Journal of Epidemiology & Community Health*, *58*(11), 917–923.

Warr, D., Feldman, P., Tacticos, T., & Kelaher, M. (2009). Sources of stress in impoverished neighbourhoods: insights into links between neighbourhood environments and health. *Australian and New Zealand Journal of Public Health*, *33*(1), 25–33.

Appendix 1

Questionnaire

CHECKLIST: SYSTEMATIC SOCIAL OBSERVATION

1 **Sampled ward:**
   a) No.:
   b) Name:
2 **Total no. of households in the ward:**
3 **Total population of the ward:**
4 **Total no. of colonies in the ward:**
5 **Name of colonies in the ward:**
   a) ....
   b) ....
   c) ....
   d) ....
   e) ....
   f) ....
6 **No. of sampled colonies in the ward:**
7 **Name of sampled colonies in the ward:**
   a) ....
   b) ....
   c) ....
   d) ....
   e) ....
   f) ....
8 **Sampled mohalla/colony:**
   a) No.:
   b) Name:
9 **Location of the ward**
   a) Core Area
   b) Fringe Area
   c) Civil line
   d) Along the river

e)   Any other
10   **Type of income group**:
a)   High
b)   Medium
c)   Low
11   **Type of housing**:
a)   New
b)   Old
c)   Planned
d)   Mixed
e)   Unplanned
f)   Private
g)   Government
h)   Authorised
i)   Jhuggi
j)   Industrial
k)   Any other
12   **Industrial/commercial unit present**
a)   Yes
b)   No
If Yes Type.....................................
13   **Open spaces/green space in the mohalla/colony**:
a)   Yes
b)   No
If yes Type.....................................
a)   Park
b)   Vacant land
c)   Any other
14   **General environment of the neighbourhood**
I)   Clean
a)   Yes
b)   No
II)   Overcrowding
a)   Yes
b)   No
III)   Road facilities
a)   *Kachcha*
b)   Pucca
c)   Both
IV)   Width of the roads
a)   Good
b)   Reasonable
c)   Narrow
d)   Congested

V)   Type of traffic flow
  a)   High
  b)   Medium
  c)   Low
VI)   Water facilities
  a)   Yes
  b)   No
  If yes
  a)   Private
  b)   Public
VII)   Drainage in the Mohalla/Ward
  a)   Exists
  b)   Does not Exist
  If exists, in which type of drainage:
  a)   Open
  b)   Closed
VIII)   Water logging conditions in the mohalla/ward:
  a)   Yes
  b)   No
  If yes
  a)   Rainwater only
  b)   Waste Water
  c)   both
IX)   Garbage in the Mohalla:
  a)   Spread everywhere
  b)   Not seen
  If spread everywhere:
  a)   In huge quantity
  b)   In small quantity
  c)   Negligible
X)   Dustbins
  a)   Adequate
  b)   Inadequate
  c)   Non-existent
  d)   Open
  e)   Covered
XI)   Street lights
  a)   Adequate
  b)   Inadequate
  c)   Non-existent
XII)   Overall maintenance
  a)   Good
  b)   Not good
XIII)   Noise
  a)   Noisy
  b)   Quiet

15 **Availability of facilities and amenities in the neighbourhoods (Table A1.1)**

Parks	Available	Not Available
Schools		
Small grocery stores		
Fruit/vegetable market		
Malls		
Health centres (Govt.)		
Health centre (Private)		
Post Office		
Religious Centres		
Cinema		
Cyber café		
Public transport		
Restaurants		
Health clubs Gyms		

NEIGHBOURHOOD ENVIRONMENTAL CONDITIONS

Ward No...............................Name..........................

A. GENERAL ENVIRONMENT

1) **General environmental condition of the ward/*Mohalla***
    I) Cleanliness
        a) Yes
        b) No
    II) Overcrowding
        a) Yes
        b) No
    III) Status of income group
        a) High
        b) Medium
        c) Mixed
        d) Low
    IV) Religious communities
        a) Hindu-dominated area
        b) Muslim-dominated area
        c) Mixed
        d) Other
    V) Caste/community domination
        a) caste........
        b) community........
        c) mixed
        d) other

B. GARBAGE

1   **Do you feel garbage collection around your house/in neighbourhood?**
   a)   Yes
   b)   No

2   **Type of garbage collected**
   a)   In bins
   b)   Spilled on ground
   c)   No garbage
   If spilled on the ground
   a)   In small amount
   b)   In large amount
   c)   In huge amount

3   **Dustbins**
   a)   Adequate
   b)   Inadequate
   c)   Non-existent
   a)   Covered
   b)   Open
   a)   Separate (for waste segregation)
   b)   Common

4   **Who collects the garbage in your ward/community?**
   a)   Municipality
   b)   Community
   c)   Household himself
   d)   Any other

5   **Collection of garbage**
   a)   Daily
   b)   Bi-weekly
   c)   Weekly
   d)   Monthly
   e)   Never

6   **Role of waste pickers in household waste collection?**
   a)   Door-to-door collection
   b)   Collection from roads
   c)   Open space/field
   d)   Any other

7   **In the absence of waste collection by municipality,**
   a)   Waste is pilfered along the roads/open space
   b)   Waste piles up
   c)   Waste collects in drain
   d)   Any other

8   **Problem of stray animals due to waste accumulated in the neighbourhood**
   a)   Yes
   b)   No

9   **Finally, where the municipality does dispose the waste?**
   a)   Dump sites/landfill sites
   b)   Outside the city
   c)   Open space/field
   d)   Any other
10   **What are the disposal methods used by municipality?**
   a)   Open dumping
   b)   Outside the city
   c)   Composting
   d)   Burial
   e)   Manual pits
   f)   Any other
11   **Are you aware of any health issue related to garbage?**
   a)   Yes
   b)   No
12   **How much do you typically pay each month to dispose your waste? Rs.........**

C. DRAINAGE AND WATER LOGGING

13   **Disposal of household waste water**
   a)   Into the *nail*
   b)   On the roads
   c)   In the field
   d)   Along roads
   e)   Any other
14   **Drainage around the house**
   a)   Exists
   b)   Doesn't exist
   If exists,
   a)   Kutcha drainage
   b)   Concrete open drainage
   c)   Concrete closed drainage
   d)   Any other, specify
15   **Are the drains clean periodically?**
   a)   Yes
   b)   No
16   **Do you experience water logging around the houses?**
   a)   Yes
   b)   No
17   **If yes, how long does it take for water to drain away?**
   a)   >2 hrs
   b)   2–8 hrs
   c)   9–15 hrs
   d)   >24 hrs

18 **Type of waterlogged**
 a) Rain water
 b) Sullage
 c) Both
 d) Other, specify
19 **Place of water logging**
 a) Around the house
 b) On the roads
 c) Open space
 d) Other, specify

D. TRANSPORT

20 **Road facilities**
 a) *Kachcha*
 b) Pucca
 c) Both
21 **Width of the roads**
 a) Good
 b) Reasonable
 c) Narrow
 d) Congested
22 **Type of traffic flow**
 a) High
 b) Medium
 c) Low
23 **Major vehicles on the roads**
 a) Rickshaw / Sometimes auto
 b) Auto Rickshaws/ cars
 c) Truck/ heavy vehicles
 d) None
 e) Other
24 **Overall characteristics of streets**
 I) Trees along the streets ……..
  a) Yes
  b) No
 II) Streets well lit at night ……..
  a) Yes
  b) No
 III) Presence of sidewalks ……..
  a) Yes
  b) No

E. AIR POLLUTION

25 **Do you feel that the air in your neighbourhood is polluted?**
   a) Yes
   b) No

26 **Source of air pollution**
   a) Indoor source
   b) Outdoor source
   If Indoor
   a) Smoke
   b) Fuel
   c) Both
   If outdoor
   a) Traffic
   b) Industry/Factory
   c) Market

F. NOISE POLLUTION

27 **Noise Pollution in neighbourhood**
   a) Yes
   b) No
   If Yes
   a) By home appliances
   b) By automobiles
   c) By train
   d) Market
   e) Any other

G. WATER POLLUTION

28 **What is the main Source of water supply in the Neighbourhood?**
   I) Private
       a) Qwn hand pump
       b) Piped water connection
       c) Own Boring
   II) Public
       a) Roadside hand pump
       b) Roadside piped water

29 **Any problem with the quality of water source for drinking and cooking?**
   a) Yes
   b) No
   If Yes
   a) Smell
   b) Taste

   c)   Colour
   d)   No problem
30 **What can be reason behind bad water quality in your neighbourhood?**
   a)   Secretion of dirty water of river
   b)   Mixing of sewage with drinking water
   c)   Can't say
   d)   Any other

H. GREEN/OPEN SPACE

31 **Open spaces/Green space in the *Mohalla*/colony**
   a)   Yes
   b)   No
   If yes Type.....................
   a)   Park
   b)   Vacant land
   c)   Any other

I. SLUMS

32 **Presence of slum in the neighbourhood**
   a)   Yes
   b)   No
   If Yes
   a)   Authorised
   b)   Unauthorised
   a)   New
   b)   Old
   Housing Type
   a)   Mud/thatched
   b)   Bricks/straw
   c)   Wood/straw
   d)   Bamboo/Plastic
   e)   Other types
   General Condition
   a)   Very Clean
   b)   Clean
   c)   Dirty
   d)   Very Dirty

J. INDUSTRIAL/COMMERCIAL UNIT

33 **Industrial/ Commercial unit present**
   a)   Yes
   b)   No
   If Yes Type......................................

34 **Distance from residential area**
   a)   0–500 m
   b)   500–1000 m
   c)   1–2 km
   d)   >2 km

35 **Problem from the industry**
   a)   Disposal of solid and liquid waste
   b)   Smoke
   c)   Industrial effluent discharged into river
   d)   Noise

36 **Effects of these Industries**
   a)   Water Pollution
   b)   Air Pollution
   c)   Noise Pollution
   d)   Garbage on the land

37 AMENITIES AND FACILITIES (Table A1.2)

Services in the neighbourhood (within 15 minute walk)	Available						Not available
	Access		Not Access				
	Satisfactory	Not satisfactory	Financial	Not aware	Not satisfactory		
					Don't use	Go for better	
Parks							
Schools							
Small grocery stores							
Fruit/vegetable market							
Malls							
Health centres (Govt.)							
Health centre (Private)							
Post Office							
Religious centres							
Cinema							
Cyber café							
Public transport							
Restaurants							
Health clubs Gyms							

38 **Do you think presence/absence of these facilities in neighbourhood affects the well-being of residents?**
   a)   Agree
   b)   Not agree
   c)   Can't say

39 **Do you see people walking, jogging or doing any exercise in your neighbourhood?**
   a)   Always
   b)   Sometimes
   c)   Never
   d)   Can't say

K. SOCIAL ENVIRONMENT

40 Are people in your neighbourhood willing to help each other?
   a) Strongly agree
   b) Agree
   c) Disagree
   d) Strongly disagree
   e) can't say

41 People in your neighbourhood can be trusted?
   a) Strongly agree
   b) Agree
   c) Disagree
   d) Strongly disagree
   e) Can't say

42 Do people in your neighbourhood visit each other and speak on streets?
   a) Strongly agree
   b) Agree
   c) Disagree
   d) Strongly disagree
   e) Can't say

L. NEIGHBOURHOOD DISORDERS (Table A1.3)

43 Thinking of the area you live in, how much of the problem is each of following:

Crime	Negligible	Minor	Somewhat serious
Theft			
Robbery			
Pickpocketing			
Drunk people			
Drug dealing			
Liquor stores			
People loitering			
People smoking			
Fighting			
Safety			
Prostitution			
Rowdy groups and street fighting			

44 Have you ever been attacked, robbed or been victim to a serious crime?
   a) Yes
   b) No

45 Have you seen something violent happen to someone (attacked, beaten, killed)?
   a) Yes
   b) No

M. SENSE OF SECURITY

46 **Do you feel a sense of security in your neighbourhood** Yes/No
If No......... then threat from
a) Thieves
b) Robbers
c) Hooligans
d) Local people

47 **Do you feel a kind of stress due to aforesaid problems in your neighbourhood?**
a) Strongly agree
b) Agree
c) Disagree

48 **Do you feel safe to let your children play in neighbourhood?**
a) Yes
b) No
If no, Reason
a) Lack of open space
b) Lack of security
c) Lack of trust
d) You are not aware of neighbours

N. ENVIRONMENTAL PROBLEMS

49 **What are the main environmental problems in your neighbourhood?**
a) Traffic congestion
b) Air pollution
c) Noise pollution
d) Water pollution
e) Solid waste
f) Sanitation
g) Water logging
h) Drainage
i) Overcrowding
j) Water supply
k) Other, specify

50 **What are major urban residential environmental issues in Azamgarh City?**
a) Shortage of water
b) Shortage of electricity
c) Poor access to education
d) Inadequate garbage removal
e) Outdoor air pollution
f) Water logging
g) Drainage problem
h) Traffic congestion
i) Lack of health facility

51 **How would you rate following characteristics of your neighbourhood? (Table A1.4)**

Characteristics	Highly Satisfactory	Satisfactory	Unsatisfactory	Highly Unsatisfactory
Reputation				
Appearance				
Cleanliness				
Streets/roads				
Quality of Life				
Social cohesion				
Safety				
Shopping facility				
Health facility				
Educational facility				

52 **How would you rate your satisfaction with following municipality services? (Table A1.5)**

Services	Highly Satisfactory	Satisfactory	Unsatisfactory	Highly Unsatisfactory
Water supply				
Sewage collection and disposal				
Waste collection				
Electricity and gas supply				
Municipal health services				
Municipal roads and storm water drainage				
Street lighting				
Municipal parks and recreation				

53 **How would you rate your neighbourhood as a place to live?**
   a)   Excellent
   b)   Good
   c)   Average
   d)   Bad
   e)   Very bad

54 **Would you like to move from this area?**
   a) Strongly agree
   b) Agree
   c) Disagree
55 **Which according to you is the best area in Azamgarh city to live........................... Why?....................**

SOCIO-ECONOMIC CONDITION OF THE RESPONDENT

Ward No..........
Ward Name...........................Colony/Mohalla............House No.

A. SOCIAL

1 **Name:**
2 **Age (years):**
   a) 15–24
   b) 25–34
   c) 35–44
   d) 45 & above
3 **Sex**
   a) Male
   b) Female
4 **Religion**
   a) Hindu
   b) Muslim
   c) Sikh
   d) Christian
   e) Others
5 **Marital status**
   a) Married
   b) Unmarried
   c) Widowed
   d) Divorced
6 **Category**
   a) General
   b) OBC............
   c) Scheduled caste............
   d) Schedule tribe............
7 **What is your migration status?**
   a) Migrant
   b) Native
   If Migrated............Reason for Migration
   a) Better housing
   b) Better environment

c)   Employment
d)   Education
e)   Other

8   **What is the nature of your family?**
a)   Joint
b)   Nuclear

9   **Total no of family members in the house**
a)   Male
b)   Female
c)   Children

10 **Educational status of the Respondent**
a)   Educated
b)   Uneducated
If educated
a)   Primary/middle
b)   High school
c)   Intermediate
d)   Graduate
e)   Postgraduate
f)   Professional
g)   Other

11 **Information about family members (Table A1.6)**

S. No.	1	2	3	4	5	6	7	8
Relation								
Age								
Sex								
Married Y/N								
Education								
Occupation								
Income								

12 **Years lived in the neighbourhood.........**
a)   0–5
b)   5–10
c)   10–15
d)   15–20
e)   More than 20

13 **Time spent by respondent/ resident in the house.......................hours/day**

B. ECONOMIC

14 **Occupational Status**
a)   Employed
b)   Unemployed

15 **Occupational Structure**
   a) Service
   b) Business
   c) Labour
   d) Other

16 **Monthly income of the Respondent**
   a) Below 5000
   b) 5001–10000
   c) 10001–20,000
   d) Above 20,000
   e) No income

17 **Total income of family**
   a) Below 5000
   b) 5001–10000
   c) 10001–20,000
   d) Above 20,000
   e) No income

18 **Employment Status**
   a) Permanent
   b) Irregular
   c) Causal
   d) Seasonal

19 **Family possessions**
   I **Ownership of vehicle**
      a) Bicycle
      b) Moped
      c) Motorcycle
      d) Car

   II. **Ownership of appliances**
      a) Fan
      b) T.V./LCD
      c) c)Washing machine
      d) Geyser
      e) Telephone
      f) Mobile
      g) Both
      h) Inverter
      i) Room Heater
      j) Water Purifier RO
      k) AC
      l) Fridge
      m) Generator
      n) LPG
      o) Exhaust fan

p) Computer without internet
q) Computer with internet

C. HOUSING CONDITION

20 **Status of house**
a) Own house
b) Rented house
c) Government house
d) Other
21 **Use of house**
a) Residential only
b) Residential and industrial
c) Residential and commercial
22 **Type of the house**
a) Kutcha
b) Pucca
c) Mixed
d) Any other
If Kutcha
a) Mud/thatched
b) Mud/brick
c) Boat/wooden
d) Any other
If Pucca
a) Bricks/concrete
b) Brick/concrete and tiles
c) Bricks asbestos
d) Any other
23 **What is the predominant material of roof?**
a) Wood/mud
b) Concrete
c) I.G. sheets
d) Any other
24 **What is the predominant material of wall?**
a) Mud/unburnt bricks
b) Concrete
c) Burnt brick
d) Any other
25 **What is predominant flooring type?**
a) Mud
b) Cemented
c) Mosaic floor tiles
d) Wood

26 **What type of floor covering?**
   a)   Carpet
   b)   hard surface
   c)   Both

27 **Total number of the rooms in a house**
   a)   One
   b)   Two
   c)   three
   d)   Above three

28 **Floor area of the house (in sq.) feet)**
   a)   <300
   b)   300–1000
   c)   1000–2000
   d)   >2000

29 **Number of persons living in a room**
   a)   One
   b)   Two
   c)   Three
   d)   >Three

30 **Do you feel your house has been cold in winter?**
   a)   Yes, always
   b)   Yes, most of time
   c)   Yes, Sometimes
   d)   No

31 **What type of heating you use in winter?**
   a)   Open fire
   b)   Gas heater
   c)   Electric heater
   d)   Other

32 **Do you notice a damp/musty smell/mould in any of the following room of the house?**
   a)   Bedroom
   b)   Kitchen
   c)   Bathroom and toilet

33 **How much mould have these rooms? (Table A1.7)**

Rooms	No	Small patches	Moderate	Large	Extensive
Living room					
Main Bedroom					
Other bedroom					
Kitchen					
Bathroom					

34 **Is there proper ventilation in the house?**
   a)   Proper
   b)   Not proper

35   **Open space**
   a)   Yes
   b)   No

36   **How old can be this house approximately? Yrs.**
   a)   0–5
   b)   5–10
   c)   10–15
   d)   15–20
   e)   20–30
   f)   >30

D. INDOOR AIR POLLUTION

37   **Place of cooking food**
   a)   Separate kitchen
   b)   Open air/varandah
   c)   Multipurpose room
   d)   don't have kitchen

38   **Type of fuel used for cooking**
   a)   Wood/coal/saw dust/dung cake/dry leaves
   b)   Kerosene
   c)   Electricity
   d)   LPG

39   **Is the cooking done under a chimney?**
   a)   Yes
   b)   No

40   **Intensity of exposure to smoke while cooking**
   a)   ½ hrs
   b)   1 hr
   c)   2 hrs
   d)   >2 hrs

41   **Ventilation in the kitchen**
   a)   Exhaust fan
   b)   Chimney
   c)   Cross ventilation
   d)   No ventilation

42   **Do you notice smoke in your house from kitchen or any source**
   a)   Yes
   b)   No

43   **Other sources of indoor air pollution?**
   a)   Fuel
   b)   Insecticide/ Pesticide
   c)   Smoking (cigarette/bidi)
   d)   Mosquito coils
   e)   Dust

44 **Main type of energy used in lightening**
   a) Electricity
   b) Kerosene
   c) Candle
   d) Other

E. HOUSEHOLD WATER SUPPLY

45 **Source of water supply**
   I   Private
       a) Own hand pump
       b) Piped water connection
       c) Own boring
   II Public
       a) Roadside hand pump
       b) Roadside piped water

46 **Duration of Water supply**
   a) 1–6 hrs
   b) 7–12 hrs
   c) 13–18 hrs
   d) 24 hrs

47 **What water source do you use if your principal water source for drinking and cooking?**
   a) Private tube well
   b) Public tube well
   c) PHE mobile water tank
   d) Surface water

48 **Any problem with the quality of water source for drinking and cooking?**
   a) Yes
   b) No
   If Yes
   a) Smell
   b) Taste
   c) Colour
   d) No problem

49 **Do you treat your water in any way to make it safer to drink?**
   a) Yes
   b) No
   If yes,
   a) Boil
   b) Use RO
   c) Add bleach/ chlorine water
   d) Other, specify

50 **Storage of water**
   a)   Yes
   b)   No
   If Yes, mode of storage
   a)   Open metal container
   b)   Closed metal container
   c)   Open Plastic container
   d)   Closed plastic container

51 **Do you clean your water container?**
   a)   Daily
   b)   Weekly
   c)   Fortnightly
   d)   Monthly

52 **How can you evaluate you're your satisfaction with the quality of service facilities?**
   a)   Highly satisfied
   b)   Satisfied
   c)   Dissatisfied
   d)   Highly dissatisfied

53 **Which areas will you want to see improvement?**
   a)   Time and duration of water served
   b)   Amount of water served
   c)   Quality
   d)   Tariff level

F. BATHROOM AND SANITATION CONDITION

54 **Toilet facility in the house**
   a)   Yes
   b)   No
   If Yes
   a)   Within premises
   b)   Outside premise
   c)   Open fields
   Within Premises
   a)   1
   b)   2
   c)   3
   If no, what do your households members use?
   a)   Public/community latrines
   b)   Roadside
   c)   Open field
   d)   Other

55 **What kind of toilet?**
  a) Flush
  b) Pit
  c) Makeshift latrines
  d) Other
  If flush,
  a) Flush to piped sewer system
  b) Flush with septic tank
  c) Flush with open drain
  d) Other specify
  If pit latrines,
  a) With slab/ventilated improved pit
  b) Open pit
  If other,
  a) Night soil disposed into open drains
  b) Night soil removed by human

56 **Means of disposal of faecal matter from manual toilet?**
  a) With garbage
  b) Open drains
  c) In the fields

57 **How many households use this toilet facility?**

58 **Is soap available at the toilet?**
  a) Yes
  b) No

59 **Is there any problem with the latrine?**
  a) Water not available for cleaning
  b) Flies/mosquitos
  c) Foul smell
  d) No problem

60 **Availability of bathing facility?**
  a) Separate Bathroom available
  b) Bathroom and toilet attached
  c) Bathing in enclosure without roof
  d) No bathroom

61 **Ventilation in the bathroom/toilet**
  a) Exhaust fan
  b) Window
  c) No ventilation

62 **Dampness and mold in the bathroom**
  a) Present
  b) Not present

G. SULLAGE AND DRAINAGE OF WATER

63 **Do you have a sewer connection?**
   a) Yes
   b) No
   If yes, is it
   a) Covered
   b) Opened

64 **Where does the sullage go?**
   a) Dumped inside the house compound
   b) Drains into natural body
   c) Into the open drain
   d) Around the house

65 **Does the waste water**
   a) Flow directly underground
   b) Into the main drain
   c) Flow slowly away from house
   d) Stagnant

H. HOUSEHOLD GARBAGE AND SOLID WASTE

66 **Type of waste**
   a) Biodegradable
   b) Non-biodegradable
   If Biodegradable then type,
   a) Kitchen waste
   b) Paper
   c) Human/animal waste
   d) Any other, specify
   If non-biodegradable or non-organic
   a) Ash
   b) Plastic
   c) Polythene bags
   d) Any other, specify
   Waste Segregation at home
   a) Yes
   b) No

67 **Collection of waste inside the house**
   a) Yes
   b) No
   If yes, how is solid waste stored in your house?
   a) Taking straight out
   b) Closed container
   c) Open container
   d) Other, specify

68 **How much solid waste do you produce a day?**
   a) 0–5 kg
   b) 1 kg
   c) 2 kg
   d) >2 kg
69 **Disposal of waste from the house?**
   a) SW bin
   b) Roadside
   c) Open field
   d) Burn
   e) Backyard
   f) Other specify
70 **Who disposes?**
   a) Self
   b) Servant
   c) Municipal worker
   d) Any other
71 **What is the distance from here to refuse dump?**...............................m
72 **Do you have your garbage collected at your home? if so how often?**
   a) Not collected
   b) Daily
   c) Twice/weeks
   d) Weekly
73 **Overall environment of your house**
   a) Highly satisfactory
   b) Satisfactory
   c) Unsatisfactory
   d) Highly unsatisfactory

I. LIFE STYLE AND BEHAVIOUR

74 **Does any member of your family take liquor?**
   a) Yes
   b) No
   If yes, how many members?
   a) 1
   b) 2
   c) 3
75 **Does any member of your family smoke?**
   a) Yes
   b) No
   If yes, how many members?
   a) 1
   b) 2
   c) 3

What do they smoke?
a) Cigarette
b) Bidi
c) Hubble-bubble

76 **Is someone in your family in the habit of taking gutkha?**
a) Yes
b) No
If yes, what do they take?
a) Pan
b) Panmasala

77 **Do you clean your house daily?**
a) Yes
b) No
If no, then when?
a) After 1 day
b) After 2 day
c) After 3 day

78 **Do you wash your hands?**
a) Before eating
b) After eating
c) Before cooking
d) After toilet

79 **Do you care about access of flies?**
a) Yes
b) No
c) Sometimes

80 **Are you careful about cleaning of your utensils, kitchen and place where you take food?**
a) Yes
b) No
c) Sometimes

81 **Do you think your neighbours/relatives will help you if you are in trouble?**
a) Yes
b) No

J. CHRONIC STRESS

82 **Do you feel any kind of stress because of? (Table A1.8)**

Problems	Always	Often	Rarely	Never
Economic condition				
Social status				
Insecure Employment				
Low control at work				
Stressful life events				

HEALTH PROFILE

A. HEALTH CARE

1 **What do you do when you find that someone in your family is not well?**
   1) Take him/her to doctor immediately
   2) Avoid
   3) Wait till the person will be fine by himself
   4) Self medication
2 **Do you go to doctor for normal health check-up?**
   1) Yes
   2) No
3 **Health insurance**
   1) Yes
   2) No

B. HEALTH AWARENESS

4 **Are you concerned about your and family's health?**
   1) Yes
   2) No
5 **Do you do any kind of exercise to keep healthy?**
   1) Yes
   2) No
   If yes, what type of exercise?
   1) Walking
   2) Jogging
   3) Cycling
   4) Member of a gym

C. HEALTH CONDITIONS

6 **In general, according to you, your health is**
   1) Excellent
   2) Very good
   3) Fair
   4) Poor
7 **Compare to one year ago, how would you rate your health in general now?**
   1) Much better now
   2) Somewhat netter
   3) About the same
   4) Somewhat worse now
   5) Much worse now

8   **What are the most prevalent diseases in your household (name 3–5 most common)**

Transient Problems (Table A1.9)

Transient Problems	Women	Men	Child
Headache			
Instant coughing			
Eye irritation			
Skin infection			
Sneezing			
Dizziness			
Mood swings			
Watering of eyes			
Sore throat			
Stomach problem			
Sleeplessness			
Sort of deafness			
High BP			
Other			

Frequently occurring Diseases

Disease	Women	Men	Child
Viral fever			
Cold/cough			
Skin infection			
Cholera			
Diarrhoea			
Malaria			
Skin infections			
Tuberculosis			
Asthma/Bronchitis			
Respiratory diseases			
Diabetes			
Sleep disturbances			
Typhoid			
Jaundice			
Anxiety			
Depression			
Shortness of breath			
Sleep disturbances			
High BP			
Heart Diseases			
Other			

D. HEALTH CARE FACILITIES

9   **Name of the health facility in your colony/ward ....**

10   **Type of facility**
   1)   Hospital
   2)   Health centre

3) Health clinic
4) Others
11 **Facility operated by**
1) Government
2) Private
3) Other
12 **Which kind of institution was last consulted?**
1) No treatment
2) Traditional healer
3) Medical personnel
4) PHC
5) Health sub centre
6) Private Clinic
7) Government hospital
8) Private hospital/nursing home
9) Self-medication
13 **Which treatment did you go for last illness case?**
1) Allopathic
2) Homeopathic
3) Ayurvedic
4) Traditional
14 **How much you or your households spend on drugs alone for the last consultation? Rs............**
15 **How far is the nearest health centre (walking hours)?............**
16 **Which type of facility is this: public or private?**
17 **What do you think about the services provided by this facility? (Table A1.10)**

Category	good	average	bad
Sufficient staff			
Qualified staff			
Ill people were well received			
Ill people are well taken care of			
Services are expensive			
Centre is well equipped			

18 **On an average how much did you pay for your last visit at this facility?**
19 **Have it ever happened that a very serious illness in your family could not be treated because of lack of money**
1) Yes
2) No
Reason....................
20 **In your opinion, which facilities provide the best services?**
1) Government
2) Private

21 **During which month of year most of the diseases occur?**
    1) December to Feb
    2) March to May
    3) June to August
    4) September to Nov
22 **Do you feel that quality of water, food and surrounding environment leads to various diseases?**
    a) Yes
    b) No
23 **What do you think is the most likely cause of environmental health problem in your area?**
    1) Road Traffic
    2) Indoor air pollution
    3) Drinking water
    4) Drainage and sanitation
    5) Solid waste
    6) Other
24 **How will you contribute to improve your household environment and neighbourhood environment?**
    1) Time effort
    2) Money effort
    3) Both
    4) Nothing
25 **To what extent are you happy with your family's health?**
    1) Very happy
    2) Happy
    3) Unhappy
    4) Very unhappy

Thank you very much for your time and effort

Appendix 2

Table A2.1 Administrative Wards of Azamgarh City (2011)

Ward No	Ward Name	Total Population	No of Households	Area (Sq. km)	Population density (Per sq.km)	Household density (Per sq.km)
1	Farashtola	1991	279	0.1429	13933	1952
2	Sidhari West	3544	526	0.5933	5973	887
3	Seetaram	4968	642	0.1598	31089	4018
4	Badarka	6405	934	0.2771	23114	3371
5	Jalandhari	3289	440	0.1076	30567	4089
6	Gurutola	3361	477	0.23	14613	2074
7	Sidhari East	5907	855	0.4836	12215	1768
8	Arazibagh	4465	651	0.3667	12176	1775
9	Bazabahadur	7411	970	0.3525	21024	2752
10	Katra	3395	512	0.1495	22709	3425
11	Asifganj	3727	523	0.1115	33426	4691
12	Harbanshpur	6383	997	2.133	2992	467
13	Ghulami ka pura	5914	865	0.5212	11347	1660
14	Mukeriganj	3764	566	0.9915	3796	571
15	Herapatti	4254	708	0.7305	5823	969
16	Sarfuddinpur	3872	608	0.7097	5456	857
17	Raidopur	2676	436	0.4315	6202	1010
18	Narauli	4067	592	0.833	4882	711
19	Matbarganj	5020	775	0.3333	15062	2325
20	Chakla Paharpur	2967	358	0.1463	20280	2447
21	Cilvil Line	9039	1464	1.6578	5452	883
22	Pandey Bazaar	2947	408	0.2076	14196	1965
23	Ailwal	3670	486	0.1909	19225	2546
24	Sadavarti	2873	416	0.2316	12405	1796
25	Madya	5047	806	0.5232	9646	1541

Source: Municipal Council, Azamgarh City, 2016–2017.

Appendix 3

Table A3.1 Colonies/Mohallas in Azamgarh City (2016–2017)

Ward No	Ward Name	Name of colonies/mohallas
1	Farashtola	Farashtola, Kaleenganj, AnshikMatbarganj, AnshikAilwal, AnshikAsifganj
2	Sidhari West	Ali Ausat colony, Babuan, Hydel colony
3	Seetaram	AnshikKot, AnshikFarashtola
4	Badarka	Friends colony, AnshikKundigarh,
5	Jalandhari	AnshikChakala
6	Gurutola	Anantpura
7	Sidhari East	Sidhari East
8	Arazibagh	Millatnagar colony, Niralanagar
9	Bazabahadur	Bazabahadur
10	Katra	Khatritola
11	Asifganj	Asifganj
12	Harbanshpur	Harbanshpur, Mission Hospital colony
13	Ghulamikapura	Rahmatnagar colony, Awasvikas colony, Harijanbasti
14	Mukeriganj	Mukeriganj, Jogiyan
15	Herapatti	Hariaudhnagar colony, Shivajinagar colony, Teachers colony
16	Sarfuddinpur	Belaisa colony, Moosepur, Palhani
17	Raidopur	Officer's colony, Pandey colony, E type colony
18	Narauli	Narauli E., Narauli W.
19	Matbarganj	purvitola
20	ChaklaPaharpur	TakiaMohalla, Rauza colony, Niswan colony
21	Cilvil Line	Nagar Palika colony, Police line colony, Judges colony
22	Pandey Bazaar	Anshikkundigarh
23	Ailwal	Lochaigali, thakurana colony
24	Sadavarti	Dalsinghar
25	Madya	Thandisadak colony, Christian's colony

Source: Municipal Council, Azamgarh City, 2016–2017.

Index

Pages in *italics* refer to figures and pages in **bold** refer to tables.

For Product Safety Concerns and Information please contact our EU
representative GPSR@taylorandfrancis.com
Taylor & Francis Verlag GmbH, Kaufingerstraße 24, 80331 München, Germany

* 9 7 8 1 0 3 2 5 8 0 8 9 0 *